Management of Elbow Trauma

Editor

GEORGE S. ATHWAL

HAND CLINICS

www.hand.theclinics.com

Consulting Editor
KEVIN C. CHUNG

November 2015 • Volume 31 • Number 4

ELSEVIER

1600 John F. Kennedy Boulevard • Suite 1800 • Philadelphia, Pennsylvania, 19103-2899

http://www.theclinics.com

HAND CLINICS Volume 31, Number 4
November 2015 ISSN 0749-0712, ISBN-13: 978-0-323-39392-8

Editor: Jennifer Flynn-Briggs
Developmental Editor: Kristen Helm

Hand Clinics (ISSN 0749-0712) is published quarterly by Elsevier Inc., 360 Park Avenue South, New York, NY 10010-1710. Months of publication are February, May, August, and November. Business and Editorial Offices: 1600 John F. Kennedy Blvd., Ste. 1800, Philadelphia, PA 19103-2899. Customer Service Office: 3251 Riverport Lane, Maryland Heights, MO 63043. Periodicals postage paid at New York, NY and at additional mailing offices. Subscription price is $390.00 per year (domestic individuals), $606.00 per year (domestic institutions), $194.00 per year (domestic students/residents), $445.00 per year (Canadian individuals), $691.00 per year (Canadian institutions), $530.00 per year (international individuals), $691.00 per year (international institutions), and $256.00 per year (international and Canadian students/residents). Foreign air speed delivery is included in all *Clinics* subscription prices. All prices are subject to change without notice. **POSTMASTER:** Send address changes to *Hand Clinics*, Elsevier Health Sciences Division, Subscription Customer Service, 3251 Riverport Lane, Maryland Heights, MO 63043. Customer Service (orders, claims, online, change of address): Elsevier Health Sciences Division, Subscription **Customer Service, 3251 Riverport Lane, Maryland Heights, MO 63043. Tel: 1-800-654-2452 (U.S. and Canada); 314-447-8871 (outside U.S. and Canada). Fax: 314-447-8029. E-mail: journalscustomerservice-usa@elsevier.com (for print support); journalsonlinesupport-usa@elsevier.com (for online support).**

Reprints. For copies of 100 or more of articles in this publication, please contact the Commercial Reprints Department, Elsevier Inc., 360 Park Avenue South, New York, New York 10010-1710. Tel.: 212-633-3874; Fax: 212-633-3820; E-mail: reprints@elsevier.com.

Hand Clinics is covered in *MEDLINE/PubMed (Index Medicus), Current Contents/Clinical Medicine, EMBASE/Excerpta Medica,* and *ISI/BIOMED.*

Contributors

CONSULTING EDITOR

KEVIN C. CHUNG, MD, MS
Charles B. G. de Nancrede Professor of
Surgery, Professor of Plastic Surgery and
Orthopaedic Surgery, Chief of Hand Surgery,
University of Michigan Health System,
Assistant Dean for Faculty Affairs, Associate
Director of Global REACH, University of
Michigan Medical School, Ann Arbor, Michigan

EDITOR

GEORGE S. ATHWAL, MD, FRCSC
Division of Orthopedic Surgery, Associate
Professor, Roth|McFarlane Hand and Upper
Limb Centre, St. Joseph's Health Center, St.
Joseph's Health Care, University of Western
Ontario, London, Ontario, Canada

AUTHORS

JOSEPH A. ABBOUD, MD
Associate Professor, Department of
Orthopaedic Surgery, The Rothman Institute,
Thomas Jefferson University Hospital,
Philadelphia, Pennsylvania

SAMUEL A. ANTUÑA, MD, PhD, FEBOT
Shoulder and Elbow Unit, Hospital
Universitario La Paz, Madrid, Spain

APRIL ARMSTRONG, MD, MSc, FRCSC
Department of Orthopedics, Bone and Joint
Institute, Penn State Hershey Medical Center,
Hershey, Pennsylvania

GEORGE S. ATHWAL, MD, FRCSC
Division of Orthopedic Surgery, Associate
Professor, Roth|McFarlane Hand and Upper
Limb Centre, St. Joseph's Health Center, St.
Joseph's Health Care, University of Western
Ontario, London, Ontario, Canada

RAUL BARCO, MD, PhD, FEBOT
Shoulder and Elbow Unit, Hospital
Universitario La Paz, Madrid, Spain

TYLER J. BROLIN, MD
Orthopaedic Resident, Department of
Orthopaedic Surgery and Biomedical
Engineering, University of
Tennessee-Campbell Clinic, Memphis,
Tennessee

KLAUS JOSEF BURKHART, MD
Department for Shoulder and Elbow
Surgery, Rhön-Clinic, Bad Neustadt,
Germany

MICHAEL J. CARROLL, MD, FRCSC
Division of Orthopedic Surgery,
Roth|McFarlane Hand and Upper Limb Centre,
St. Joseph's Health Center, University of
Western Ontario, London, Ontario, Canada

EMILIE V. CHEUNG, MD
Associate Professor, Chief of Shoulder
Elbow Service, Orthopedic Surgery,
Stanford University, Redwood City,
California

KEVIN C. CHUNG, MD, MS
Charles B. G. de Nancrede Professor of
Surgery, Professor of Plastic Surgery and
Orthopaedic Surgery, Chief of Hand Surgery,
University of Michigan Health System,
Assistant Dean for Faculty Affairs, Associate
Director of Global REACH, University of
Michigan Medical School, Ann Arbor, Michigan

BENJAMIN J. COTTRELL, BS
Foundation for Orthopaedic Research and
Education, Tampa, Florida

JOSHUA S. DINES, MD
Associate Attending, Sports Medicine and
Shoulder Service, Hospital for Special Surgery,
Associate Professor of Orthopaedic Surgery,
Weill Cornell Medical College, New York,
New York

KENNETH J. FABER, MD, MPHE, FRCSC
Division of Orthopedic Surgery,
Roth|McFarlane Hand and Upper Limb Centre,
St. Joseph's Health Center, University of
Western Ontario, London, Ontario, Canada

LESLIE A. FINK BARNES, MD
Fellow, Shoulder and Elbow Surgery, Leni and
Peter W. May Department of Orthopaedics,
Icahn School of Medicine at Mount Sinai
Medical Center, New York, New York

CHARLES L. GETZ, MD
Associate Professor, Department of
Orthopaedic Surgery, The Rothman Institute,
Thomas Jefferson University Hospital,
Philadelphia, Pennsylvania

FRANK E. GOHLKE, MD
Department for Shoulder and Elbow Surgery,
Rhön-Clinic, Bad Neustadt, Germany

RUBY GREWAL, MD, MSc, FRCSC
Associate Professor, Roth|McFarlane Hand
and Upper Limb Centre, London, Ontario,
Canada

LUKE S. HARMER, MD, MPH, FRCSC
Department of Orthopedic Surgery, Mayo
Clinic, Rochester, Minnesota

MICHAEL HAUSMAN, MD
Robert K. Lippmann Professor and Chief of
Hand and Elbow Surgery, Leni and Peter W.
May Department of Orthopaedics, Icahn
School of Medicine at Mount Sinai Medical
Center, New York, New York

JOHN HAVERSTOCK, MD, FRCSC
Fellow, Roth|McFarlane Hand and Upper Limb
Centre, London, Ontario, Canada

JAY D. KEENER, MD
Associate Professor, Department of
Orthopaedic Surgery, Washington University,
St Louis, Missouri

BRIAN P. KELLEY, MD
House Officer, Section of Plastic Surgery,
The University of Michigan Health System,
Ann Arbor, Michigan

GRAHAM J.W. KING, MD, MSc, FRCSC
Division of Orthopedic Surgery,
Roth|McFarlane Hand and Upper
Limb Centre, St. Joseph's Health Center,
University of Western Ontario, London,
Ontario, Canada

DAVID KOVACEVIC, MD
Department of Orthopaedic Surgery,
Clinical Fellow, The Center for Shoulder,
Elbow, and Sports Medicine, New York
Presbyterian/Columbia University Medical
Center, New York, New York

WILLIAM N. LEVINE, MD
Frank E. Stinchfield Professor and
Chairman of Orthopaedic Surgery,
Department of Orthopaedic Surgery,
The Center for Shoulder, Elbow, and Sports
Medicine, New York Presbyterian/Columbia
University Medical Center, New York,
New York

LARS P. MÜLLER, MD
Department for Trauma, Hand and Elbow
Surgery, University of Cologne, Cologne,
Germany

MARK A. MIGHELL, MD
Board Examiner, The American Board of
Orthopaedic Surgery, Chapel Hill, North
Carolina; Associate Professor,
Department of Orthopaedic Surgery,
University of South Florida; Co-Director,
Shoulder and Elbow Fellowship Program,
Florida Orthopaedic Institute, Tampa,
Florida; Instructor of Surgery, Uniformed
Services University of the Health Sciences,
F. Edward Hébert School of Medicine,
Bethesda, Maryland

ANAND M. MURTHI, MD
Editor, Department of Orthopaedic Surgery,
MedStar Union Memorial Hospital, Baltimore,
Maryland

BRADFORD O. PARSONS, MD
Chief of Shoulder Surgery, Associate
Professor and Residency Program Director,
Leni and Peter W. May Department of
Orthopaedics, Icahn School of Medicine
at Mount Sinai Medical Center, New York,
New York

MIGUEL A. RAMIREZ, MD
Department of Orthopaedic Surgery,
MedStar Union Memorial Hospital,
Baltimore, Maryland

LAUREN H. REDLER, MD
Fellow, Hospital for Special Surgery, New York,
New York

JOAQUIN SANCHEZ-SOTELO, MD, PhD
Consultant and Professor, Department of
Orthopedic Surgery, Mayo Clinic, Rochester,
Minnesota

ERIC J. SARKISSIAN, MD
Department of Orthopaedic Surgery, Stanford
University Hospital and Clinics, Stanford,
California

PAUL M. SETHI, MD
The ONS Sports and Shoulder Service,
Greenwich, Connecticut

JASON A. STEIN, MD
Department of Orthopaedic Surgery, MedStar
Union Memorial Hospital, Baltimore, Maryland

BRENT STEPHENS, MD
Florida Orthopaedic Institute, Tampa, Florida

GEOFFREY P. STONE, MD
Florida Orthopaedic Institute, Tampa, Florida

THOMAS THROCKMORTON, MD
Associate Professor, Department of
Orthopaedic Surgery and Biomedical
Engineering, University of
Tennessee-Campbell Clinic, Memphis,
Tennessee

LAURA A. VOGEL, MD
Resident, Department of Orthopaedic Surgery,
The Center for Shoulder, Elbow, and Sports
Medicine, New York Presbyterian/Columbia
University Medical Center, New York, New York

KILIAN WEGMANN, MD
Department for Trauma, Hand and Elbow
Surgery, University of Cologne, Cologne,
Germany

JUSTIN C. WONG, MD
Fellow, Department of Orthopaedic Surgery,
Thomas Jefferson University Hospital,
Philadelphia, Pennsylvania

Contents

faster, easier rehabilitation compared with internal fixation; and overall good outcomes reported in terms of both pain relief and function. Implant failure leading to revision surgery does happen, and patients must comply with certain limitations to extend the longevity of their implant. Development of high-performance implants may allow expanding the indications of elbow arthroplasty for fractures.

Capitellar and Trochlear Fractures

Michael J. Carroll, George S. Athwal, Graham J.W. King, and Kenneth J. Faber

Fractures of the capitellum and trochlea account for a small proportion of elbow trauma. Clinicians need to be vigilant in their assessment as they are commonly associated with other injuries about the elbow. To optimize outcomes, the goals of management include a stable, anatomic reduction and early range of motion. Closed reduction of noncomminuted fractures may be successful but requires close follow-up. Open reduction and internal fixation is the preferred management of displaced capitellum-trochlear fractures. Elbow stiffness is the most commonly reported complication in operatively treated fractures. Arthroscopic-assisted reduction and internal fixation and arthroplasty are evolving management options.

Distal Biceps Injuries

John Haverstock, George S. Athwal, and Ruby Grewal

A review of distal biceps tendon injuries is presented. Notable and recent studies on the incidence, presentation, diagnosis, and treatment are outlined. The benefits and risks of 1- and 2-incision techniques for repair are discussed, and classic studies are reviewed.

Distal Triceps Tendon Injuries

Jay D. Keener and Paul M. Sethi

Acute triceps ruptures are an uncommon entity, occurring mainly in athletes, weight lifters (especially those taking anabolic steroids), and following elbow trauma. Accurate diagnosis is made clinically, although MRI may aid in confirmation and surgical planning. Acute ruptures are classified on an anatomic basis based on tear location and the degree of tendon involvement. Most complete tears are treated surgically in medically fit patients. Partial-thickness tears are managed according to the tear severity, functional demands, and response to conservative treatment. We favor an anatomic footprint repair of the triceps to provide optimal tendon to bone healing and, ultimately, functional outcome.

Arthroscopic Management of Elbow Fractures

Leslie A. Fink Barnes, Bradford O. Parsons, and Michael Hausman

Several types of elbow fractures are amenable to arthroscopic or arthroscopic-assisted fracture fixation, including fractures of the coronoid, radial head, lateral condyle, and capitellum. Other posttraumatic conditions may be treated arthroscopically, such as arthrofibrosis or delayed radial head excision. Arthroscopy can be used for assessment of stability or intra-articular fracture displacement. The safest portals are the midlateral (soft spot portal), proximal anteromedial, and proximal anterolateral. Although circumstances may vary according to the injury pattern, a proximal anteromedial portal is usually established first. Arthroscopy enables a less invasive surgical exposure that facilitates visualization of the fracture fragments in select scenarios.

In caring for athletes, the physician must be able to accurately diagnose and appro-priately treat all forms of elbow injuries. Traumatic injuries to the elbow are common in the athlete. The late cocking phase of throwing produces tremendous valgus stress on the elbow that can lead to medial epicondyle avulsion fractures in ado-lescents or rupture of the medial ulnar collateral ligament in skeletally mature over-head throwers, such as baseball pitchers and javelin throwers. Common traumatic elbow injuries suffered by athletes, surgical techniques for operative repair of these injuries, as well as postoperative rehabilitation protocols and the clinical results are presented.

The elbow is a highly congruent trochoginglymoid joint allowing motion in both flexion-extension and pronosupination across 3 articulations. Therefore, treatment of fractures of the elbow can be technically challenging to manage, even after initial surgery. The posttraumatic elbow is prone to complications such as stiffness asso-ciated with heterotopic ossification, instability or subluxation (posterolateral rotatory instability and varus posteromedial instability patterns), and wound complications. This article discusses the pathoanatomy, prevention, and treatment of these complications.

The elbow is particularly prone to trauma, and soft-tissue reconstruction can be challenging given the inherent motion, pressure, and lack of local tissue laxity. Small wounds and those without exposure of vital structures may be amenable to primary repair. Large wounds and those requiring more substantial structural or anatomic repair may require local, regional or free flap-based reconstruction. A comprehen-sive review of soft-tissue reconstruction of the elbow is provided to offer surgeons alternative options in complicated upper extremity wounds.

HAND CLINICS

HAND CLINICS

RELATED INTEREST

Orthopedic Clinics of North America, July 2015 (Vol. 46, Issue 3)
Asif Ilyas, Saqib Rehman, Giles R. Scuderi, Felasfa M. Wodajo, Editors
Available at: http://www.orthopedic.theclinics.com/

Preface
Elbow Trauma—It's All in the Details

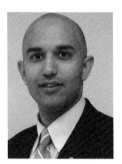

George S. Athwal, MD, FRCSC
Editor

The past decade has brought substantial change to the understanding, evaluation, and treatment of elbow trauma. This issue of *Hand Clinics*, dedicated to elbow trauma, discusses these current developments and provides guidance on clinical and technical applications.

It is an exciting time for elbow surgery with the advent of advanced imaging, new surgical approaches, precontoured fracture-specific plates, and third-generation implants. Just as important, the development of disease-specific, patient-specific, and limb-specific outcome measures will objectively determine the value of these advances. It is the intention of this issue to provide the physician/fellow/resident with a resource to appreciate the foundations and advances in elbow trauma management.

This issue was only made possible through the efforts of the contributing authors, an internationally renowned group. I am truly indebted to these esteemed clinicians and researchers. They have taken time out of their busy clinical, research, and family lives to complete this issue—my sincerest thanks!

I would also like to thank my mentors at Queen's University, the Hospital for Special Surgery, the Mayo Clinic, and the University of Western Ontario for their support and guidance. I would specifically like to thank Drs Jim Roth, Graham King, and Jim Johnson for their mentorship, support, and "protection." In addition, I would like to thank my wife, Lorraine, my sister Sonia, and my children, Marcus, Victoria, and Simon, for their support, understanding, and love. I would like to dedicate this issue to my mother and father, who instilled in me the values of hard work, dedication, precision, and perseverance.

George S. Athwal, MD, FRCSC
Roth|McFarlane Hand and
Upper Limb Centre
St Joseph's Health Care
University of Western Ontario
268 Grosvenor Street
London, Ontario N6A 4L6, Canada

E-mail address:
gathwal@uwo.ca

hand.theclinics.com

Management of Elbow Trauma: Anatomy and Exposures

Raul Barco, MD, PhD, FEBOT*, Samuel A. Antuña, MD, PhD, FEBOT

KEYWORDS

- Anatomy • Exposures • Surgical approaches • Elbow • Fracture • Dislocation

KEY POINTS

- When managing elbow fractures, selecting the most convenient approach is essential to perform an adequate surgical technique and avoid unexpected complications.
- When lateral approaches are done to treat radial head and capitellum fractures, the posterior interosseous nerve and the lateral collateral ligament must be protected.
- Medial approaches for coronoid fracture fixation may result in ulnar nerve–related complications. Extensive nerve dissection should be avoided.
- Posterior approaches to treat distal humerus fractures may be through the olecranon or the triceps tendon. Whenever possible, a paratricipital approach (Alonso-Llames) is preferred.

RELEVANT ELBOW ANATOMY

The elbow is a complex anatomic area in which key neurovascular, tendinous, ligamentous, and osseous structures are in close vicinity. Any traumatic episode to the elbow alters the anatomy and increases the difficulty in identifying and using the usual planes of dissection. A deep knowledge of the anatomy is desirable to diminish the risk of complications and to increase confidence with the most commonly used surgical approaches.

The elbow contains three separate articulations. The ulnohumeral joint is a modified hinge joint that allows flexion and extension. The radiohumeral joint is a combined hinge and pivot joint that permits flexion and extension, and rotation of the head of the radius on the capitellum of the humerus. The proximal radioulnar joint facilitates rotation during supination and pronation.

The distal humerus can be described as comprised of the capitellum and the trochlea, supported by lateral and medial columns. The distal humeral articular segment is projected 30° anteriorly from the long axis of the humerus, so that the anterior cortex of the humeral diaphysis crosses the ulnohumeral joint at approximately its center of rotation (**Fig. 1**). The radial head articulates with both the lesser sigmoid notch of the proximal ulna and the capitellum and it is covered with cartilage superiorly and around 280° of its circumference. Most of the fractures affecting the radial head include the lateral or anterolateral fragment lacking cartilage and subchondral bone (**Fig. 2**). The proximal ulna has a complex anatomy with an average dorsal angulation of 6° and an axial angulation of 10°, which both should be considered when fixing proximal ulna fractures.[1] The coronoid acts as a buttress against posterior, posterolateral, and posteromedial displacement. Its anteromedial part is a medial projection of the proximal ulna overhanging the diaphysis, and serves as the insertion of the anterior bundle of the medial collateral ligament (aMCL), buttressing also against varus posteromedial displacement (**Fig. 3**).[2,3]

The elbow has medial and lateral ligamentous structures that provide stability to the elbow reinforcing the anatomic congruity of the osseous

Disclosure: The authors have not received any financial benefit from the completion of this article.
Shoulder and Elbow Unit, Hospital Universitario La Paz, Paseo de la Castellana 261, Madrid 28046, Spain
* Corresponding author.
E-mail address: raulbarco@hotmail.com

hand.theclinics.com

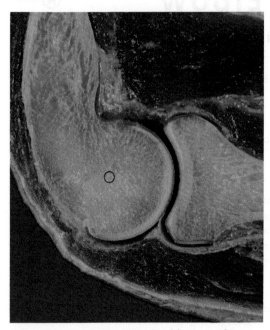

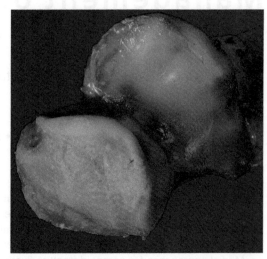

Fig. 3. Superior view of the proximal ulna showing the overhanging of the medial coronoid in relation to the ulnar shaft.

Fig. 1. When reconstructing distal humerus fractures it is important to understand that the capitellum is flexed with respect to the long axis of the humerus and that the axis of flexoextension of the elbow is in line with the anterior humeral cortex. O, axis of rotation.

anatomy (**Fig. 4**). The MCL complex comprises an anterior, a posterior, and a transverse bundle. The aMCL originates in the medial epicondyle and inserts in the sublime tubercle providing stability against valgus displacement. The posterior bundle of the MCL originates from the medial epicondyle and inserts on the olecranon and when contracted may limit elbow flexion. The transverse band connects the aMCL with the posterior bundle of the MCL and its function is unknown. The lateral

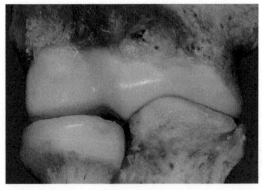

Fig. 2. The anterolateral portion of the radial head lacks cartilage and is the weakest part that usually is involved in radial head fractures.

collateral ligament (LCL) complex, especially the lateral ulnar collateral ligament, confers rotational and varus stability. Unlike the medial side, distinct fascicles cannot be clearly individualized, but according to the origin and insertion its different components are the radial collateral ligament, the annular ligament, and the ulnar collateral ligament.[4]

Four muscle groups act on the elbow. The major flexors are the biceps brachialis (which also supinates the forearm), brachioradialis, and brachialis muscles; the extensors are the triceps and anconeus muscles. The supinators consist of the supinator and biceps brachialis muscles. The pronator quadratus, pronator teres, and flexor carpi radialis muscles accomplish pronation.

The elbow also has a complex innervation, and all the nerves that cross the elbow may be at risk during certain surgical procedures (**Fig. 5**). The median nerve crosses the elbow anteromedially and passes through the two heads of the pronator teres, a potential site of entrapment. The ulnar nerve runs along the medial arm and posterior to the medial epicondyle through the cubital tunnel, a likely site of compression. The nerve then travels between the ulnar and humeral heads of the flexor carpi ulnaris (FCU). It is important to recognize that the floor of the cubital tunnel is actually the superficial aspect of the MCL; this anatomic reference should be taken into consideration when dealing with pathology on the medial compartment of the elbow. The radial nerve descends the arm laterally, dividing into superficial (sensory) and deep (motor, or posterior interosseous) branches. The deep branch passes through the arcade of Frohse, a fibrous arch formed by the proximal margin of

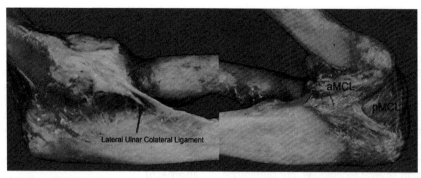

Fig. 4. Lateral and medial ligamentous complexes. pMCL, posterior band of the medial collateral ligament.

the superficial head of the supinator muscle, where it is most susceptible to injury, especially when developing lateral approaches to the elbow joint, or when using retractors.

GENERAL PRINCIPLES

The correct diagnosis of the elbow injury leads to an understanding of the natural history of the injury pattern, and the associated injuries and potential complications. A surgical plan is then developed, which includes exposure, expected and potentially unexpected findings, repair, and rehabilitation. Previous scars must be taken into consideration and although a previous mobile scar may be obviated, it is probably better if it is included in the new surgical plan. When a separate incision must be made, an appropriate skin bridge must be respected to avoid skin ischemia. Full-thickness subcutaneous flaps are favored because they respect the skin circulation.

Prior operative notes are especially useful when approaching the medial side of the elbow regarding previous handling of the ulnar nerve. Whenever possible, internervous anatomic planes should be used because they are safer, cause less bleeding, and are probably less painful. The authors also recommend a tourniquet for most procedures around the elbow.[5]

APPROACHES

There are many approaches described for elbow surgery but only a few are really required to perform the most common surgical procedures related to elbow trauma. We present surgical approaches that are versatile for the whole spectrum of elbow pathology.

Distal Humerus Fractures

Any approach to the distal humerus must balance the degree of triceps tendon detachment and the

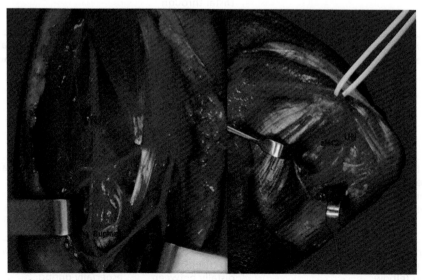

Fig. 5. Knowing the three-dimensional location of nerves around the elbow is critical to avoid complications. The radial nerve is at risk in the anterior part of the elbow as it enters the supinator. The ulnar nerve should be protected with any posterior or medial approach to the elbow. RN, radial nerve; UN, ulnar nerve.

amount of exposure achieved. Additionally, appropriate management of the ulnar nerve must be considered. A universal posterior skin incision, with full-thickness flaps, is used in all different approaches (**Table 1**).

Leaving the triceps attachment intact has obvious advantages and we tend to use an Alonso-Llames approach for fractures with minimal involvement of the joint surface. We prefer the olecranon osteotomy for the more complex distal humerus fractures. Even though fixation of the olecranon osteotomy may be performed with several techniques, our preference is a tension band wire fixation.

Most simple fractures of the capitellum may be approached arthroscopically or through a modified Kocher approach with slight proximal extension. Complex fractures extending into the trochlea, however, may benefit from an olecranon osteotomy to allow better joint exposure. When treating a distal humerus fracture with high proximal extension, the surgeon needs to identify the radial nerve laterally and posteriorly, and the ulnar nerve medially, to avoid nerve damage during plate fixation.

The best way to manage the ulnar nerve is controversial. Iatrogenic nerve injury is not infrequent and seems to be reduced by leaving the ulnar nerve in place.[6] However, if the nerve has any tendency to subluxate anteriorly or if it lies directly on top of the medial plate, we do not hesitate to transpose it anteriorly into a subcutaneous pocket.

The Alonso-Llames approach (bilaterotricipital approach)

This approach was originally described to treat supracondylar fractures in children. Its main advantage is that it leaves the triceps intact.[7]

A posterior skin incision is used and full-thickness subcutaneous flaps are developed (**Fig. 6**). Once identified, the medial and lateral borders of the triceps are incised and dissected free from the posterior part of the humerus. Ulnar nerve dissection and protection is recommended during the approach and during any manipulation of the forearm to avoid

Table 1
Surgical approaches for fractures of the distal humerus according to fracture type

Indication	Approach	Extension	Commentary	Nerves in Danger
Extrarticular Simple intrarticular	Alonso-Llames (bilaterotricipital)	Proximal with protection of radial and ulnar nerve on the lateral and medial side, respectively. Distal through ECU-anconeous interval	Easy conversion to olecranon osteotomy	Ulnar nerve, radial nerve
All distal humeral fractures	Triceps splitting	Proximally limited by the radial nerve	May be performed in the midline or slightly medially Slightly less exposure for internal fixation compared with olecranon osteotomy	Ulnar nerve, radial nerve
All distal humeral fractures, articular distal humeral fractures	Olecranon osteotomy	Proximally until radial nerve	The workhorse for internal fixation of the distal humerus Fixation with multiple options	Ulnar nerve
Comminuted distal humerus fractures (elbow arthroplasty)	Bryan-Morrey	Proximal medial (to triceps) and distally between ECU and FCU	Must protect the ulnar nerve, especially during dislocation of the joint	Ulnar nerve

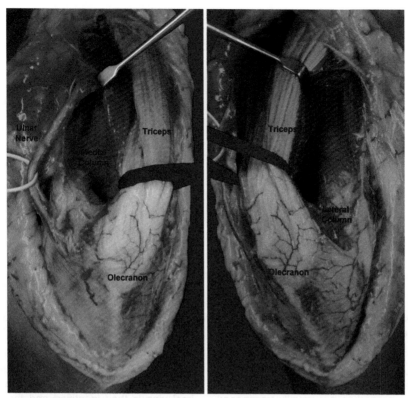

Fig. 6. The Alonso-Llames approach allows access to the posterior part of the elbow joint without triceps detachment.

traction injuries to the nerve. If the lateral border needs to be extended proximally the radial nerve can be identified and protected. The nerve is typically located approximately at the level of the proximal end of the tendinous portion of the triceps.

The distal exposure achieved with this approach is limited, so it is not suitable for complex intra-articular distal humerus fractures.

Posterior triceps-splitting approaches

The triceps tendon and muscle are incised at its midline exposing the humerus and dissecting each half of the triceps to either side (**Fig. 7**).[8,9] Ulnar nerve identification and protection is advised. Distally, the incision runs over the olecranon and separates the anconeus laterally and the FCU medially. Access to the posterior and posterolateral aspect of the humerus is readily available but positioning of true lateral plates can be cumbersome. Meticulous closure of the triceps with side-to-side sutures and additional transosseous sutures at the level of the olecranon is recommended.

Olecranon osteotomy

This is probably the most used approach to treat distal humerus fractures because it provides great access to the articular surface and the supracondylar columns (**Fig. 8**). The chevron osteotomy is favored over transverse osteotomy because of added intrinsic stability.

After the olecranon is identified, the ulnar nerve should be located and protected. The ulnohumeral joint is opened laterally to the olecranon and protected with a sponge when performing the osteotomy.

A distal chevron is made at the level of the bare spot of the greater sigmoid notch of the ulna. The cut is started with a saw and finished with an osteotome. The proximal olecranon and tendon are retracted proximally and separated from capsular attachments and collateral ligaments. The dissection can be carried out proximally as in a bilatero-tricipital approach. At the end of the procedure the olecranon is reduced and fixed with a cerclage and K-wires, a lag screw, an intramedullary nail, or a plate.

To avoid denervation of the anconeus, some authors favor dissecting the anconeus distally, reflecting it from the ulna without detaching it from the triceps to preserve its innervation.[10]

Bryan-Morrey approach

A posterior skin incision is performed just slightly lateral to the tip of the olecranon. After elevating

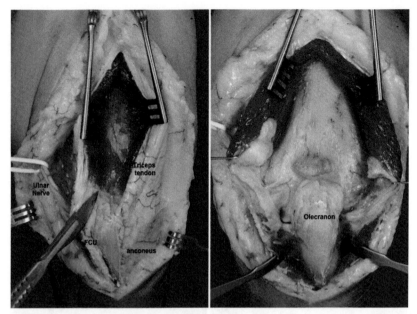

Fig. 7. Triceps-splitting approach. As seen in the picture, this approach gives good exposure and allows distal extension by retracting the FCU and the anconeus.

the cutaneous flaps, the ulnar nerve is dissected and protected throughout the procedure and at the end of the procedure it is usually transposed anteriorly into a subcutaneous pouch.

The triceps is released from the entire posterior aspect of the distal humerus (**Fig. 9**). The forearm fascia and ulnar periosteum are elevated from the medial margin toward the lateral side of the ulna. The triceps tendon is carefully detached from the tip of the olecranon by sharp dissection of Sharpey fibers. The lateral margin of the proximal ulna is then identified and the anconeus is elevated from its ulnar bed. Finally, the extensor mechanism is reflected laterally from the margin of the lateral epicondyle.[11]

Repair of the extensor mechanism is an integral part of the procedure and it includes performing two oblique and one transverse bone tunnels in

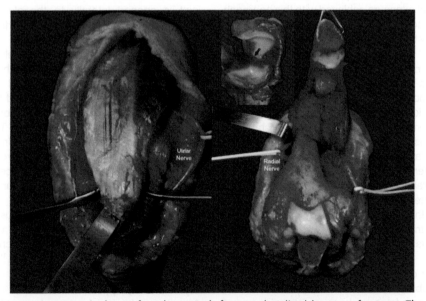

Fig. 8. Olecranon osteotomy is the preferred approach for complex distal humerus fractures. The osteotomy should be done through the bare area of the greater sigmoid notch (*arrow*).

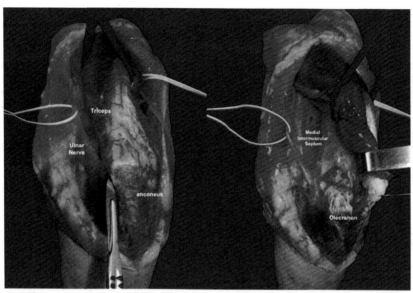

Fig. 9. Bryan-Morrey approach was originally described for implantation of elbow arthroplasty and is rarely used for trauma.

the olecranon. A Krackow stitch is passed through the triceps tendon and then passed in a criss-cross manner through the proximal ulna bone tunnels. Postoperative protection of extension against resistance is recommended.

Fractures of the Radial Head and Capitellum

Access to the lateral aspect of the elbow can be done through a direct lateral skin incision or with a posterior "universal" skin incision and elevation of a thick cutaneous flap until the lateral epicondyle is reached. This decision is made based on the presence of associated injuries that might also need to be addressed.

Most simple radial head fractures can be treated through a Kaplan or a limited Kocher exposure with a direct lateral skin incision. More complex cases may need a posterior skin incision (**Table 2**). In patients with intact lateral ligaments, an extensor digitorum comminus splitting approach may also be used.

Capitellar fractures need to be carefully assessed to rule out significant posterior comination and extension into the trochlea that may be better visualized through an olecranon osteotomy. Simple capitellar fractures may be fixed arthroscopically but if not feasible or the surgeon does not have experience with elbow arthroscopy, a Kocher approach provides the best access to fix these injuries.

Kaplan approach

This approach is mostly used for isolated fractures of the radial head, specifically those involving the anterior half, without associated bony or ligamentous injury leading to instability. A skin incision extending from the lateral epicondyle toward the Lister's tubercle of the distal radius is performed and the superficial interval between the extensor carpi radialis and the extensor digitorum muscle is developed (**Fig. 10**).[12]

The interval between the extensor carpi radialis brevis and the supinator is located by noting that the fibers of the supinator muscle are oblique to the fibers of the extensor carpi radialis brevis. The proximal aspect of the origin of the supinator is detached and the capsule over the radial head is incised longitudinally. The posterior interosseous nerve is in close vicinity to the distal part of this incision and it is advisable to work with the forearm in pronation.[13]

Kocher approach

The Kocher approach uses the interval between the anconeus and the extensor carpi ulnaris (ECU) (**Fig. 11**). It can be extended proximally and is safe because the ECU protects the radial nerve. However, in this approach care must be taken to identify, preserve, or repair if necessary the lateral ligamentous complex. This approach is used for radial head fractures associated with elbow instability and for capitellar fractures without significant comination or medial extension.

The interval between the anconeus and the ECU can be identified by subtle palpation: by moving your finger from posterior to anterior you can feel the anterior margin of the anconeus. Additionally, a thin strip of fat is usually present in this interval.

Table 2
Surgical approaches for fractures involving the radial head

Indication	Approach	Extension	Commentary	Nerves in Danger
All radial head fractures including associated LCL injuries, coronoid fractures, and capitellar fractures	Kocher	ECU-anconeous interval. Proximal and distal extension is possible and can be improved further with detachment of one-third triceps tendon (Mayo modified Kocher approach).	Limited part of the Kocher may be used for the more simple fractures but it is the most expandable lateral approach.	Radial nerve in proximal extension.
Radial head fractures	Kaplan	Proximally. Distally limited by the PIN.	Ideal for radial head fractures without LCL involvement (fixation or arthroplasty).	PIN. Beware of retraction using anterior Hohman retractor around the radial neck.

Abbreviation: PIN, posterior interosseous nerve.
Data from Kocher T. Text-book of operative surgery. London: Adam and Charles Black; 1911; and Kaplan EB. Surgical approaches to the proximal end of the radius and its use in fractures of the head and neck of the radius. J Bone Joint Surg 1941;23:86.

It is better defined distally, because more proximally the fascia of both muscles coalesces toward the insertion.[14]

After the intermuscular plane is opened, the lateral capsule and ligaments are identified and incised to enter the joint. The LCL originates from the lateral epicondyle and inserts on the crista supinatoris of the ulna. These fibers must be recognized and protected when opening the capsule. It is usually safe to open the capsule just anterior to the ligament if it is intact. If the ligament is torn, its proximal stump should be dissected and tagged for final reattachment at the end of the operation.

Complex radial head fractures may need an associated LCL and extensor muscle repair and this is easier accessed through a Kocher approach rather than a Kaplan approach. Dissection must avoid extending the original damage to the ligaments. In terrible triad cases where the radial head has a simple fracture pattern and only needs to be fixed, access to the coronoid is performed

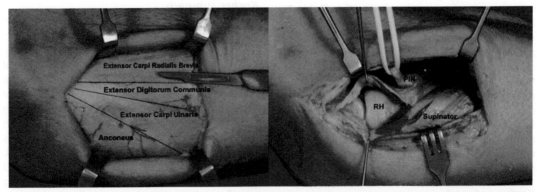

Fig. 10. Kaplan approach is more anterior than the Kocher approach and is used for fixation of simple radial head fractures. The access to the radial head (RH) is easy, but care should be taken to avoid distal extension that may jeopardize the posterior interosseous nerve (PIN).

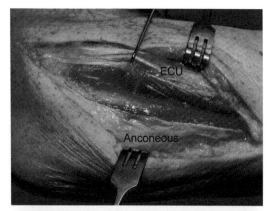

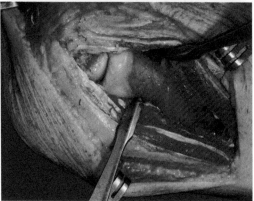

Fig. 11. Kocher approach allows access to the lateral ligament complex and to the radial head and capitellum. Proximal extension by detaching the brachioradialis anteriorly and the triceps posteriorly allows better exposure for difficult capitellum fractures or fracture sequelae.

When fixing a capitellar fracture, the Kocher approach may be slightly extended proximally to improve visualization of the reduction and orientation of the screws. Some complex capitellar fractures with medial extension can be fixed through a Kocher approach if there is no severe comminution. Occasionally the fracture line includes the lateral epicondyle and the repair can be done by elevating this fragment and reflecting the lateral ligament complex with it and fixing it at the end of the procedure. This maneuver permits opening the joint hinging on the medial side of the elbow. Otherwise, an olecranon osteotomy is favored.

Fractures of the Coronoid and Medial Epicondyle

When approaching the medial aspect of the elbow, a posterior midline skin incision might be preferred because it reduces the risk of damaging the medial antebrachial cutaneous nerve. To avoid painful neuromas, the nerve must be identified and protected, especially in the distal part of the incision where it usually arborizes.

The ulnar nerve must also be identified and protected. Decompression in the ulnar tunnel is occasionally needed in medial epicondyle fractures, fractures of the anteromedial coronoid facet, or when plate fixation is needed. Extensive medial dissection should be avoided in anteromedial coronoid fractures with a very small fragment precluding safe fixation. Under these circumstances, applying a lateral external fixator and lateral ligament reconstruction may be a better option.[3]

Flexor carpi ulnaris interval approach

This approach uses the interval between the humeral and the ulnar heads of the FCU (**Fig. 12**). The ulnar nerve lies in this interval and has a direct

before fixation of the radial head by extending the Kocher approach proximally, detaching the extensors from the humerus and elevating the anterior capsule.

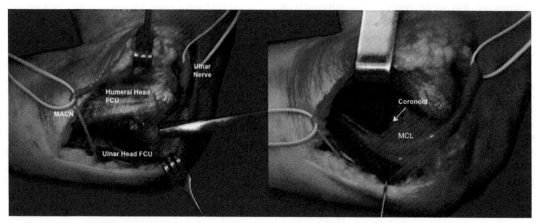

Fig. 12. Medial approach to the elbow. Note the situation of the medial antebrachial cutaneous nerve (MACN), crossing the surgical field. The approach goes in between both heads of the FCU. MCL, medial collateral ligament.

relationship with the MCL. Identification and proper protection of the nerve is necessary. In some cases the ulnar nerve needs to be fully mobilized to work safely. At the end of the procedure the nerve can be left in place or transposed anteriorly depending on its tendency to subluxate and its position relative to metallic implants. In cases of anterior transposition, resection of the intermuscular septum must be performed to avoid compression at the site where the nerve courses from the posterior to the anterior compartment of the arm.

To gain exposure into the joint, the sublime tubercle is located by palpation. The humeral head of the FCU is split in line with its fibers 1 cm distally to the sublime tubercle and dissected to bone. With a scalpel blade placed parallel to the bone we progress proximally as we encounter the sublime tubercle leaving the MCL insertion below the scalpel blade and the FCU above it. The brachialis muscle is seen in the deep aspect of this exposure with its fibers inserting distally to the coronoid with an angulation of 60°. The dissection may need to progress toward the epicondyle until we obtain an adequate exposure of the capsule. The capsule is incised in line with the MCL and just anterior to it, exposing the ulnohumeral joint and extending the approach proximally by elevating the capsule up to the medial epicondyle.

Coronoid tip fractures are readily visible and in patients with an anteromedial fracture, the fracture line is typically just underneath the most anterior part of the MCL. If the exposure needs to be extended distally, the brachialis and the FCU are dissected from the ulna, protecting the ulnar nerve and its branches.

For fractures of the tip of the coronoid a transmuscular approach through the humeral head of the FCU may be used with or without prior transposition of the ulnar nerve. This approach is more anterior to the previous described one and can improve the angle of vision and limit the dissection required.[15,16]

Fractures of the Olecranon and Proximal Ulna

These fractures are approached from a posterior skin incision. After subcutaneous dissection, olecranon fractures are readily accessible and can be fixed accordingly. Complex fractures of the olecranon and proximal ulna generally need plate fixation that can be dorsally or laterally applied. It is important to understand that the proximal ulna can have a variable bony anatomy when applying a precontoured plate, including dorsal angulation and axial alignment. An approach between the FCU and the ECU is used to achieve proper reduction and plate fixation. Extension of the fracture into the coronoid may include an anteromedial fragment that may need additional plating or specific screw targeting for open reduction and internal fixation. Reduction can be accomplished by extending the FCU-ECU approach medially reflecting the flexor-pronator mass.[17] Again, the ulnar nerve must be identified and protected. Decompression or transposition of the ulnar nerve is left to the discretion of the surgeon.

SUMMARY

Elbow trauma presents with a diverse range of injury patterns. Each injury pattern has a typical mechanism and discrete elements that may require surgical management. When managing elbow trauma surgically, many operative approaches exist. As such, surgeons should have a good working knowledge of elbow anatomy and the advantages and disadvantages of the available approaches.

ACKNOWLEDGMENTS

We would like to acknowledge the work of Drs J. Ballesteros, M. LLusá and P. Forcada for the surgical preparations that appear throughout the chapter.

REFERENCES

1. Rouleau DM, Canet F, Chapleau J, et al. The influence of proximal ulnar morphology on elbow range of motion. J Shoulder Elbow Surg 2012;21(3):384–8.
2. O'Driscoll SW, Jupiter JB, Cohen MS, et al. Difficult elbow fractures: pearls and pitfalls. Instr Course Lect 2003;52:113–34.
3. Pollock JW, Brownhill J, Ferreira L, et al. The effect of anteromedial facet fractures of the coronoid and lateral collateral ligament injury on elbow stability and kinematics. J Bone Joint Surg Am 2009;91(6):1448–58.
4. Cohen MS, Bruno RJ. The collateral ligaments of the elbow: anatomy and clinical correlation. Clin Orthop Relat Res 2001;(383):123–30.
5. Harty M, Joyce JJ III. Surgical approaches to the elbow. J Bone Joint Surg Am 1964;46:1598–606.
6. Vazquez O, Rutgers M, Ring DC, et al. Fate of the ulnar nerve after operative fixation of distal humerus fractures. J Orthop Trauma 2010;24(7):395–9.
7. Alonso-Llames M. Bilaterotricipital approach to the elbow. Its application in the osteosynthesis of supracondylar fractures of the humerus in children. Acta Orthop Scand 1972;43(6):479–90.
8. Campbell WC. Arthroplasty of the elbow. Ann Surg 1922;76(5):615–23.

9. Shahane SA, Stanley D. A posterior approach to the elbow joint. J Bone Joint Surg Br 1999;81(6):1020–2.

10. Cheung EV, Steinmann SP. Surgical approaches to the elbow. J Am Acad Orthop Surg 2009;17(5): 325–33.

11. Bryan RS, Morrey BF. Extensive posterior exposure of the elbow. A triceps-sparing approach. Clin Orthop Relat Res 1982;(166):188–92.

12. Kaplan EB. Surgical approaches to the proximal end of the radius and its use in fractures of the head and neck of the radius. J Bone Joint Surg 1941;23:86.

13. Strachan JC, Ellis BW. Vulnerability of the posterior interosseous nerve during radial head resection. J Bone Joint Surg Br 1971;53(2):320–3.

14. Kocher T. Text-book of operative surgery. London: Adam and Charles Black; 1911.

15. Smith GR, Altchek DW, Pagnani MJ, et al. A muscle-splitting approach to the ulnar collateral ligament of the elbow. Neuroanatomy and operative technique. Am J Sports Med 1996;24(5):575–80.

16. Thompson WH, Jobe FW, Yocum LA, et al. Ulnar collateral ligament reconstruction in athletes: muscle-splitting approach without transposition of the ulnar nerve. J Shoulder Elbow Surg 2001;10(2): 152–7.

17. Taylor TK, Scham SM. A posteromedial approach to the proximal end of the ulna for the internal fixation of olecranon fractures. J Trauma 1969;9:594–602.

Simple Elbow Dislocation

April Armstrong, MD, MSc, FRCSC

KEYWORDS

- Elbow • Instability • Dislocation • Medial collateral ligament • Lateral collateral ligament

KEY POINTS

- Most simple elbow dislocations may be treated nonoperatively.
- The three primary static stabilizers of the elbow are the ulnohumeral articulation, the anterior bundle of the medial collateral ligament, and the lateral collateral ligament complex.
- The extent of soft tissue injury following a simple elbow dislocation can vary and one must be vigilant about assessing postreduction radiographs to ensure congruent reduction of the elbow.
- Forearm rotation affects the stability of the elbow.
- Any muscle that crosses the elbow joint provides compressive stability to the elbow, and therefore rehabilitation programs should stress active range of motion programs.

ELBOW STABILITY

The elbow's stability is provided by static and dynamic constraints. The static constraints include the bony architecture and the capsuloligamentous structures. The dynamic stabilizers, which are muscles that cross the elbow joint, provide a compressive stability to the elbow during active muscular contraction. A "fortress of elbow stability" has been previously described that highlights the importance of the primary and secondary stabilizers of the elbow (**Fig. 1**).[1] The three primary stabilizers of the elbow include (1) the ulnohumeral articulation, (2) the anterior bundle of the medial collateral ligament (MCL), and (3) the lateral collateral ligament (LCL) complex.

Practically, if these three primary elbow structures are intact, then for the most part the elbow is stable. The important secondary stabilizers of the elbow are the radial humeral articulation, the common flexor pronator tendon, and the common extensor tendon. In a simple elbow dislocation, there is not bony disruption of the ulnohumeral articulation; however, there is disruption of the LCL complex and possibly the anterior bundle of the MCL. It is generally accepted that the LCL complex is universally disrupted with any elbow

dislocation; however, less agreed on is the degree of involvement of the medial soft tissues. Some authors believe that the MCL is disrupted 100% of the time,[2] whereas others have reported that there is a sequential disruption of the soft tissues starting laterally and then eventually progressing to the medial side depending on the magnitude of the elbow dislocation.[3] The important point is that each of these soft tissue stabilizers play an important role about the elbow and that radiographic analysis and clinical examination can help to determine the degree of involvement to dictate the treatment plan. The question is, if two out of the three primary stabilizers are involved with a simple elbow dislocation, then why can the elbow still remain reduced? This is because the ulnohumeral articulation has a highly constrained bony anatomy and there are compressive forces generated by the muscles that cross the elbow joint during active motion of the elbow.[4–6]

MECHANISM OF INJURY

The classic mechanism for injury is a fall on an outstretched arm. The classic mechanism proposed for a typical posterolateral elbow dislocation is an elbow that has been loaded axially in a valgus

Disclosure: Paid consultant for Zimmer.
Department of Orthopedics, Bone and Joint Institute, Penn State Hershey Medical Center, 30 Hope Drive, Hershey, PA 17033, USA
E-mail address: aarmstrong@hmc.psu.edu

Hand Clin 31 (2015) 521–531
http://dx.doi.org/10.1016/j.hcl.2015.06.002
0749-0712/15/$ – see front matter © 2015 Elsevier Inc. All rights reserved.

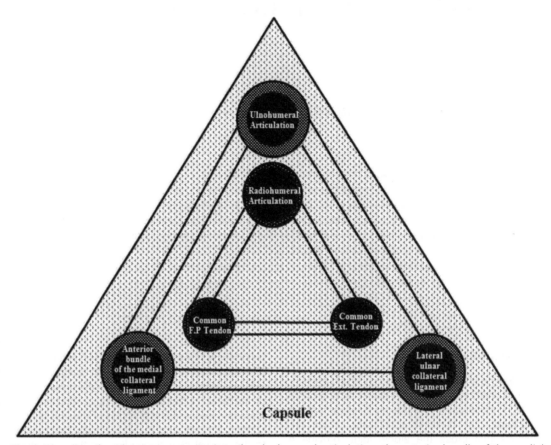

Fig. 1. The elbow has three primary restraints: the ulnohumeral articulation, the anterior bundle of the medial collateral ligament, and the lateral collateral ligament complex. The secondary constraints are the radiocapitellar joint, the common flexor, and extensor tendons. (*Adapted from* O'Driscoll SW, Jupiter JB, King GJ, et al. The unstable elbow. Instr Course Lect 2001;50:91; with permission.)

position with the forearm supinated.[3] It is believed that the soft tissues are disrupted in a circular fashion from lateral to medial with this mechanism.[7] Other mechanisms for elbow dislocation have been described[8] that are important for clinicians to appreciate because the degree of soft tissue disruption can be mechanism dependant, which may require a change in treatment protocol. The bottom line is that not all simple elbow dislocations are treated alike and understanding the principles of treatment is important.

CASE EXAMPLES
Case #1

Fig. 2 shows a posterolateral dislocation of an elbow in a 17-year-old man. He was involved in a skateboarding injury and landed on his outstretched arm. His postreduction lateral film is shown in **Fig. 3**, which shows incongruence of the elbow joint and gapping at the ulnohumeral articulation. The forearm was positioned in

supination when this radiograph was taken. The elbow is appropriately positioned close to 90°, which takes advantage of the high congruency of the ulnohumeral joint. Therefore, the persistent joint incongruity could be because the forearm is not rotationally reduced or something is interposed between the bones not allowing for full reduction, which could be bone, cartilage, muscle, or nerve, such as the ulnar nerve. The forearm may be simply repositioned to see if one is dealing with a rotationally unstable elbow. There is the option of positioning the forearm in pronation, neutral, or supination. Because the LCL complex is universally torn in elbow dislocations, typically the choice is between forearm pronation or neutral positioning. If repositioning the forearm does not provide stability to the elbow, the next consideration is to investigate further for an interposed fragment. Physical examination of the neurovascular structures and possibly an MRI or a computed tomography scan to look for any type of bone or cartilage lesion that is preventing the reduction of

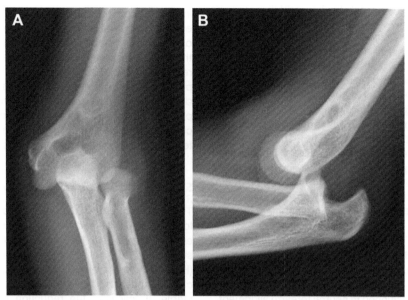

Fig. 2. Case #1: Anteroposterior (*A*) and lateral (*B*) image of posterolateral elbow dislocation.

the elbow joint is required. In **Fig. 4**, the forearm was repositioned into pronation, which allowed for a congruent reduction of the elbow joint. The persistent ulnohumeral gapping shown in **Fig. 3** represented persistent rotational instability of the elbow. By simply repositioning the forearm, a concentric radiographic reduction was obtained. This case demonstrates an important concept regarding the effect of forearm rotation in an LCL-deficient elbow. The LCL complex is an important varus and rotational stabilizer of the elbow.[5] It has been shown that an LCL-deficient elbow can be rendered stable with passive pronation of the forearm and active muscle contraction.[5] The classic teaching point with a posterolateral elbow dislocation is to place the forearm in pronation to render it stable to offload the disruption of the LCL.

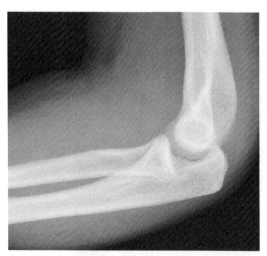

Fig. 3. Case #1: Postreduction lateral film shows incongruence at the ulnohumeral articulation. The forearm was positioned in supination.

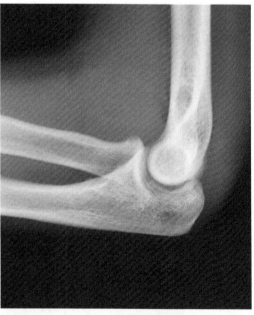

Fig. 4. Case #1: Forearm repositioned in pronation that shows congruent reduction of the elbow joint.

Case #2

Not all elbow dislocations have similar soft tissue disruption. This is a case of a 24-year-old man who fell skiing and was referred for inability to maintain a reduction of the elbow joint. This patient had sustained a direct lateral elbow dislocation as shown in **Fig. 5**. Following closed reduction of the elbow the patient was placed in 90° of elbow flexion with the forearm pronated. The postreduction films demonstrated persistent ulnohumeral joint gapping on the lateral image and on the anteroposterior film one can appreciate gapping at the medial joint line (**Fig. 6**). This case demonstrates an important concept regarding the effect of forearm rotation with a significant medial-sided injury. It has been shown that an MCL-deficient elbow can be rendered stable with passive supination of the forearm and active muscle contraction.[6] **Fig. 7** shows postreduction images after the forearm was repositioned in neutral forearm alignment. The forearm was repositioned in neutral to offload the stress on the medial and lateral structures, which allows for joint congruency on the anteroposterior and lateral images. These two case examples highlight the important concept that not all simple elbow dislocations are treated alike and it is important to be vigilant about the radiographic assessment and treatment plan.

There are instances in which one may see a slight widening of the ulnohumeral joint but not necessarily asymmetric in alignment. This has been referred to as the "drop sign."[9,10] This can be a warning sign of persistence of instability and should be followed closely. In most cases this corrects itself within a week, likely related to increased muscle contraction by the patient and increased compression forces at the joint. However, if it persists then this is concerning for risk of recurrent instability. It is recommended that the patient continue to be immobilized until it corrects itself. Also, a gravity-loaded rehabilitation program is recommended for a patient with a drop sign. Active rehabilitation with the patient supine and overhead elbow flexion and extension can also take advantage of the compressive effects of gravity on the elbow (**Fig. 8**).

SYSTEMATIC TREATMENT APPROACH

There are some instances when simple elbow dislocations are not effectively treated with a nonoperative approach. In these circumstances a systematic surgical approach is recommended (**Fig. 9**). After an elbow is reduced, the treating clinician must decide if the elbow is stable or unstable. If following the reduction it is believed that the elbow is stable through the reasonable arc of elbow flexion and extension, and the radiographs show a congruent joint, then the patient may be placed in a sling and advanced to an active rehabilitation program. There is limited research about immediate motion following posterior dislocations of the elbow and this approach requires a very compliant patient.[11] Most often patients are immobilized for a short period of time rather than mobilized immediately. If the elbow is radiographically congruent and stable through an arc of motion from 45 to 60° of elbow flexion then a more conservative approach is to immobilize the patients for 5 to 7 days at 90° of flexion in the stable forearm position, typically neutral or pronation. Following a short period of immobilization the

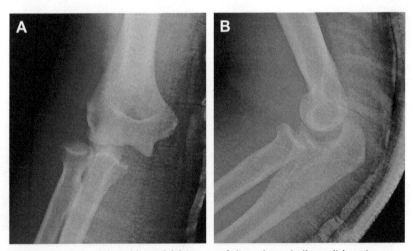

Fig. 5. Case #2: Anteroposterior (*A*) and lateral (*B*) image of direct lateral elbow dislocation.

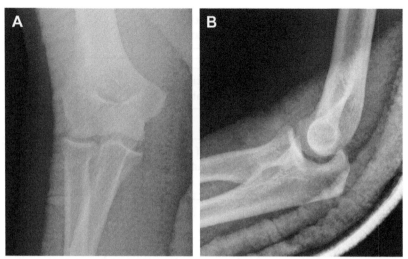

Fig. 6. Case #2: Anteroposterior (*A*) and lateral (*B*) postreduction films show persistent ulnohumeral gapping, forearm is positioned in pronation. The anteroposterior (*A*) image demonstrates gapping at the medial joint line.

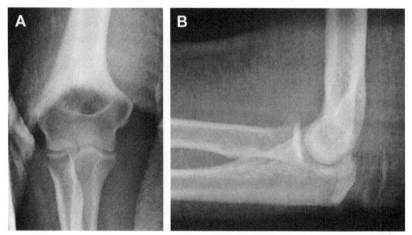

Fig. 7. Case #2: Anteroposterior (*A*) and lateral (*B*) films with the forearm repositioned in neutral alignment. The ulnohumeral gapping and gapping at the medial joint line on the anteroposterior (*A*) image is no longer evident.

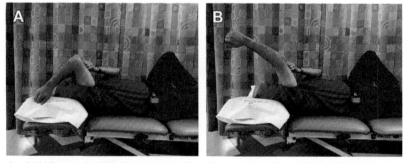

Fig. 8. Gravity-loaded elbow rehabilitation program for elbow flexion (*A*) and extension (*B*) is effective for treating simple elbow dislocations.

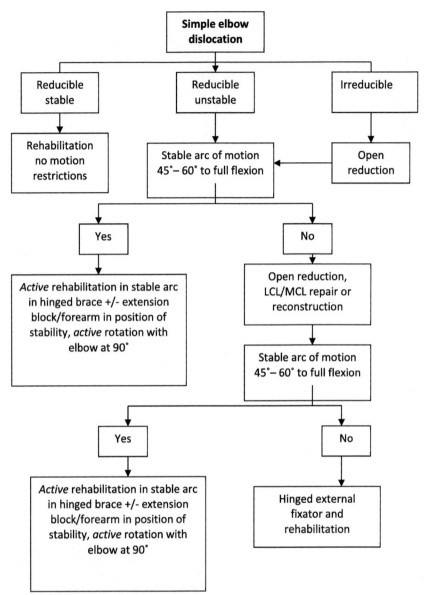

Fig. 9. A systematic approach to simple elbow dislocations. (*From* Armstrong A. Acute, current and chronic elbow instability. In: Galatz LM, editor. Orthopedic knowledge update 3: shoulder and elbow. Rosemont (IL): American Academy of Orthopedic Surgeons, 2008; with permission.)

patient is then placed in a removable splint with or without an extension block depending on the stability of the elbow on examination. If the patient is apprehensive as one moves further into extension then an extension block splint is preferred for a short period of time. It is recommended that the extension block be removed at 3 to 4 weeks' time to gradually allow for the patient to extend into full extension range of motion and prevent a flexion contracture. This is a situation where a gravity-loaded active rehabilitation program can help the patient by taking advantage of not just

the compressive forces of the muscles but also gravity (see **Fig. 8**).

The patient is then allowed to advance to an active rehabilitation program where they do active range of motion exercises through their stable arc of motion and also work on active full pronation and supination of the forearm with the elbow at 90° to prevent a rotational contracture. The goal is to achieve close to full active range of motion by 6 to 8 weeks following their injury. If patients still have residual stiffness at that time, then consideration should be given to a static progressive splinting program, typically around 8 to 10 weeks following the injury when the elbow is no longer swollen. A strengthening program may start 8 to 12 weeks following the injury. During the rehabilitation program, the patient is also asked to prevent varus positioning of the elbow. For instance, when elevating the arm, the patient should elevate with their elbow down by their side instead of away from their body to minimize varus loading of the elbow (**Fig. 10**). Frequent weekly radiographs in the first 2 to 3 weeks following an elbow dislocation are required to confirm concentric reduction of the elbow. Following 3 weeks of concentric radiographic reduction the frequency of images may be reduced. Typically a repeat image is performed at 6 weeks and then again at 3 months.

If the elbow is not reducible or considered to have an incongruent reduction, then the patient requires an open reduction. Typically this is approached surgically through a posterior midline incision or a combined medial and lateral approach as needed. The joint is first approached through a lateral Kocher interval between the anconeus and the extensor carpi ulnaris. The LCL is typically avulsed proximally but can be avulsed at the crista supinatoris, or rarely disrupted because of a cristae supinatoris fracture. The joint is opened to inspect for any bony fragments or cartilage fragments, or other structures preventing reduction. The next step is to repair the LCL. The ligament should be repaired at the anatomic site of insertion on the humerus, which is located at the center of the lateral surface of the capitellum, which is also the center of the axis of rotation of the elbow. Posteriorly there can be an impression fracture of the capitellum and this area should not be used to judge the anatomic insertion point.[12] A drill hole is created at the isometric point, which is identified by finding the center point from the anterior and inferior portion of the capitellum, and then the ligament is either repaired to the bone with a suture anchor or bone tunnels. The common extensor origin should also be repaired because it is an important secondary elbow stabilizer. The elbow is then assessed under fluoroscopic imaging to determine a stable arc of motion (45–60° flexion minimum) and to determine positioning of the forearm, either neutral or pronation. Occasionally, the forearm may be placed in supination if the LCL ligament repair is robust in good bone and it is believed that this positioning is important to offload a medial-sided injury, but this could put the LCL complex repair at risk.

If the elbow continues to be unstable, then consideration should be given to repairing the MCL complex. Often there is already a split in the flexor pronator mass, which takes one right down to the anterior bundle of the MCL. The anterior bundle of the MCL can be ruptured off of the humerus but can also show an intrasubstance tear or rupture from the sublime tubercle on the ulna. For a humeral avulsion, the ligament is repaired to the isometric point of insertion on the humerus, with anchors or bone tunnels. The approximate isometric point is located at the anterior inferior portion of the medial epicondyle, close to the center of the trochlea, which falls in line with the axis of rotation of the elbow. Avulsion of the ligament from the distal insertion at the sublime tubercle on the ulna may also be repaired with bone tunnels or suture anchor. Intrasubstance tearing is usually very difficult to repair and in this situation, the common flexor should be repaired. If the elbow continues to be unstable then consideration should be given to external fixation, which is typically maintained for 4 to 6 weeks. Static or hinged external fixation is appropriate and at the surgeon's discretion. In some situations, a hinged external fixator may be considered. Placement of the axis pin for alignment of the external fixator is critical and needs to be placed at the anatomic axis of rotation.

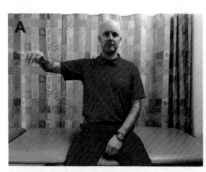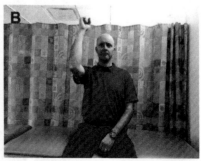

Fig. 10. During the first 4 to 6 weeks of recovery from a simple elbow dislocation, it is recommended that the patient avoid the varus loaded position shown in (*A*) and instead elevate the arm as shown in (*B*), which offloads the lateral collateral ligament injury.

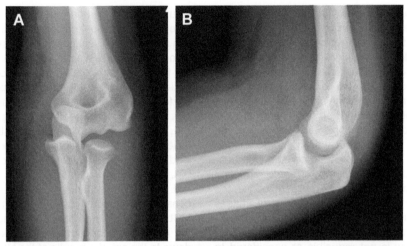

Fig. 11. Case #3: Anteroposterior (*A*) and lateral (*B*) image of a recurrent direct medial elbow dislocation.

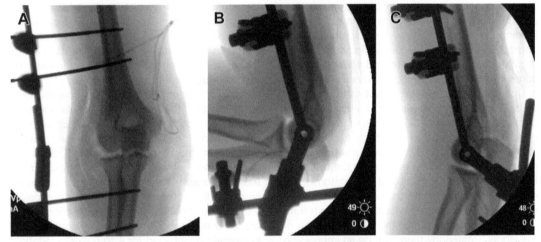

Fig. 12. Case#3: Anteroposterior (*A*), lateral in 90° flexion (*B*), and lateral in extension (*C*) images of the elbow following placement of hinged external fixator show congruent elbow joint.

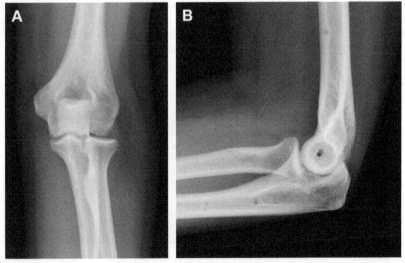

Fig. 13. Case #3: Final anteroposterior (*A*) and lateral (*B*) image of the elbow 6 months after injury showing a stable and congruent elbow.

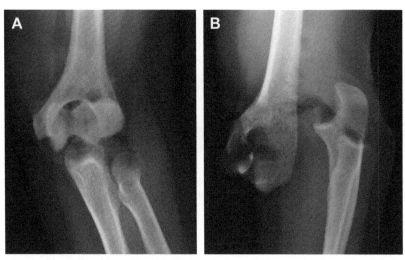

Fig. 14. Case #4: Anteroposterior (*A*) and lateral (*B*) elbow images of an open elbow dislocation.

CASE EXAMPLES
Case #3

This is a case of a 42-year-old woman who presented 3 weeks after undergoing a closed elbow reduction at an outside facility for a direct medial elbow dislocation. She was placed in a sling and

was allowed immediate elbow range of motion and no further follow-up had been arranged. **Fig. 11** shows her elbow radiographs at the time of presentation at 3 weeks and shows a recurrent elbow dislocation. After following the systematic approach to open reduction of the elbow (see **Fig. 9**), her elbow could not be stabilized and she was then subsequently placed in a hinged external fixator (**Fig. 12**). Six months after her injury, the patient had regained near full stable range of motion of her elbow (**Fig. 13**). Jockel and colleagues[13] recently reported four cases of recurrent instability following medial elbow dislocation. They proposed that the soft tissue injury may be more

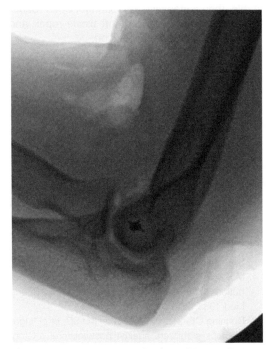

Fig. 15. Case #4: Intraoperative lateral image showing an anatomically reduced elbow joint and a suture anchor for repair of the lateral collateral ligament complex.

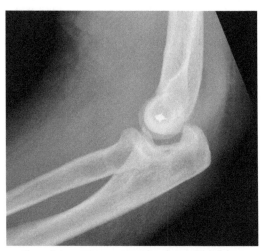

Fig. 16. Case #4: Lateral image of the elbow 1 week after index procedure shows recurrent elbow instability.

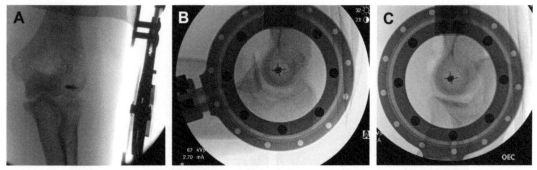

Fig. 17. Case #4: Anteroposterior (*A*), lateral in 90° flexion (*B*), and lateral in extension (*C*) images of the elbow following placement of hinged external fixator show congruent elbow joint.

significant with this instability pattern and therefore it is recommended that there be an increased vigilance when following this injury pattern for recurrent instability.

Case #4

Fig. 14 shows radiographs of an open dislocation of an elbow sustained by a 57-year-old woman who fell from a horse. She also had an acute median neurapraxia and an angiogram for an assessment of a potential arterial injury was negative. She underwent an immediate LCL repair with a bone anchor, which was stable intraoperatively (**Fig. 15**). Unfortunately, within 1 week she showed recurrent instability of the elbow (**Fig. 16**). She was then placed in a hinged external fixator (**Fig. 17**). The important lesson learned from this case, however, was that because the anchor for LCL repair was correctly placed at the center of rotation of the elbow at the index procedure, it then made placement of the axis pin for alignment of the hinged fixator difficult. It is recommended that a transosseous technique be considered for fixation of the lateral ligament if there is a potential that an external fixator may be used. For static external fixation this is not a concern.

CLINICAL RESULTS IN THE LITERATURE

Long-term outcome studies have shown that the risk for recurrent instability following a simple elbow dislocation is low. However, slight early degenerative changes have also been reported 10 to 20 years following simple elbow dislocation. Fortunately, these degenerative changes rarely cause functional problems or significant symptoms.[14–16] It has been shown that greater restoration of flexion and extension motion of the elbow following a simple elbow dislocation predicted better pain and function for the patient.[16]

SUMMARY

Effective treatment of simple elbow dislocations requires a detailed clinical assessment and sequential radiographic follow-up. A simple elbow dislocation that is rotationally unstable can be stabilized by simply repositioning the forearm. It is important to follow these patients on a weekly basis for the first 3 weeks to monitor for recurrent instability. The joint must be reduced concentrically and a systematic protocol should be followed to ensure that the elbow is rendered stable. The rehabilitation program stresses early active range of motion through the stable arc of motion and forearm rotation. If the elbow cannot be rendered stable, then a stepwise approach for open reduction is recommended with soft tissue repair and the possibility of external fixation.

REFERENCES

1. O'Driscoll SW, Jupiter JB, Cohen MS, et al. Difficult elbow fractures: pearls and pitfalls. Instr Course Lect 2003;52:113–34.
2. Josefsson PO, Gentz CF, Johnell O, et al. Surgical versus non-surgical treatment of ligamentous injuries following dislocation of the elbow joint. A prospective randomized study. J Bone Joint Surg Am 1987;69(4):605–8.
3. O'Driscoll SW, Morrey BF, Korinek S, et al. Elbow subluxation and dislocation. A spectrum of instability. Clin Orthop Relat Res 1992;(280):186–97.
4. Morrey BF, An KN. Articular and ligamentous contributions to the stability of the elbow joint. Am J Sports Med 1983;11(5):315–9.
5. Dunning CE, Zarzour ZD, Patterson SD, et al. Ligamentous stabilizers against posterolateral rotatory instability of the elbow. J Bone Joint Surg Am 2001;83-A(12):1823–8.
6. Armstrong AD, Dunning CE, Faber KJ, et al. Rehabilitation of the medial collateral ligament-deficient

elbow: an in vitro biomechanical study. J Hand Surg Am 2000;25(6):1051–7.

7. O'Driscoll SW, Bell DF, Morrey BF. Posterolateral rotatory instability of the elbow. J Bone Joint Surg Am 1991;73(3):440–6.

8. Deutch SR, Jensen SL, Olsen BS, et al. Elbow joint stability in relation to forced external rotation: an experimental study of the osseous constraint. J Shoulder Elbow Surg 2003;12(3):287–92.

9. Coonrad RW, Roush TF, Major NM, et al. The drop sign, a radiographic warning sign of elbow instability. J Shoulder Elbow Surg 2005;14(3):312–7.

10. Duckworth AD, Kulijdian A, McKee MD, et al. Residual subluxation of the elbow after dislocation or fracture-dislocation: treatment with active elbow exercises and avoidance of varus stress. J Shoulder Elbow Surg 2008;17(2):276–80.

11. Ross G, McDevitt ER, Chronister R, et al. Treatment of simple elbow dislocation using an immediate motion protocol. Am J Sports Med 1999;27(3):308–11.

12. Faber KJ, King GJ. Posterior capitellum impression fracture: a case report associated with posterolateral rotatory instability of the elbow. J Shoulder Elbow Surg 1998;7(2):157–9.

13. Jockel CR, Katolik LI, Zelouf DS. Simple medial elbow dislocations: a rare injury at risk for early instability. J Hand Surg Am 2013;38(9):1768–73.

14. Josefsson PO, Johnell O, Gentz CF. Long-term sequelae of simple dislocation of the elbow. J Bone Joint Surg Am 1984;66(6):927–30.

15. Mehlhoff TL, Noble PC, Bennett JB, et al. Simple dislocation of the elbow in the adult. Results after closed treatment. J Bone Joint Surg Am 1988; 70(2):244–9.

16. Anakwe RE, Middleton SD, Jenkins PJ, et al. Patient-reported outcomes after simple dislocation of the elbow. J Bone Joint Surg Am 2011;93(13):1220–6.

Fractures of the Radial Head

Klaus Josef Burkhart, MD[a],*, Kilian Wegmann, MD[b], Lars P. Müller, MD[b],
Frank E. Gohlke, MD[a]

KEYWORDS

- Radial head • Fracture • ORIF • Locking plate • Arthroplasty • Outcome

KEY POINTS

- Radial head fractures are associated with a high rate of concomitant ligament tears. The authors recommend viewing radial head fractures not merely as osseous lesions but as osteoligamentous lesions.
- Simple fractures displaced less than 2 mm can be treated nonoperatively. Prolonged rehabilitation should raise suspicion of complicating additional injuries.
- The treatment of choice for 2 to 5 mm displaced partial articular fractures remains debatable. Several investigators report good results of nonoperative treatment comparable to open reduction and internal fixation (ORIF) but with lower complication rates. However, rate of osteoarthritis seems to be higher with nonoperative treatment.
- ORIF is preferred whenever an anatomic and stable reduction can be achieved. Modern implants and techniques, such as radial head–specific low-profile locking plates, extend the indications for ORIF.
- If anatomic and stable reduction cannot be achieved, radial head arthroplasty remains the treatment of choice.

INTRODUCTION AND ANATOMIC PRINCIPALS

The elbow joint plays a critical role in the functionality of the human upper extremity. It facilitates complex actions of the hand that are indispensable to daily activities. Injuries of the elbow joint are accompanied by pain and a limited range of motion (ROM), resulting in restriction of the aforementioned tasks. This has also been shown for fractures of the radial head.[1,2] The outcome of these fractures depends largely on the severity of the injury. Though undisplaced stable fractures

have a good prognosis with nonoperative treatment, it is necessary to identify the displaced unstable fractures and determine whether reduction and fixation is possible, or whether replacement must be performed to prevent pain, stiffness, and secondary arthrosis.

The vulnerability of the elbow joint is based on its intricate anatomy in which 3 separate articulations are functionally combined and rely on distinct active and passive stabilizers such as muscles, bony structures, and ligaments. The radial head is related to the functionality and

Disclosures: The biomechanical laboratory of the Department of Trauma, Hand, and Elbow Surgery of the University of Cologne is supported by a yearly grant by Medartis but not specifically for this study. K.J. Burkhart and L.P. Müller were involved in the development of the Medartis Aptus 2.0 proximal radius plates. K. Wegmann, K.J. Burkhart, and L.P. Müller serve as consultants for Medartis. No benefits in any form have been received or will be received related directly or indirectly to the subject of this article.
^a Department for Shoulder Surgery, Rhön-Clinic, Bad Neustadt, Salzburger Leite 1, 97616 Bad Neustadt/Saale, Germany; ^b Department for Trauma, Hand and Elbow Surgery, University of Cologne, Kerpener Straße 62, 50937 Köln, Germany
* Corresponding author. Shoulder and Elbow Surgery, Department for Shoulder Surgery, Rhön-Clinic, Salzburger Leite 1, Bad Neustadt 97616, Germany.
E-mail address: klaus.j.burkhart@gmail.com

Hand Clin 31 (2015) 533–546
http://dx.doi.org/10.1016/j.hcl.2015.06.003
0749-0712/15/$ – see front matter © 2015 Elsevier Inc. All rights reserved.

influences the biomechanics of all 3 of these separate articulations.

The lateral aspect of the elbow joint is represented by the articulation of the radial head with the capitellum. Its stability comes from the opposite congruity of the convex capitellum and the concave radial head. Moreover, the lateral collateral ligament (LCL) prevents varus angulation.[3] The lateral ulnar collateral ligament (LUCL), together with the lateral bony prominence of the proximal ulna, the supinator crest, resist posterior subluxation of the radial by acting as a hammock. A deficiency of these structures may result in posterolateral rotatory instability (PLRI).[4]

In the center of the elbow joint, the radial head articulates with the lesser sigmoid notch of the proximal ulna to form the proximal radioulnar joint (PRUJ). The joint is stabilized by the annular ligament. Elbow fractures are often associated with injuries to the annular ligament; however, the clinical relevance has not been clarified.[5]

The radial head acts as the main stabilizer of longitudinal forearm stability because it resists proximalization of the radius in axial loading of the forearm.[6] At the elbow, approximately 60% of the mechanical load goes through the radial column. Loss of the radial head shifts 100% of the loading onto the ulnar column (**Fig. 1**). Thus, sole resection of the radial head due to unreconstructable fractures should not be performed, particularly not in an acute setting. Doing so could lead to early erosion of the ulnar joint and proximal migration of the radius, or to possible pain and limited function (**Fig. 2**).[7]

Further relevant stabilizers of the elbow joint are found at the medial aspect of the elbow, as represented by the trochlea and the proximal ulna. The 2 bony components show an anatomic fit and close joint congruency, offering stability and guidance during movement. Ligamentous stability is given by the medial collateral ligament (MCL), of which the anterior bundle acts as the main stabilizer against valgus stress.[8] The radial head plays the role of the secondary valgus stabilizer. Thus, MCL and radial head integrity influence each other. This should be acknowledged when dealing with radial fractures, which are often accompanied by lesions of the collateral ligaments.

EPIDEMIOLOGY

Fractures of the radial head are the most common elbow injuries, accounting for approximately 30% of all elbow fractures in adult patients. Duckworth and colleagues[9] reported an incidence in Scotland of 55 of every 100,000 inhabitants. Though the investigators did not find a significant difference

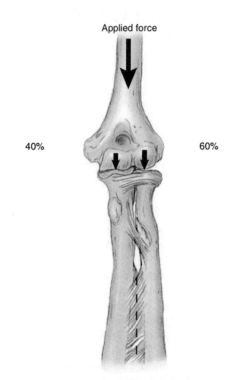

Fig. 1. Force transmission through the elbow. (*From* An K, Zobitz ME, Morrey BF. Biomechanics of the elbow. In: Morrey BF, Sanchez-Sotelo J, editors. The elbow and its disorders. 4th edition. Philadelphia: Elsevier; 2009. p. 39–63; with permission.)

specifically by gender, they discovered a bimodal distribution of patient age and mechanism of trauma at the time of injury according to gender. The fracture incidence in men peaked at 37 years of age with high-energy traumas, whereas simple falls were dominant in women at 52 years. This observation was corroborated by Kaas and colleagues[10] in 2010. Both study groups reported no significant differences by gender or age in the type of fracture or the incidence of accompanying ligamentous or osseous lesions. However, differences were observed for the injury mechanism. Hence, the investigators stated that the incidence of accompanying lesions increased proportionally to the type of fracture according to the Mason classification.

CLASSIFICATION

The Mason classification system, reported in 1954, is the accepted classification system for fractures of the radial head.[11] The classification distinguishes undisplaced fractures (type I), displaced fractures (type II), and fractures that are displaced with comminution (type III). A fourth type was added by Johnston[12] in 1962, describing

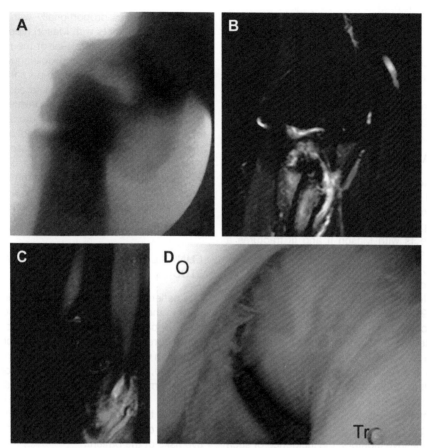

Fig. 2. Radial head resection was performed after early failed open reduction and internal fixation. Persistent ulnar instability visualized under fluoroscopy (*A*). MRI scans show osteoarthritis primarily in the radial part of the ulnohumeral joint (*B, C*). The patient was referred for management due to constant pain and joint locking 8 times per day. Arthroscopic debridement was performed. View from the high dorsoradial portal shows deep grooves in the lateral part of the trochlea (*D*). O, olecranon; Tr, trochlea.

a fracture of the radial head accompanied by elbow dislocation. Moreover, in 1987, Broberg and Morrey[13] added a metric definition of displacement (<2 mm or >2 mm) and an area of involvement of the articular surface (>30%) to differentiate between Mason I and II (**Fig. 3**).

The Mason classification, however, has shown low interobserver and intraobserver reliability;

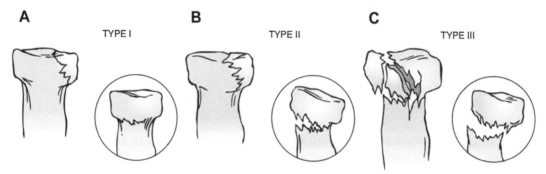

Fig. 3. Mason classification of uncomplicated radial head fractures. (*A*) Type I. (*B*) Type II; the exact definition is often difficult to determine. (*C*) Type III. Type IV is not included because it represents a complicated fracture. (*From* van Riet RP, Van Glabbeek F, Morrey BF. Radial head fracture. In: Morrey BF, Sanchez-Sotelo J, editors. The elbow and its disorders. 4th edition. Philadelphia: Elsevier; 2009. p. 359–81; with permission.)

hence, it is difficult to derive conclusive treatment algorithms.[14,15] The use of 3-dimensional computed tomography (CT) imaging significantly improves the interobserver reliability compared with 2-dimensional imaging but there is still only moderate agreement in the field.[15] Thus, a conclusive system that determines the correct treatment method is required.

ACCOMPANYING LESIONS

Several studies have reported a high incidence of associated lesions of the soft tissue of the elbow with fractures of the radial head. In 2005, Itamura and colleagues[16] demonstrated in an MRI study of 24 subjects with Mason II and III fractures a rate of 54% injuries of the MCL and 80% injuries of the LUCL. Both ligaments injured were found in 50% of cases. Moreover, associated capitellar chondral defects and loose bodies occurred in 30% and 91% of cases, respectively. Recently, Kaas and colleagues[17] reported 8 LCL lesions in 17 subjects with radial head fracture, including those with a Mason I fracture. These studies emphasize the need to carefully investigate the ligamentous and osteocartilaginous lesions of patients with radial head fractures. Accompanying injuries of the interosseous membrane have also been reported by McGinley and colleagues.[18] According to the investigators, the incidence of such

injuries increases proportionally with the type of fracture. All subjects with Mason type III fractures had suffered a complete tear of the interosseous membrane. Hausmann and colleagues[19] investigated subjects with Mason type I fractures and found a partial lesion of the interosseous membrane in 9 of 14 individuals, even in such presumed low-grade fractures. With the increasing severity of the causal injury, the likelihood of injuries to the wrist or shoulder joint rises, and emphasis must be placed accordingly.[20]

In summary, the authors recommend viewing radial head fractures not merely as osseous lesions but as osteoligamentous lesions (**Fig. 4**).

CLINICAL INVESTIGATIONS AND IMAGING STUDIES

The patient's history must be considered with regard to the trauma mechanism and the perceived areas of pain. In many radial head fracture cases, patients report a fall on the outstretched arm in pronation with sudden pain around the elbow joint. Therefore, prior injuries or surgical procedures to the joint must be elucidated when taking the history. The medical history is of great importance because the indication for surgical interventions depends on the general condition and perioperative risks of the patient.

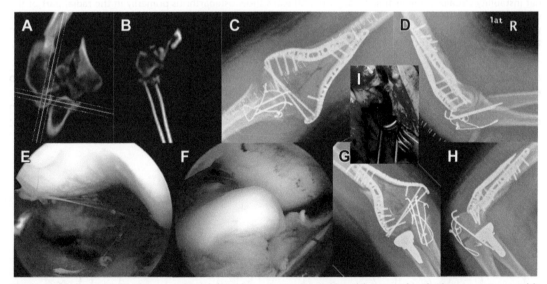

Fig. 4. A 25-year-old man with a combined distal humerus and radial head fractures (*A*, *B*). The unreconstructable radial head was excised. As the elbow was considered stable by the index trauma surgeon, radial head arthroplasty was not performed (*C*, *D*). During the early postoperative period, the patient developed a painful and stiff elbow. Arthroscopic view on the site after radial head excision showing a good reconstruction of the distal humeral articular surface (*E*, *F*). The loss of ulnohumeral contact revealed significant instability (*F*). After arthroscopic anterior capsulectomy, an open implantation of a radial head prosthesis (*G*, *H*) was performed through the former dorsal skin incision via the Boyd approach (*I*).

It is of primary importance to check for open fractures and to document the neurovascular status. Depending on the injury, swelling, hematoma, and deformity can also be located. Then, via palpation, the point of maximum tenderness should be defined and correlated with possible injuries to the according anatomic regions (**Fig. 5**). The bony formations of the radial head (pronation or supination), the medial and lateral epicondyle, and the olecranon can easily be palpated. To identify associated lesions of the forearm and wrist, subtle palpation along the interosseous membrane should be performed, and the distal radioulnar joint should be checked for tenderness or instability compared with the healthy contralateral side. Moreover, active and passive ROM must be determined and documented. Great attention must be given to potential crepitus within the joint when moving the extremity, and the clinician must check for joint instability. Varus and valgus stability should be investigated in full extension and 30° of flexion, and, if possible, documented under fluoroscopy. PLRI can be tested using the pivot shift test or posterolateral rotatory drawer test. However, these tests are difficult to perform, particularly in a painful, tender, acutely injured patient.

The clinician must determine whether imaging studies are necessary. Clinical tests that exclude relevant injury and avoid the need for radiographs, following the Ottawa ankle rules in the treatment of lower extremity injuries, are currently being sought.[21] When imaging is indicated, radiographs, including the anteroposterior (AP), oblique, and lateral projection are the basic measures. Subtle fractures are often difficult to see on radiographs. Soft tissue findings typical of occult fractures include the presence of the anterior or posterior fat pad sign. In addition, a slight irregularity of the transition of the radial head to the neck may be visible on radiographic studies, even in low-grade fractures with minimal displacement. Adequate articulation of the joint must also be determined, including the presence of a drop-sign or posterolateral subluxation of the radial head suspicious for PLRI. Additional information provided by radiographs is the presence and quantity of free bony fragments. According to Rineer and colleagues,[22] the complete loss of cortical contact of at least 1 radial head fracture fragment is strongly correlated with a complex injury pattern. The interobserver reliability of this observation is moderate.[23] Moreover the degree of displacement of fracture fragments (>2 mm) can be judged, although the reliability of such predications should be better on CT scans. With modern technology, 2-dimensional and 3-dimensional reconstructions of the radial head are possible but still do not reduce interobserver variation.[15] The presence of small free intraarticular fragments or the presence of impacted fractures can be judged much better on CT scans, following which the decision of whether surgery is indicated can be made.[24]

Using MRI scans, the clinician is able to assess the state of the soft tissues, visualizing even the slightest fracture line within bone and detecting intraosseous edema.[17,25] The routine use of MRI scans is not necessary because the impact of MRI scans on the selected treatment has not been established in the literature.[26]

THERAPY
Mason I

Undisplaced or minimally displaced 2-part fractures of the radial head can usually be treated nonoperatively. A mechanical block to rotation is an indication for surgery. The diagnosis of mechanical blocks can be facilitated via the aspiration of the trauma hematoma and injection of local anesthetics. This may lead to faster rehabilitation but is not obligatory. Good results can be expected in 80% to 95% of patients with short-term immobilization in a cast with 90° flexion and neutral

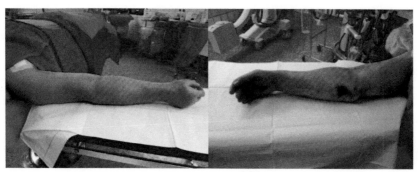

Fig. 5. Setting in the operating room for surgery of a Mason IV fracture. Soft tissue damage is worse on the ulnar side.

rotation, or a sling for a maximum of 7 to 10 days followed by early physiotherapy.[11,12,27–29]

Nevertheless, Mason I fractures should not be underestimated. These patients should be followed and routinely reexamined to recognize potential complications early. In the authors' experiences, patients with a simple Mason I fracture will present an uneventful short-term course because a stable elbow is not overly painful. Most often patients recover within 4 weeks, with a rapid decrease of symptoms and a noticeable increase in ROM. Persistent pain or a difficult rehabilitation course may indicate additional injuries that complicate this simple fracture, such as dynamic PLRI. The authors surveyed a cohort of subjects with neglected Mason I fractures suffering stiffness, osteoarthritis, and rotatory instability that was both medial and posterolateral. These cases demonstrated that even undisplaced radial head fractures may be caused by a dislocation mechanism.[30] Therefore, the authors recommend reexamination and, potentially, an early MRI for patients with complicated courses following Mason I fractures.

Mason II

Whether Mason II fractures need open reduction and internal fixation (ORIF) is controversial. Good results with few complications are usually achieved with ORIF of partially displaced fractures of the radial head. Since Akesson and colleagues[29] first reported good long-term results of nonsurgically treated 2 to 5 mm displaced Mason II fractures, the indication for surgery is again in question. In their retrospective study, they reported that 40 of 49 subjects declared that they had no symptoms after a mean follow-up of 19 years. Only minimal differences between the injured and uninjured elbow were noted. Six of these 49 subjects had undergone radial head excision within 4 to 6 months, due to an unfavorable outcome. Conversely, Lindenhovius and

colleagues[31] reported a positive outcome in their retrospective case series of 16 subjects with a surgically treated Mason II fracture after a mean follow-up of 22 years. Because they did not find clearly better results for ORIF compared with those undergoing Akesson and colleagues[29] nonsurgical treatment, Lindenhovius and colleagues[31] questioned whether ORIF is justified for these fractures because ORIF may result in further complications.

In the authors' practices, isolated partial fractures of the radial head with a displacement of more than 2 mm present an indication for surgery with screws (**Fig. 6**) or resorbable pins, although there is a lack of evidence in the literature for this opinion. Partial radial head fractures represent articular fractures. Therefore, restoration of the articular congruence is a main factor in the prevention of posttraumatic arthritis (**Fig. 7**). Of the 34 nonsurgically treated subjects who had long-term radiographic follow-up in Akesson and colleagues[29] study, 28 showed clear signs of posttraumatic arthritis. On the contrary, Lindenhovius and colleagues[31] found only slight degenerative changes in 2 of 16 subjects in their operative series. In a retrospective comparison of 10 surgically with 16 nonsurgically treated Mason II fractures, Khalfayan and colleagues[32] reported a higher incidence of degenerative changes in the nonoperative group. Overall, 90% of the surgically treated subjects versus only 44% of the nonoperatively treated subjects reached a good outcome. Conversely, Akesson and colleagues[29] reported that most of the degenerative changes remained asymptomatic, an observation that has been confirmed by similar, recently published studies.[28,33] Yoon and colleagues[33] retrospectively compared nonoperative treatment and ORIF in subjects with isolated radial head fractures with displacement of 2 to 5 mm. They could not find a clinical benefit of ORIF because the subject-rated elbow evaluation score, ROM, and grip strength did not show a significant difference.

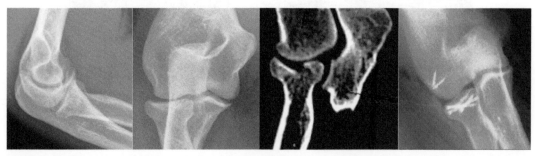

Fig. 6. Mason II fracture. The CT-scan discloses the step of the articular surface. ORIF was performed using headless compression screws. LCL and CEO were refixed using suture anchors.

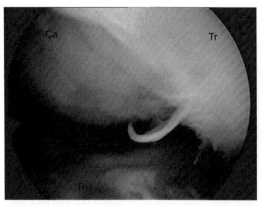

Fig. 7. Arthroscopic view of a nonsurgically treated Mason I-II fracture with a step of 2 mm. The irregularity of the articular surface led to a complete loss of capitellar cartilage within 6 months. For comparison, note the original thickness of the trochlear cartilage.

However, the Mayo Elbow Performance Score (MEPS) was higher in the nonoperative group. Unfortunately, the presence of degenerative changes was not reported and differences in age and follow-up disadvantaged the ORIF group and were reported as weaknesses of this study.

Simon and colleagues[34] reported primarily good results for percutaneous reduction of Mason II fractures. At a mean follow-up of 21 months, 22 of 26 subjects had good results, with a mean MEPS of 93.8. Of the 4 subjects who did not reach a good result, 2 subjects secondarily lost the reduction and 2 had persistent pain though an anatomic reduction. Radiographic results were only reported concerning the quality of reduction but not concerning follow-up osteoarthritis. In addition to the 2 subjects with complete secondary loss of reduction, 2 other subjects showed a slight loss without subjective impairment.[34] This approach might be an interesting alternative because it combines the advantage of anatomic

reduction of ORIF with the lower complication rate of nonsurgical treatment.

At present, no randomized controlled trials exist to guide treatment. Therefore, it remains unclear how to best manage displaced partial articular fractures of the radial head.[35]

Mason III and IV

The surgical treatment of multifragmentary radial head fractures is technically challenging. Optimal treatment decisions remain controversial. Multifragmentary fractures that are amenable to anatomic and stable ORIF should be fixed (**Fig. 8**). The restoration of the lateral column enables physiologic load transmission. Arthroplasty is indicated for comminuted unreconstructable fractures with concomitant ligamentous injuries (**Fig. 9**). Resection of the radial head without prosthetic replacement should only be considered in the case of a stable elbow. Elbow stability must be examined after resection of the radial head to exclude valgus instability and longitudinal instability of the forearm (**Fig. 10**). Varus, valgus, posterolateral rotatory, and axial stress examination should be performed carefully under fluoroscopic control. Significant instability can almost always be found in these cases because unreconstructable Mason III fractures are accompanied by a high percentage of associated ligament tears. Therefore, radial head resection is rarely indicated because it does not sufficiently accommodate these capsuloligamentous injuries. If stability is disputable, radial head replacement should be performed.

Although biomechanical data predict that radial head excision alters elbow kinematics significantly, even in a stable elbow, good long-term clinical results of primary radial excision have been published in the recent literature. Antuna and colleagues[36] reported that, in a series of 26 subjects treated with primary radial head excision for isolated Mason II and III fractures, good results

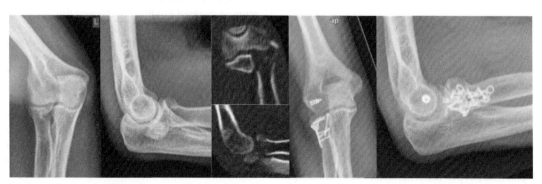

Fig. 8. ORIF of a multifragmentary radial head fracture with a radial head–specific low-profile locking plate.

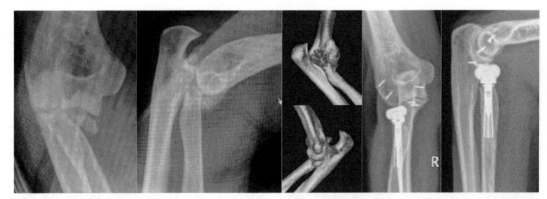

Fig. 9. Unreconstructable radial head fracture Mason IV treated with radial head arthroplasty. LCL and MCL were refixed using suture anchors.

were achieved in 24 subjects, with a mean MEPS of 95 and a follow-up of 15 years. No correlation between a high rate of degenerative changes and subject disorders was found. Comparing acute radial head excision with ORIF, Lindenhovius and colleagues[31] reported a better DASH-score and a lower rate of posttraumatic arthritis for the ORIF group. Ikeda and colleagues[37] found superior results for ORIF in a retrospective comparison of ORIF and acute radial head resection for comminuted radial head fractures.

These clinical data support biomechanical data that show the benefit of restoring the radial column either by ORIF or arthroplasty. Because 60% of the axial loads are transmitted through the humeroradial column, the ulnohumeral joint must bear 100% of the load after radial head excision. Therefore, the rate of radiographic osteoarthritis is high after radial head excision (see **Fig. 2**).[38] These findings are in agreement with in vitro biomechanical studies that indicate changes in kinematics and greater laxity after radial head resection compared with the intact, repaired, and replaced radial head.[39–42] This might be an advantage of radial head arthroplasty compared with resection,

even in isolated unreconstructable radial head fractures, although there are no clinical studies supporting this assumption. Therefore, radial head replacement is considered the treatment of choice for the unreconstructable radial head fracture. Many types of radial head prostheses are commercially available. Modern concepts include monopolar versus bipolar and cemented versus cementless designs. Monobloc and bipolar metal implants, both cemented and cementless, have proven to restore elbow stability, even in unstable elbow fracture-dislocations.[39,40,42–44] Therefore, in the setting of unstable fracture-dislocations, radial head replacement is the treatment of choice for unreconstructable fractures.[45] Promising short-term and midterm results have been reported; however, the long-term results are unknown.[46–53]

In addition to several advantages, there are disadvantages and complications of radial head arthroplasty. The radial head's anatomy is complex and highly variable. The currently available implants do not replicate the radial head's anatomy perfectly. This becomes clear when recognizing that most implants are round, whereas the radial head is elliptical. Furthermore, implantation of a radial head prosthesis is a technically demanding procedure. Yian and colleagues[44] showed that even in optimal in vitro conditions, the anatomic implantation of a radial head prosthesis was not reproducible. Biomechanical studies have shown that different sizes and orientations influence elbow kinematics and load transmission. To achieve good clinical and radiographic results, the implant and implantation should restore anatomy and kinematics as accurately as possible. One of the most important points is the choice of implant size and implantation height. This might be difficult to achieve, particularly in an unstable elbow due to rupture of the MCL or interosseous membrane. The lesser sigmoid notch has been

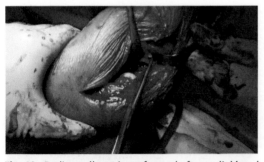

Fig. 10. Radius pull test is performed after radial head resection to exclude longitudinal forearm instability.

validated as a reference for correct implantation height. The prosthesis should be level with the lateral rim of the coronoid process or slightly deeper. Therefore, Kocher's approach between the anconeus and extensor carpi ulnaris muscle is chosen because this approach allows for the visualization of the PRUJ (**Fig. 11**). Placing the radial head prosthesis too high might lead to capitellar erosion due to increased contact pressure. Biomechanical data illustrate that an overlengthening of 2.5 mm leads to a significant increase in radiocapitellar contact pressure.[54,55]

The detection of overlengthening of the radial head is difficult. Frank and colleagues[56] showed in an in vitro study that overlengthening cannot be ruled out by a loss of parallelism of the ulnar ulnohumeral joint line on AP radiographs until there is 6 mm of overstuffing for monopolar implants in the MCL-sufficient elbow. Athwal and colleagues[57] recently presented a method that allows for the reliable determination of an overlengthening of 1 mm for monopolar implants by comparing the AP radiograph with the uninjured elbow. Although this method may be too time-consuming for intraoperative assessment, it is a good tool to exclude overlengthening during outpatient clinic assessment. No method has been described regarding the diagnostics of overlengthening in MCL-deficient elbows and overlengthening of bipolar implants.

Because implants and implantation technique are imperfect, human anatomy cannot be precisely imitated. These imperfections may lead to decreased joint contact areas in the radiohumeral joint and PRUJ, thus increasing the risk of cartilage wear (**Fig. 12**).[58,59] Though most of the degenerative changes reported in outcome studies after radial head arthroplasty are asymptomatic, they might become symptomatic within the course of time because most patients suffering a radial head fracture are young and may have to cope with fracture sequelae for 30 to 50 years.

It is still a matter of debate which radial head fractures to fix versus replace. In 2002, Ring and colleagues[60] found worse clinical results and higher complication rates of ORIF in radial head fractures with more than 3 fragments and, therefore, recommended that the radial head should be replaced in these cases. However, new techniques and implants, such as radial head–specific plates were developed and provided enhanced primary stability.[61,62] In the current literature, several papers have been published regarding the results of ORIF for comminuted radial head fractures with mostly good outcomes.[37,63–65] What had once been common complications, such as secondary loss of fixation, implant failure, nonunion, and radial head necrosis, were not relevant issues in these cohorts at short-term follow-up. Burkhart and colleagues[66] experience with a low-profile locking radial head plate revealed good results in 18 of 21 subjects. None of the previously mentioned complications were observed, with 4- or 5-fragment radial head fractures. One partial necrosis was observed in a 3-part fracture case. Presently, 2 retrospective studies exist comparing ORIF to radial head arthroplasty and neither found significant differences in outcomes at short-term follow-up.[67,68] Oversizing of the

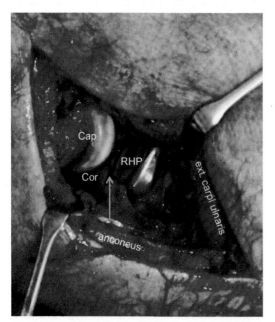

Fig. 11. Visualization of the PRUJ (*arrow*) through Kocher's approach allowing the correct leveling of a radial head prosthesis.

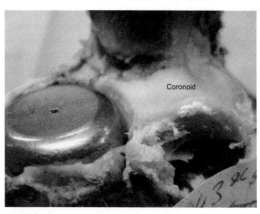

Fig. 12. Decreased contact area of a modular monopolar radial head prosthesis in the PRUJ.

prosthesis was a main reason for a poor clinical result.[67] Although 2 prospective randomized controlled trials have been published reporting superior results of radial head arthroplasty compared with ORIF for Mason III fractures,[69,70] Gao and colleagues[71] concluded in their Cochrane review that there is insufficient data for evidence-based treatment decisions because the available studies may be biased, only provide short-term results, and do not include radial head–specific implants.

In the authors' opinions, the development of new fixation techniques and devices extended the indications for ORIF of comminuted radial head fractures. If the fracture morphology and bone quality of a comminuted radial head fracture allow for anatomic and stable fixation, ORIF may be performed. Nevertheless, radial head arthroplasty is still the treatment of choice for those fractures that do not allow anatomic and stable fixation.

SURGICAL TECHNIQUE

Preoperative planning: AP, lateral, and oblique radiographs, CT scan.

Preparation and patient positioning: supine positioning with the arm on an arm table is preferred. Alternatively, the arm can be placed over the chest using a bolster. Prone positioning may be used in case of a concomitant proximal ulna fracture. Usually, a nonsterile tourniquet is used.

Surgical approach: several approaches exist for the surgical management of radial head fractures. The approaches described by Kaplan[72] and Kocher[73] are most commonly used. These can be reached via a lateral or posterior skin incision. Some surgeons prefer a dorsal superficial approach to reach the deep lateral and medial approaches with only 1 skin incision. The advantage of a posterior skin incision is better protection of the medial and lateral cutaneous nerves. The disadvantage is the production of large skin flaps, which increases the risk of hematoma and seroma. In the authors' practices, we prefer the lateral approach. If the MCL or coronoid must be addressed, a second medial incision is used.

A posterior skin incision is sometimes used in case of concomitant proximal ulna fractures. The radial head is then addressed via the Boyd approach by elevating the anconeus subperiosteally from the ulna.

The Kaplan approach is a muscle-tendon splitting approach through the common extensor origin (CEO) anterior to the LCL. The described interval is between the extensor carpi radialis longus and the extensor digitorum communis. Splitting the CEO reveals the capsule. Capsule and annular ligament are split to reach the radial head. The Kaplan approach allows the best exposure of the anterior part of the radial head. Therefore, in the authors' practices, this approach is primarily used for the ORIF of anterior radial head fragments.

The Kocher approach is developed between the anconeus and extensor carpi ulnaris muscles and, therefore, lies posterior compared with the Kaplan approach. The Kocher approach allows for better visualization of the posterior parts of the radial head and direct view on the PRUJ. Therefore, we prefer this approach for multifragmentary radial head fractures when considering radial head arthroplasty to determine the correct height of the prosthesis. Both approaches can be extended proximally and distally. With extension of the approaches, the differences in the vantages provided by each approach decrease because both can provide a good visualization up to the ulnar part of the joint.[74] In case of an LCL injury, the Kocher approach should be used because it allows the best visualization of the lateral ligament. If the LCL is partially torn, it may be fully released to provide sufficient visualization without the excessive use of retractors, which might harm the radial nerve.

SURGICAL PROCEDURE
Open Reduction and Internal Fixation

After opening the joint, the fracture site is inspected and washed out. Any interposing tissue is removed from the fracture gap. In case of a partial articular fracture, the fragments can be reduced against the intact part of the radial head's articular surface (**Fig. 13**). Care is taken to spare the periosteum, which provides blood supply.

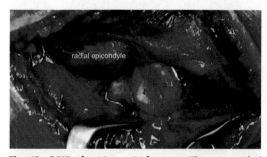

Fig. 13. ORIF of a Mason IV-fracture: The trauma led to a complete disruption of the LCL and CEO from the radial epicondyle. The dislocation simplifies anatomic reduction of the 3 free fragments (1–3) against the intact part (4) of the radial head. Countersunk free screws were used for preliminary fixation. A buttress plate was added to enhance stability.

The reduction can be secured with Kirschner wires, which are exchanged with 1.5 to 2.5 mm cortical screws according to the sizes of the fracture fragments. Alternatively, resorbable pins or cannulated headless compression screws can be used. Screw heads should be countersunk beneath the cartilage. Screw penetration of the far cortex must be carefully avoided. Depending on the fracture morphology and bone quality, a buttress plate may be beneficial in achieving sufficient stability.

In case of complete articular fractures, the head is first anatomically reconstructed with free screws. The reconstructed head is then fixed to the shaft using a plate or crossed screws. Crossed screws pose a good option for fractures without metaphyseal comminution. Plates provide higher stability in case of metaphyseal defects. Because these defects are often found due to valgus impaction load during trauma, we prefer low-profile locking radial head plates (**Fig. 14**). Plates should be placed in the safe zone to avoid restricting forearm rotation. The fracture morphology may occasionally necessitate placing the plate outside the safe zone. In such cases, the plate should be removed as soon as healing has occurred, together with a surgical release of the PRUJ.

Arthroplasty

The exact surgical technique depends on the specific implant being implanted. After inspection of the fracture site, bony fragments are removed and the radial neck is osteotomized. This is followed by stability testing, to assess the interosseous membrane and the MCL. The fragments of the radial head are used to determine the correct implant size (**Fig. 15**). When sizing of the radial head is between implant sizes, the smaller sized implant is used. The radial shaft is prepared according to the implant manual. The height of the

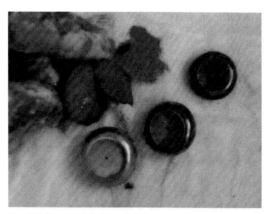

Fig. 15. Determination of the correct component size using the main parts of the fractured radial head.

prosthesis is leveled at the PRUJ (see **Fig. 11**). The deepest point of the native radial head should be used as a reference. It should be considered that most radial head prostheses do not replicate the radial head's articular concavity. After insertion of the trial implants, ROM is examined, as is the alignment of the implant with the capitellum and PRUJ. Stability and implant position are checked by fluoroscopy. Mild overlengthening cannot be adequately ruled out by fluoroscopy. Nevertheless, the medial ulnohumeral joint space is checked for parallelism to exclude major overlengthening and ulnar variance at the wrist. Definitive implantation is performed according to the manufacturer's recommendations.

Ligament Repair

The ruptured LCL is refixed anatomically with transosseous sutures or suture anchors. Stability is then checked again. If there is still significant medial instability leading to subluxation of the elbow, the MCL should be repaired through a

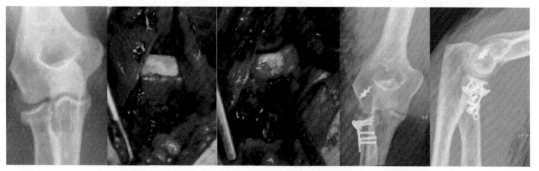

Fig. 14. ORIF on a valgus impacted radial neck fracture. The slight angulation leads to the complete loss of radiocapitellar contact. Reduction of the fragment restores joint congruence. The metaphyseal defect is addressed with a buttress plate.

medial approach or by mounting a hinged or static external fixator.

POSTOPERATIVE REHABILITATION

Uncomplicated Mason II fractures usually can be moved right away without limitations. In the case of more complex injuries, the time of splinting depends on the fracture type and the stability of fixation. Active and active-assisted physiotherapy are initiated on the second day after surgery to regain full ROM and train the active stabilizers. Varus and valgus stresses as well as resistive exercises should be omitted for 6 weeks. Forearm rotation should be performed in 90° of elbow flexion to protect the collateral ligaments. During extension exercises, the LCL is protected in pronation and the MCL in supination. If both ligaments are injured, extension exercises are performed in the neutral rotation or in the position that provided the highest stability during intraoperative testing.

REFERENCES

1. Furey MJ, Sheps DM, White NJ, et al. A retrospective cohort study of displaced segmental radial head fractures: is 2 mm of articular displacement an indication for surgery? J Shoulder Elbow Surg 2013;22:636–41.
2. Ring D. Displaced, unstable fractures of the radial head: fixation vs replacement–what is the evidence? Injury 2008;39:1329–37.
3. de Haan J, Schep NW, Eygendaal D, et al. Stability of the elbow joint: relevant anatomy and clinical implications of in vitro biomechanical studies. Open Orthop J 2011;5:168–76.
4. Reichel LM, Milam GS, Sitton SE, et al. Elbow lateral collateral ligament injuries. J Hand Surg Am 2013; 38:184–201 [quiz: 201].
5. Mak S, Beltran LS, Bencardino J, et al. MRI of the annular ligament of the elbow: review of anatomic considerations and pathologic findings in patients with posterolateral elbow instability. AJR Am J Roentgenol 2014;203:1272–9.
6. Wegmann K, Dargel J, Burkhart KJ, et al. The Essex-Lopresti lesion. Strategies Trauma Limb Reconstr 2012;7:131–9.
7. Loeffler BJ, Green JB, Zelouf DS. Forearm instability. J Hand Surg Am 2014;39:156–67.
8. Hassan SE, Parks BG, Douoguih WA, et al. Effect of distal ulnar collateral ligament tear pattern on contact forces and valgus stability in the posteromedial compartment of the elbow. Am J Sports Med 2015; 43(2):447–52.
9. Duckworth AD, Clement ND, Jenkins PJ, et al. The epidemiology of radial head and neck fractures. J Hand Surg Am 2012;37:112–9.
10. Kaas L, van Riet RP, Vroemen JP, et al. The epidemiology of radial head fractures. J Shoulder Elbow Surg 2010;19:520–3.
11. Mason ML. Some observations on fractures of the head of the radius with a review of one hundred cases. Br J Surg 1954;42:123–32.
12. Johnston GW. A follow-up of one hundred cases of fracture of the head of the radius with a review of the literature. Ulster Med J 1962;31:51–6.
13. Broberg MA, Morrey BF. Results of treatment of fracture-dislocations of the elbow. Clin Orthop Relat Res 1987;(216):109–19.
14. Sheps DM, Kiefer KR, Boorman RS, et al. The interobserver reliability of classification systems for radial head fractures: the Hotchkiss modification of the Mason classification and the AO classification systems. Can J Surg 2009;52:277–82.
15. Guitton TG, Ring D, Science of Variation Group. Interobserver reliability of radial head fracture classification: two-dimensional compared with three-dimensional CT. J Bone Joint Surg Am 2011;93: 2015–21.
16. Itamura J, Roidis N, Mirzayan R, et al. Radial head fractures: MRI evaluation of associated injuries. J Shoulder Elbow Surg 2005;14:421–4.
17. Kaas L, Turkenburg JL, van Riet RP, et al. Magnetic resonance imaging findings in 46 elbows with a radial head fracture. Acta Orthop 2010;81:373–6.
18. McGinley JC, Gold G, Cheung E, et al. MRI detection of forearm soft tissue injuries with radial head fractures. Hand (N Y) 2014;9:87–92.
19. Hausmann JT, Vekszler G, Breitenseher M, et al. Mason type-I radial head fractures and interosseous membrane lesions–a prospective study. J Trauma 2009;66:457–61.
20. Kaas L, van Riet RP, Vroemen JP, et al. The incidence of associated fractures of the upper limb in fractures of the radial head. Strategies Trauma Limb Reconstr 2008;3:71–4.
21. Jie KE, van Dam LF, Verhagen TF, et al. Extension test and ossal point tenderness cannot accurately exclude significant injury in acute elbow trauma. Ann Emerg Med 2014;64:74–8.
22. Rineer CA, Guitton TG, Ring D. Radial head fractures: loss of cortical contact is associated with concomitant fracture or dislocation. J Shoulder Elbow Surg 2010;19:21–5.
23. Bruinsma WE, Guitton T, Ring D, Science of Variation Group. Radiographic loss of contact between radial head fracture fragments is moderately reliable. Clin Orthop Relat Res 2014;472:2113–9.
24. Sormaala MJ, Sormaala A, Mattila VM, et al. MDCT findings after elbow dislocation: a retrospective study of 140 patients. Skeletal Radiol 2014;43: 507–12.
25. Timmerman LA, Schwartz ML, Andrews JR. Preoperative evaluation of the ulnar collateral ligament by

magnetic resonance imaging and computed tomography arthrography. Evaluation in 25 baseball players with surgical confirmation. Am J Sports Med 1994;22:26–31 [discussion: 32].

26. Kaas L, van Riet RP, Turkenburg JL, et al. Magnetic resonance imaging in radial head fractures: most associated injuries are not clinically relevant. J Shoulder Elbow Surg 2011;20:1282–8.

27. Smits AJ, Giannakopoulos GF, Zuidema WP. Long-term results and treatment modalities of conservatively treated Broberg-Morrey type 1 radial head fractures. Injury 2014;45:1564–8.

28. Duckworth AD, Wickramasinghe NR, Clement ND, et al. Long-term outcomes of isolated stable radial head fractures. J Bone Joint Surg Am 2014;96:1716–23.

29. Akesson T, Herbertsson P, Josefsson PO, et al. Primary nonoperative treatment of moderately displaced two-part fractures of the radial head. J Bone Joint Surg Am 2006;88:1909–14.

30. Burkhart KJ, Franke S, Wegmann K, et al. [Mason I fracture - a simple injury?]. Unfallchirurg 2014;118(1):9–17 [in German].

31. Lindenhovius AL, Felsch Q, Ring D, et al. The long-term outcome of open reduction and internal fixation of stable displaced isolated partial articular fractures of the radial head. J Trauma 2009;67(1):143–6.

32. Khalfayan EE, Culp RW, Alexander AH. Mason type II radial head fractures: operative versus nonoperative treatment. J Orthop Trauma 1992;6:283–9.

33. Yoon A, King GJ, Grewal R. Is ORIF superior to nonoperative treatment in isolated displaced partial articular fractures of the radial head? Clin Orthop Relat Res 2014;472:2105–12.

34. Simon P, Unterhauser F, von Roth P, et al. Treatment of Mason type II radial head fractures by percutaneous reduction. Unfallchirurg 2014;117:341–7 [in German].

35. Bruinsma W, Kodde I, de Muinck Keizer RJ, et al. A randomized controlled trial of nonoperative treatment versus open reduction and internal fixation for stable, displaced, partial articular fractures of the radial head: the RAMBO trial. BMC Musculoskelet Disord 2014;15:147.

36. Antuna SA, Sanchez-Marquez JM, Barco R. Long-term results of radial head resection following isolated radial head fractures in patients younger than forty years old. J Bone Joint Surg Am 2010;92:558–66.

37. Ikeda M, Sugiyama K, Kang C, et al. Comminuted fractures of the radial head. Comparison of resection and internal fixation. J Bone Joint Surg Am 2005;87:76–84.

38. Mikic ZD, Vukadinovic SM. Late results in fractures of the radial head treated by excision. Clin Orthop Relat Res 1983;(181):220–8.

39. Beingessner DM, Dunning CE, Gordon KD, et al. The effect of radial head excision and arthroplasty on elbow kinematics and stability. J Bone Joint Surg Am 2004;86-A:1730–9.

40. Johnson JA, Beingessner DM, Gordon KD, et al. Kinematics and stability of the fractured and implant-reconstructed radial head. J Shoulder Elbow Surg 2005;14:195S–201S.

41. King GJ, Zarzour ZD, Rath DA, et al. Metallic radial head arthroplasty improves valgus stability of the elbow. Clin Orthop Relat Res 1999;(368):114–25.

42. Pomianowski S, Morrey BF, Neale PG, et al. Contribution of monoblock and bipolar radial head prostheses to valgus stability of the elbow. J Bone Joint Surg Am 2001;83-A:1829–34.

43. King GJ, Patterson SD. Metallic radial head arthroplasty. Tech Hand Up Extrem Surg 2001;5:196–203.

44. Yian E, Steens W, Lingenfelter E, et al. Malpositioning of radial head prostheses: an in vitro study. J Shoulder Elbow Surg 2008;17:663–70.

45. Rief H, Raven TF, Lennert A, et al. Ist die posttraumatische Radiuskopfresektion noch zeitgemäß? Obere Extremität 2014;9:121–7.

46. Burkhart KJ, Mattyasovszky SG, Runkel M, et al. Mid- to long-term results after bipolar radial head arthroplasty. J Shoulder Elbow Surg 2010;19:965–72.

47. Dotzis A, Cochu G, Mabit C, et al. Comminuted fractures of the radial head treated by the Judet floating radial head prosthesis. J Bone Joint Surg Br 2006;88:760–4.

48. Frosch KH, Knopp W, Dresing K, et al. A bipolar radial head prosthesis after comminuted radial head fractures: indications, treatment and outcome after 5 years. Unfallchirurg 2003;106:367–73 [in German].

49. Grewal R, MacDermid JC, Faber KJ, et al. Comminuted radial head fractures treated with a modular metallic radial head arthroplasty. Study of outcomes. J Bone Joint Surg Am 2006;88:2192–200.

50. Moro JK, Werier J, MacDermid JC, et al. Arthroplasty with a metal radial head for unreconstructible fractures of the radial head. J Bone Joint Surg Am 2001;83-A:1201–11.

51. Popovic N, Gillet P, Rodriguez A, et al. Fracture of the radial head with associated elbow dislocation: results of treatment using a floating radial head prosthesis. J Orthop Trauma 2000;14:171–7.

52. Shore BJ, Mozzon JB, MacDermid JC, et al. Chronic posttraumatic elbow disorders treated with metallic radial head arthroplasty. J Bone Joint Surg Am 2008;90:271–80.

53. Wick M, Lies A, Muller EJ, et al. Prostheses of the head of the radius. What outcome can be expected? Unfallchirurg 1998;101:817–21 [in German].

54. Van Glabbeek F, Van Riet RP, Baumfeld JA, et al. Detrimental effects of overstuffing or understuffing with a radial head replacement in the medial collateral-ligament deficient elbow. J Bone Joint Surg Am 2004;86-A:2629–35.

55. Cohn M, Glait SA, Sapienza A, et al. Radiocapitellar joint contact pressures following radial head arthroplasty. J Hand Surg 2014;39:1566–71.

56. Frank SG, Grewal R, Johnson J, et al. Determination of correct implant size in radial head arthroplasty to avoid overlengthening. J Bone Joint Surg Am 2009; 91:1738–46.

57. Athwal GS, Rouleau DM, MacDermid JC, et al. Contralateral elbow radiographs can reliably diagnose radial head implant overlengthening. J Bone Joint Surg Am 2011;93:1339–46.

58. Wegmann K, Hain MK, Ries C, et al. Do the radial head prosthesis components fit with the anatomical structures of the proximal radioulnar joint? Surg Radiol Anat 2014. [Epub ahead of print].

59. Liew VS, Cooper IC, Ferreira LM, et al. The effect of metallic radial head arthroplasty on radiocapitellar joint contact area. Clin Biomech 2003;18:115–8.

60. Ring D, Quintero J, Jupiter JB. Open reduction and internal fixation of fractures of the radial head. J Bone Joint Surg Am 2002;84-A:1811–5.

61. Burkhart KJ, Mueller LP, Krezdorn D, et al. Stability of radial head and neck fractures: a biomechanical study of six fixation constructs with consideration of three locking plates. J Hand Surg Am 2007;32: 1569–75.

62. Koslowsky TC, Mader K, Dargel J, et al. Reconstruction of a Mason type-III fracture of the radial head using four different fixation techniques. An experimental study. J Bone Joint Surg Br 2007;89: 1545–50.

63. Businger A, Ruedi TP, Sommer C. On-table reconstruction of comminuted fractures of the radial head. Injury 2009;41(6):583–8.

64. Koslowsky TC, Mader K, Gausepohl T, et al. Reconstruction of Mason type-III and type-IV radial head fractures with a new fixation device: 23 patients followed 1-4 years. Acta Orthop 2007;78:151–6.

65. Nalbantoglu U, Kocaoglu B, Gereli A, et al. Open reduction and internal fixation of Mason type III radial head fractures with and without an associated elbow dislocation. J Hand Surg 2007;32:1560–8.

66. Burkhart KJ, Gruszka D, Frohn S, et al. Locking plate osteosynthesis of the radial head fractures: clinical and radiological results. Unfallchirurg 2014 [in German; Epub ahead of print].

67. Schnetzke M, Aytac S, Deuss M, et al. Radial head prosthesis in complex elbow dislocations: effect of oversizing and comparison with ORIF. Int Orthop 2014;38:2295–301.

68. Watters TS, Garrigues GE, Ring D, et al. Fixation versus replacement of radial head in terrible triad: is there a difference in elbow stability and prognosis? Clin Orthop Relat Res 2014;472:2128–35.

69. Chen X, Wang SC, Cao LH, et al. Comparison between radial head replacement and open reduction and internal fixation in clinical treatment of unstable, multi-fragmented radial head fractures. Int Orthop 2011;35:1071–6.

70. Ruan HJ, Fan CY, Liu JJ, et al. A comparative study of internal fixation and prosthesis replacement for radial head fractures of Mason type III. Int Orthop 2009;33:249–53.

71. Gao Y, Zhang W, Duan X, et al. Surgical interventions for treating radial head fractures in adults. Cochrane Database Syst Rev 2013;(5):CD008987.

72. Kaplan EB. Surgical approaches to the proximal end of the radius and its use in fractures of the head and neck of the radius. J Bone Joint Surg 1941;23:86.

73. Kocher T. Textbook of Operative Surgery. 3rd edition. London: Adam and Charles Black; 1911.

74. Desloges W, Louati H, Papp SR, et al. Objective analysis of lateral elbow exposure with the extensor digitorum communis split compared with the Kocher interval. J Bone Joint Surg Am 2014;96:387–93.

Complex Elbow Instability
Radial Head and Coronoid

David Kovacevic, MD[a], Laura A. Vogel, MD[a],
William N. Levine, MD[b],*

KEYWORDS

- Complex elbow instability • Radial head • Coronoid • Surgical technique • Rehabilitation
- Clinical outcomes

KEY POINTS

- Complex elbow dislocations associated with coronoid or radial head fractures must be identified and typically require surgical treatment so as to avoid recurrent instability, posttraumatic arthritis, and arthrofibrosis.
- The treatment goals are to obtain a concentric reduction with adequate elbow stability to allow for early range of motion.
- Radial head management should include osteosynthesis or radial head replacement with a metal, modular prosthesis because excision alone can lead to elbow instability, chronic wrist pain, and the longitudinal instability of the distal radioulnar joint.
- Lateral ulnar collateral ligament complex repair is required to allow for early motion and to prevent late posterolateral rotatory instability.
- Managing patient expectations and educating the patient on the need to adhere to postoperative rehabilitation and exercises will allow for the desired clinical outcome—a pain-free functional elbow.

INTRODUCTION: NATURE OF THE PROBLEM

Elbow fracture dislocations occur during falls onto an outstretched hand, falls from a height, motor vehicle accidents, or other high-energy trauma, and the typical mechanism of dislocation is hyperextension and valgus stress applied to the pronated forearm. In particular, complex elbow dislocations associated with radial head or coronoid fractures have a poor natural history. Subluxation or recurrent dislocation events are likely with closed treatment. Treatment of the radial head fracture by excision alone in the setting of an elbow dislocation is associated with a high rate of failure due to recurrent instability. Recurrent instability episodes, posttraumatic arthrosis, and severe stiffness lead to poor functional outcomes.[1]

Source of Funding: No external funding was used for this investigation.
Disclosure: Dr W.N. Levine is an unpaid consultant for Zimmer Holdings, Inc (Warsaw, IN, USA), is a board or committee member for the American Board of Orthopaedic Surgery and the American Orthopaedic Association, and is on the editorial or governing board for the Journal of the American Academy of Orthopaedic Surgeons.
[a] Department of Orthopaedic Surgery, The Center for Shoulder, Elbow, and Sports Medicine, New York Presbyterian/Columbia University Medical Center, 622 West 168th Street, PH-11, New York, NY 10032, USA;
[b] Department of Orthopaedic Surgery, The Center for Shoulder, Elbow, and Sports Medicine, New York Presbyterian/Columbia University Medical Center, 622 West 168th Street, PH-1130, New York, NY 10032, USA
* Corresponding author.
E-mail address: wnl1@columbia.edu

SURGICAL TECHNIQUE
Cornerstones of Surgical Management

- First, restore the ulnohumeral joint by reduction of the intact joint or coronoid fracture fixation.
- Second, the radial head should be fixed or replaced if the ulnohumeral joint has been injured because the former is an important secondary stabilizer to both valgus and posterolateral rotatory stability.
- The lateral ulnar collateral ligament (LUCL) complex should be repaired in all cases.
- If the medial ulnar collateral ligament (MUCL) complex is deficient, then the complex should be primarily repaired or stabilized by an external fixator if instability persists after fixation of the coronoid, radial head, and LUCL.
- Elbow subluxation or luxation within 45° of extension warrants reassessment to ensure that both primary and secondary constraints have been appropriately addressed.

- A meticulous and systematic approach to management of an acute complex elbow dislocation will maximize clinical outcomes.

Preoperative Planning

Orthogonal radiographs in the anteroposterior and lateral plane are obtained before and after closed reduction, and advanced imaging with three-dimensional (3D) reconstruction is helpful for defining the fracture pattern and in planning for surgical treatment (**Fig. 1**). The surgeon should plan to have the proper equipment and implants available. Intraoperative fluoroscopy is required during surgery to ensure proper implant placement and to confirm concentric reduction during a flexion-extension arc of motion. Final intraoperative films should be obtained before leaving the operating room. Coronoid fractures can be repaired with sutures, small fragment osteosynthesis, or cannulated screws of appropriate size. Osteosynthesis of radial head fractures is

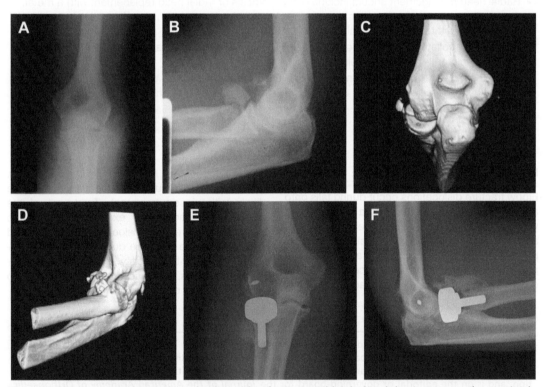

Fig. 1. (*A, B*) Anteroposterior and lateral radiographs of a 52-year-old right-hand-dominant man who sustained a right closed posterolateral elbow dislocation associated with a comminuted fracture of the radial head and avulsion fracture of the lateral epicondyle. (*C, D*) Preoperative 3D reconstruction images demonstrated a comminuted radial head fracture with a small displaced lateral epicondyle avulsion fracture. The coronoid was intact. (*E, F*) Postoperative radiographs after radial head replacement and LUCL complex repair with a suture anchor. An MUCL complex repair was not required because the coronoid was intact and the elbow was stable at the completion of the procedure. At 6 years following surgery, the patient is satisfied with the result and his range of motion is 10° to 135° with flexion-extension and prosupination of 110°. (*Courtesy of* Columbia University Center for Shoulder, Elbow, and Sports Medicine, New York, NY; with permission.)

preferred and can be executed with small fragment plates and screws. Countersunk Herbert screws (ie, headless, 1.0 mm–2.4 mm) can be used to fix articular head fragments. A metallic, modular radial head implant system should be available if the radial head or neck is not repairable. In cases where bony and ligamentous repair does not restore elbow stability (ie, maintained concentric reduction during flexion-extension arc of motion), then the surgeon should plan to use a dynamic, hinged external fixator. Application can be technically demanding, and in such instances, a static external fixator or patient referral is an appropriate treatment alternative.

Preparation and Patient Positioning

Typically, the patient is positioned supine on the operative table, placed under general endotracheal anesthesia or regional anesthesia, and the operative limb is supported on a hand table. An examination under anesthesia should be performed to assess for gross ulnohumeral instability as well as varus and valgus instability. A sterile tourniquet is applied to the upper arm after sterile preparation and draping. Alternatively, a lateral decubitus position can be used with the operative extremity supported by a padded bolster, especially if the surgeon plans to use a hinged external fixator.

Surgical Approach

The senior author's preferred approach to access both sides of the elbow includes a posterior-based skin incision with elevation of full-thickness skin flaps at the fascial level. For this approach, the patient is typically in the lateral decubitus position with the operative extremity placed on a padded bolster. Alternatively, the lateral approach can be used to address injuries of the coronoid, radial head, and LUCL complex by creating a direct lateral incision along the lateral supracondylar humeral ridge curving at the lateral epicondyle toward the radial head and neck.

Regardless of approach, full-thickness skin flaps are created and elevated permitting insertion of a self-retaining retractor. The common extensor origin is then split in line with its fibers, although it is avulsed two-thirds of the time, allowing the surgeon to use the traumatic dissection plane to gain exposure of the elbow.[2] The LUCL complex will have avulsed from its origin of the distal humerus, leaving a bare spot (**Fig. 2**A). Surgical reconstruction occurs in a systematic fashion from deep to superficial.

If the radial head is to be replaced, its excision provides excellent exposure of the coronoid through the lateral approach (see **Fig. 2**B). Alternatively, if the radial head is to be fixed, then the fractured fragments are covered in a damp sterile gauze and placed in a sterile basin to provide access to the coronoid. When the coronoid fracture fragments cannot be fixed through the lateral approach because screw fixation is not possible or visualization is difficult because of an intact radial head, then plating of a coronoid fracture as well as MUCL complex repair can be accomplished via a medial approach to the elbow. A fascial incision along the medial supracondylar ridge is created. The ulnar nerve is at risk in this approach and should be identified, protected, and tagged with a vessel loop. The common flexor origin is split distal to the medial epicondyle to expose the coronoid medially. From the medial side, a buttress or spring plate can be used to secure a comminuted fracture.

Surgical Procedure

Fix the coronoid fracture
For type I coronoid fractures, suture fixation with a nonabsorbable braided suture passed through the anterior elbow capsule and above the coronoid fragment is recommended. Two parallel drill holes

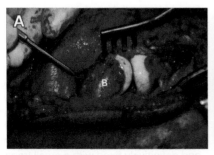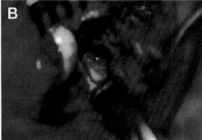

Fig. 2. (*A*) The LUCL complex avulsed from its proximal humeral origin revealing the resultant bare spot. (*B*) Removing the radial head from the surgical field permits exposure of the coronoid fracture through a lateral approach. Asterisk, coronoid fracture; B, bare spot. (*Courtesy of* Columbia University Center for Shoulder, Elbow, and Sports Medicine, New York, NY; with permission.)

are made from the dorsal surface of the proximal ulna through a separate percutaneous incision and directed toward the coracoid tip with either a small drill (ie, 2-mm drill bit) or Kirschner wire (K-wire). An anterior cruciate ligament (ACL) drill guide placed on the dorsal ulna greatly facilitates accurate placement of the drill holes. Then, no. 2 braided suture is passed through the anterior elbow capsule above the coronoid in a mattress fashion, and the suture limbs are retrieved through the drill holes using a Hewson suture retriever (Smith & Nephew, Memphis, TN, USA), transosseous suture passer (Arthrex, Naples, FL, USA), or Keith needle (Aspen Surgical Products, Caledonia, MI, USA). The suture limbs are tied over the dorsal surface of the proximal ulna to plicate the anterior elbow capsule. This type of fixation is used when the coronoid fragment is too small to accept a screw.[3]

Type II and III coronoid fractures can be fixed with either 1 or 2 screws (ie, cannulated, regular, partially threaded, or cancellous screws) after debriding the fracture site and anatomically reducing the fragment with a pointed instrument, such as a dental pick. With anatomic reduction confirmed by direct visualization, an ACL drill guide can be used to place a K-wire from the dorsal surface of the proximal ulna, across the fracture bed, and into the fracture fragment (**Fig. 3**). A second K-wire is inserted across the fracture site with the ACL drill guide for rotational control. With the K-wires in place, the fracture fragment is first drilled and then tapped. It is very important to drill and tap the fracture fragment before screw placement to avoid splitting the fragment on screw insertion. After screw placement, the K-wires are removed and coronoid stability is evaluated throughout a full range of motion with fluoroscopy. Coronoid fractures that are comminuted are managed by fixing the largest fragment with articular cartilage.

Fix or replace the radial head

The radial head fracture is addressed after treatment of the coronoid injury because, once the proximal radius is fixed or replaced, access to the coronoid from the lateral approach is significantly limited. The decision to fix a radial head is based on the fracture configuration and severity of comminution. Osteosynthesis is typically undertaken when only 2 or 3 head fragments are present. Otherwise, fractures that are severely comminuted (ie, >3 fragments) or with articular surface damage require radial head replacement.

The radial head and neck are exposed as necessary for fracture reduction and fixation by extending the Kaplan interval (ie, extensor digitorum communis and extensor carpi radialis longus). The posterior interosseous nerve is at risk during

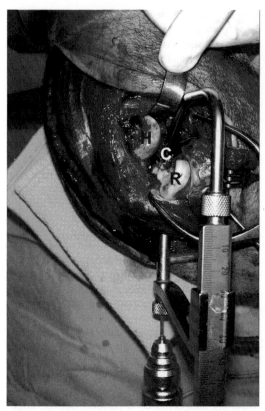

Fig. 3. An ACL drill guide is placed on the dorsal surface of the proximal ulna and the coronoid fracture fragment to allow controlled placement of a K-wire across the fracture bed. C, coronoid fracture fragment; H, distal humerus; R, radial head. (*Courtesy of* Columbia University Center for Shoulder, Elbow, and Sports Medicine, New York, NY; with permission.)

distal radial neck exposures, and its distance from the surgical field can be maximized by keeping the forearm in full pronation, by dissecting the supinator bluntly, and by avoiding retractor placement over the radial neck.[4] A study showed that with pronation, the posterior interosseous nerve is an average of 38 mm distal to the articular surface of the radial head.[5]

When osteosynthesis is used, the radial head fragments are initially reduced and held with a pointed reduction clamp. Then, the fragments are temporarily fixed with a 2-mm K-wire and replaced with a Herbert screw for fragment fixation. It is important to countersink the screw head if it is inserted through articular cartilage. As for radial neck fractures, they are reduced with a pointed reduction clamp, provisionally held with a K-wire, and definitively fixed with a small fragment T-plate in the "safe zone." Smith and Hotchkiss[6] characterized the nonarticular portion of the radial head based on reference points made in the operative wound. If the radial head is bisected in the anteroposterior plane with the elbow in neutral, full pronation, and full supination, the "safe zone" can be defined as half the distance between the middle and posterior marks and about two-thirds the distance between the middle and anterior marks. Alternatively, a more distal referencing system can be used. Caputo and colleagues[7] have approximated this zone based on landmarks between the radial styloid and Lister tubercle. Being aware of the position of the posterior interosseous nerve is imperative to avoid injury while exposing the radial neck and shaft or by trapping it under the plate distally. If the radial head cannot be reconstructed, then it is replaced.

Metallic radial head prostheses should be used because silicone implants are biomechanically inferior and biologically reactive.[8] A modular prosthesis is used because it permits intraoperative flexibility with sizing of the stem diameter independent of the radial head diameter and thickness. A microsagittal saw can be used, if necessary, to osteotomize the proximal radius at the level of the neck. The intramedullary canal of the proximal radius is reamed by hand to the endosteal cortical bone with sequentially larger reamers. Radial head size is judged by assembling the fracture fragments that have been removed, and downsizing the radial head is recommended to avoid overstuffing of the elbow joint.[9,10] A trial implant is then inserted to test stability and check elbow flexion-extension and forearm rotational range of motion. Under direct visualization, symmetry of the proximal radioulnar joint articulation is assessed to determine if the radial head diameter seems appropriate. In particular, intraoperative visualization of a gap in the lateral ulnohumeral joint is a reliable indicator of overlengthening following the insertion of a radial head prosthesis. Once optimal sizing is obtained with the trial implants, the definitive implant is inserted in a press-fit manner.

Repair the lateral ulnar collateral ligament complex

After addressing the coronoid and radial head pathologic condition, attention is turned to the LUCL complex. The LUCL complex is a distinct structure that can be easily identified in the acutely injured elbow, and failure to repair this structure allows the radial head to subluxate into a posterolateral position with forearm supination. The LUCL complex is commonly avulsed from the distal humerus. Its anatomic origin is slightly posterior to the lateral epicondyle at the center of the capitellar arc that lies deep to the common extensor origin and continues distally to insert on the supinator crest of the ulna.

The LUCL complex is then reattached to the distal humerus through bone tunnels or suture anchors. The former is preferred when a hinged external fixator may need to be used. In such a scenario, a drill, K-wire, or a pointed towel clip is used to create holes in the distal humerus above the lateral epicondyle. Suture limbs are passed through the bony tunnels and snapped. Alternatively, a suture anchor (ie, 2.0 mm or 2.4 mm) can be placed in the lateral epicondyle at the LUCL origin. Irrespective of fixation method, a nonabsorbable, no. 2 braided suture is used for repair of the LUCL complex by passing the suture through the ligament and capsule in a running, locked fashion (ie, Krackow) (**Fig. 4**A). Next, the common extensor tendon origin is repaired separately with a running, locked stitch using the same type of suture for the ligament and capsule repair (see **Fig. 4**B). The elbow is held in 90° of flexion and full forearm pronation before tying the sutures. The wound is irrigated and then closed in a layered fashion.

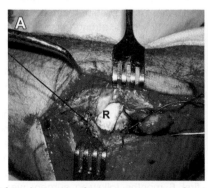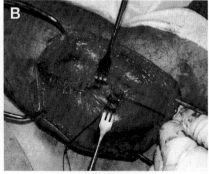

Fig. 4. (*A*) After placement of a 2.4-mm suture anchor in the lateral epicondyle at the origin of the LUCL, one no. 2 suture limb from the anchor was passed in a running Krakow fashion up to the LUCL complex and capsule and then back down before tying the sutures. (*B*) No. 2 braided suture was run in a locking fashion to repair the common extensor tendon origin after separately repairing the LUCL complex and capsule. Both repairs were performed with the forearm in pronation. R, radial head.

Assess elbow stability within 30°–130° degrees of flexion-extension arc with the forearm in full pronation

At this point, the elbow is taken through a functional arc of motion to assess dynamic stability with intraoperative fluoroscopy. The lateral view is assessed to ensure concentric reduction of the elbow joint through a functional arc of motion. If asymmetry is present during dynamic testing, then additional efforts are required to obtain sufficient elbow stability so early motion may be initiated in the postoperative period.

Repair the medial ulnar collateral ligament complex if elbow is unstable

MUCL complex repair is performed through a separate medial incision. A deep approach to the medial elbow puts the ulnar nerve at risk, and it needs to be identified and protected during the procedure. Usually the MUCL is torn in its midsubstance, and suture repair with a nonabsorbable, no. 2 braided suture is used. Dynamic elbow stability is then reassessed once again during a functional arc of motion using fluoroscopy. If stability remains insufficient, then applying a hinged external fixator is the final option.[11] If the hinged fixator is not available or the surgeon is not familiar with its use, then a static external fixator can be applied to maintain elbow reduction.

Apply hinged external fixator for persistent elbow instability despite medial ulnar collateral ligament complex repair to maintain concentric reduction and initiate early range of motion

A guide pin is inserted from medial to lateral by starting at the medial epicondyle and should be directed through the center of elbow rotation (ie, center of capitellum). After guide pin insertion, the elbow is held reduced while the frame is assembled around it. The hinge is placed over the guide pin on either side of the elbow such that it can slide. Three-quarter rings are then attached proximal and distal to the elbow. Two half-pins are then inserted in the humerus above the elbow through small incisions over the posterior surface by bluntly dissecting the triceps fibers with a snap or Adson clamp. Two half-pins are then inserted in the proximal ulna over its subcutaneous border dorsally. At this point, the pins are attached to the rings before tightening all components of the hinged external fixator. Using fluoroscopy, concentric elbow reduction in the frame is verified through 30° to 130° of motion and forearm pronation to protect the LUCL complex repair. The elbow is locked at 90° degrees in the hinged external fixator for the initial postoperative course,

and final films are obtained in the operating room before conclusion of the procedure.

REHABILITATION AND RECOVERY

Using intraoperative fluoroscopy, orthogonal views of the elbow are obtained to verify appropriate hardware placement and confirm congruent reduction. After confirmation of a stable, surgically repaired construct, the elbow is placed in a hinged elbow brace, and the involved upper extremity is placed in a sling for comfort.

The patient is typically admitted to the hospital overnight for pain control, completion of 24 hours of prophylactic antibiotics, swelling control, as well as clinical assessment of motor and sensory status of the operated limb. Heterotopic ossification prophylaxis is routinely not initiated unless the patient sustained a concomitant head injury at the time of the initial injury. In this case, indomethacin is prescribed (ie, 25 mg by mouth 3 times daily for 3 weeks).

Once discharged from the hospital, the patient returns for office follow-up at 7 to 10 days following surgery for wound check and suture removal, if necessary. The patient is instructed and educated on the importance of formal physical therapy for obtaining a pain-free and functional limb, and range-of-motion exercises are initiated at this time under the direct supervision of a physical therapist. Active and active-assisted flexion-extension between 30° and 130° and forearm prosupination with the elbow at 90° of flexion is started. Abduction and excessive internal/external rotation of the shoulder should be avoided for the first 4 to 6 weeks to avoid placing varus/valgus stress on the healing LUCL complex repair.[12]

The patient returns for follow-up at 4, 8, and 12 weeks after surgery for clinical assessment and review of elbow radiographs. At 8 weeks, the patient is allowed unrestricted range of motion, and at 12 weeks, strengthening exercises are undertaken. Evidence of fracture union on radiographs is usually seen 6 and 8 weeks following surgery. After 12 weeks, the patient can be seen at the 6- and 12-month mark, followed by a final office visit at 2 years.

It is important to counsel the patient that regaining full motion is slow and progressive and does not plateau up to 12 months following surgery. In a prospective cohort that underwent surgical treatment of complex elbow instability, the authors found that the first 6 months following surgery were critical to obtain functional elbow range of motion, with 70% (53 of 76 patients) and 80% (61 of 76 patients) recovering a functional arc of motion between 3 and 6 months and at 12 months, respectively.[13]

CLINICAL RESULTS

Complex elbow instability with fractures of the radial head and coronoid are referred to as "terrible triad" injuries because of the difficulty in management and frequent complications of stiffness, recurrent instability, posttraumatic arthritis, and pain. They are relatively infrequent injuries and the available literature largely comprises heterogenous treatment algorithms and small sample sizes. The rate of secondary procedures for stiffness, heterotopic ossification, and ulnar neuropathy ranges in the literature from 15% to 25%.[14] A study by Kalicke and colleagues[15] found that moderate and poor outcomes were associated with immobilization greater than 3 weeks; thus, early operative treatment is advisable.

A retrospective review by Ring and colleagues[1] included 11 patients with elbow dislocations and concomitant radial head and coronoid fractures treated by different surgeons of varying training levels and no standardized treatment protocol. One patient with severe peripheral neuropathy was treated with immobilization only; 1 patient underwent only debridement of a traumatic wound, and 9 patients underwent definitive surgical treatment. Of those 9 patients, 5 underwent radial head osteosynthesis and 4 underwent radial head resection. Three patients had LUCL complex repair. No patients had coronoid fracture repair. Five patients experienced recurrent dislocations postoperatively, including all 4 treated with radial head resection. Four of the 5 patients who had a recurrent dislocation were treated successfully with ulnohumeral joint transfixation with smooth Steinmann pins for 3 to 6 weeks; one patient had multiple failed secondary procedures and was ultimately treated with a total elbow replacement. One patient developed a proximal radioulnar synostosis and underwent subsequent capsular release. The mean flexion-extension of their patients was 31° to 123°, mean supination 60°, and mean pronation 66°. The 4 patients in this series that had satisfactory early results all had successful internal fixation of the radial head. Posttraumatic arthritis was present in 9 of 10 patients that retained their native elbow; the degree of arthritis was less severe in patients treated successfully with radial head internal fixation with a concentric joint reduction.

A recent retrospective review by Gupta and colleagues[14] attempted to eliminate heterogeneity by investigating a standard protocol at a single institution with 4 fellowship-trained orthopedic trauma

Table 1
Mean flexion-extension arc of motion and rotational arc of motion

Author		Flexion	Extension	Flexion Arc	Pronation	Supination	Rotational Arc
		\multicolumn{6}{c}{Mean Range of Motion (Degrees)}					
Ring et al,[1] 2002	—	123	31	92	66	60	126
Pugh et al,[17] 2004	—	131	19	112	—	—	136
Egol et al,[18] 2007	—	—	—	109	—	—	128
Forthman et al,[19] 2007	—	134	17	117	75	62	137
Lindenhovius et al,[20] 2008	—	135	17	119	78	63	141
Zeiders & Patel,[21] 2008	—	130	12	100	—	—	—
Gupta et al,[14] 2014	Primary procedures	128	17	110	77	72	148
	Secondary procedures, preoperatively	108	51	57	28	27	55
	Secondary procedures, postoperatively	122	26	96	57	68	124

Values omitted when not reported.
Data from Refs.[1,14,17–21]

Table 2
Complications and postoperative sequelae requiring secondary surgical procedures

Author	Stiffness	Nerve Transposition or Neurolysis	Tenolysis	Infection	Instability	Hardware Removal	Conversion Radial Head Prosthesis	Interposition Arthroplasty	Total Elbow Arthroplasty	Total
				Secondary Procedures						
Ring et al,[1] 2002	1	—	—	—	4	—	—	—	1	6
Pugh et al,[17] 2004	2	—	—	1	1	4	—	—	—	8
Egol et al,[18] 2007	2	—	—	—	1	1	2	—	—	6
Forthman et al,[19] 2007	4	4	—	—	—	—	—	1	—	9
Lindenhovius et al,[20] 2008	2	3	—	1	—	—	—	—	—	6
Zeiders & Patel,[21] 2008										
Gupta et al,[14] 2014	9	8	2	—	1	—	1	—	1	22
Total	20	15	2	2	7	5	3	1	2	57

Dash marks, no procedures were reported, except in study by Zeiders & Patel, where no secondary procedures were reported.
Data from Refs.[1,14,17–21]

surgeons. Their series included 34 patients with a minimum 6-month radiographic and clinical follow-up evaluating the recurrent dislocation rate, range of motion, patient-perceived stiffness, and secondary procedures. The surgical protocol called for (1) treatment of large coronoid fractures with screws and small fragments with suture repair of the anterior joint capsule; (2) radial head osteosynthesis or arthroplasty for comminuted fractures in which primary repair that was not anticipated to allow physiologic loads through a functional arc of motion; (3) repair of the LUCL complex and common extensor origin; and (4) repair of the MUCL complex if ulnohumeral stability and a concentric reduction are not achieved after addressing steps 1 through 3. External fixation was never used. Their postoperative regimen included immobilization in a posterior plaster splint for a maximum of 2 days, at which point active and active-assisted range of motion was started. Terminal extension in supination was avoided for 3 weeks postoperatively. No heterotopic ossification prophylaxis was used. One patient had a recurrent dislocation 33 days after surgery resulting from a fall onto the affected extremity and underwent LUCL reconstruction and removal of heterotopic ossified bone; the patient was later lost to follow-up and excluded from subsequent analysis. In patients who underwent only a single primary index procedure, mean flexion-extension was 17° to 128° degrees; mean supination was 72°, and pronation was 77°. In patients who underwent secondary procedures (9 of 34, 26%), range of motion before the secondary procedure included mean flexion-extension of 51° to 108° degrees, mean supination of 27°, and mean pronation of 28°. After the secondary procedure, the mean range of motion improved to flexion-extension of 26° to 122°, supination of 68°, and pronation of 57°. The investigators concluded that the postoperative dislocation rate was low, and although postoperative arthrofibrosis was common, most patients were able to obtain a functional range of motion after undergoing a secondary procedure.

A systematic review by Rodriguez-Martin and colleagues[16] analyzed the results from 5 studies using standard treatment protocols in the operative treatment of 137 terrible triad injuries of the elbow. The treatment protocols included coronoid fracture fixation, fixation or replacement of the radial head, repair of the LUCL complex, and MUCL complex repair and external fixator placement in cases of residual instability. The range-of-motion outcomes of the pooled data included a mean flexion-extension arc of 111.4° and a rotational arc of 135.5°. Mean postoperative range of motion and the reasons for revision surgery secondary to complications and fracture sequelae for the 7 clinical studies[17–21] are summarized in **Tables 1** and **2**.

SUMMARY

Patients who sustain a complex elbow dislocation involving the radial head and coronoid can achieve adequate pain relief and a functional arc of motion with a standardized surgical treatment protocol. Meticulous and thoughtful preoperative planning, including advanced imaging, is required to create a stable construct that can withstand early postoperative rehabilitation. Intraoperatively, the systematic approach first calls for coronoid fracture fixation, then radial head osteosynthesis or replacement, followed by LUCL complex repair before assessing elbow stability within a functional flexion-extension arc of motion. If the elbow is deemed unstable, then MUCL complex repair is undertaken, followed by application of an external fixator for persistent elbow instability to maintain concentric reduction and initiate early range of motion.

REFERENCES

1. Ring D, Jupiter JB, Zilberfarb J. Posterior dislocation of the elbow with fractures of the radial head and coronoid. J Bone Joint Surg Am 2002;84-A(4):547–51.
2. Morrey BF, Tanaka S, An KN. Valgus stability of the elbow. A definition of primary and secondary constraints. Clin Orthop Relat Res 1991;(265):187–95.
3. McKee MD, Pugh DM, Wild LM, et al. Standard surgical protocol to treat elbow dislocations with radial head and coronoid fractures. Surgical technique. J Bone Joint Surg Am 2005;87(Suppl 1(Pt 1)):22–32.
4. Hotchkiss RN. Displaced fractures of the radial head: internal fixation or excision? J Am Acad Orthop Surg 1997;5(1):1–10.
5. Diliberti T, Botte MJ, Abrams RA. Anatomical considerations regarding the posterior interosseous nerve during posterolateral approaches to the proximal part of the radius. J Bone Joint Surg Am 2000; 82(6):809–13.
6. Smith GR, Hotchkiss RN. Radial head and neck fractures: anatomic guidelines for proper placement of internal fixation. J Shoulder Elbow Surg 1996;5(2 Pt 1):113–7.
7. Caputo AE, Mazzocca AD, Santoro VM. The nonarticulating portion of the radial head: anatomic and clinical correlations for internal fixation. J Hand Surg 1998;23(6):1082–90.
8. Moro JK, Werier J, MacDermid JC, et al. Arthroplasty with a metal radial head for unreconstructible fractures of the radial head. J Bone Joint Surg Am 2001;83-A(8):1201–11.

9. Athwal GS, Frank SG, Grewal R, et al. Determination of correct implant size in radial head arthroplasty to avoid overlengthening: surgical technique. J Bone Joint Surg Am 2010;92(Suppl 1 Pt 2):250–7.

10. Frank SG, Grewal R, Johnson J, et al. Determination of correct implant size in radial head arthroplasty to avoid overlengthening. J Bone Joint Surg Am 2009; 91(7):1738–46.

11. McKee MD, Bowden SH, King GJ, et al. Management of recurrent, complex instability of the elbow with a hinged external fixator. J Bone Joint Surg Br 1998;80(6):1031–6.

12. Pipicelli JG, Chinchalkar SJ, Grewal R, et al. Rehabilitation considerations in the management of terrible triad injury to the elbow. Tech Hand Up Extrem Surg 2011;15(4):198–208.

13. Giannicola G, Polimanti D, Bullitta G, et al. Critical time period for recovery of functional range of motion after surgical treatment of complex elbow instability: prospective study on 76 patients. Injury 2014; 45(3):540–5.

14. Gupta A, Barei D, Khwaja A, et al. Single-staged treatment using a standardized protocol results in functional motion in the majority of patients with a terrible triad elbow injury. Clin Orthop Relat Res 2014;472(7):2075–83.

15. Kalicke T, Muhr G, Frangen TM. Dislocation of the elbow with fractures of the coronoid process and radial head. Arch Orthop Trauma Surg 2007; 127(10):925–31.

16. Rodriguez-Martin J, Pretell-Mazzini J, Andres-Esteban EM, et al. Outcomes after terrible triads of the elbow treated with the current surgical protocols. A review. Int Orthop 2011;35(6):851–60.

17. Pugh DM, Wild LM, Schemitsch EH, et al. Standard surgical protocol to treat elbow dislocations with radial head and coronoid fractures. J Bone Joint Surg Am 2004;86-A(6):1122–30.

18. Egol KA, Immerman I, Paksima N, et al. Fracture-dislocation of the elbow functional outcome following treatment with a standardized protocol. Bull NYU Hosp Jt Dis 2007;65(4):263–70.

19. Forthman C, Henket M, Ring DC. Elbow dislocation with intra-articular fracture: the results of operative treatment without repair of the medial collateral ligament. J Hand Surg 2007;32(8):1200–9.

20. Lindenhovius AL, Jupiter JB, Ring D. Comparison of acute versus subacute treatment of terrible triad injuries of the elbow. J Hand Surg 2008;33(6):920–6.

21. Zeiders GJ, Patel MK. Management of unstable elbows following complex fracture-dislocations–the "terrible triad" injury. J Bone Joint Surg Am 2008; 90(Suppl 4):75–84.

Varus Posteromedial Instability

Miguel A. Ramirez, MD, Jason A. Stein, MD, Anand M. Murthi, MD*

KEYWORDS

- Elbow • Instability • Coronoid fracture • Radial collateral ligament • Anteromedial facet
- Varus instability

KEY POINTS

- The medial facet of the coronoid is a major ulnohumeral joint stabilizer providing stability against posteromedial forces.
- The medial facet of coronoid fractures is often associated with avulsion of the lateral collateral ligament, which contributes to rotatory instability.
- Gravity-assisted varus stress test is the physical examination of choice; however, findings may be subtle in delayed cases.
- The standard management of these injuries is surgical; studies have shown persistent varus instability and poor outcomes with nonsurgical treatment.
- Reconstruction requires fixation of the coronoid fracture, reconstruction, or repair of the lateral collateral ligament, with possible external fixation in cases of persistent instability.

INTRODUCTION

Varus posteromedial instability of the elbow is the result of a traumatic injury to the major elbow stabilizers, the anteromedial facet of the coronoid, and the lateral collateral ligament (LCL).[1,2] Treatment of these injuries involves surgically addressing the anteromedial facet of the coronoid and repairing the LCL.[1–3] The purpose of this article is to describe the mechanism for varus posteromedial instability and discuss the authors' approach to addressing these injuries.

ANATOMY

The coronoid process of the elbow is a major ulnohumeral joint stabilizer. Several studies have shown that the function of the coronoid is to resist posterior ulnar subluxation and posteromedial and posterolateral rotatory forces.[4–6] The anteromedial facet of the coronoid in particular lengthens the articular surface of the elbow and prevents varus instability. Because approximately 60% of the coronoid is unsupported by the ulna metaphysis, it is prone to fracture, as seen in terrible triad injuries.[7] The O'Driscoll classification of coronoid fractures is helpful to identify fractures associated with varus posteromedial rotatory instability (VPMRI). Type II fractures involve the medial facet of the coronoid and thus render the elbow susceptible to varus stress. These injuries are usually the result of elbow subluxation and not frank dislocation. Therefore, the radial head is usually intact and commonly there is an associated LCL avulsion from the lateral epicondyle.[8,9]

Repair of larger coronoid fractures is critical in restoring elbow stability.[4,10] Surgical management of these fractures with open reduction and internal fixation (ORIF) has increased in popularity during the past few years.[7] Previously, these fractures

Financial Disclosures: The authors report no potential conflict of interest related to this report.
Department of Orthopaedic Surgery, MedStar Union Memorial Hospital, 3333 North Calvert Street, Suite 400, Baltimore, MD 21218, USA
* Corresponding author.
E-mail address: lyn.camire@medstar.net

were treated with excision or benign neglect, but outcomes were poor.[8,11] As a result, there is new interest in developing procedures to reconstruct the coronoid and therefore restore biomechanical stability. A study by Doornberg and Ring[9] showed that 6 of 18 patients who lost reduction after ORIF of a coronoid fracture had varus subluxation of the elbow and radiographic arthrosis 26 months after injury. All patients whose fracture healed in adequate alignment had good or excellent results.

The LCL has 4 major components—the lateral ulnar collateral ligament (LUCL), the radial collateral ligament (RCL), the annular ligament, and the accessory collateral ligament. Although rupture of these structures does not directly cause VPMRI, coronoid medial facet fractures are often associated with the LCL tears, and these tears must be addressed at the time of surgery to restore stability to the elbow.

The LCL complex has a common origin on the lateral epicondyle, deep to the extensor muscles. The ligaments separate distally to form individual structures. The LUCL attaches on the supinator crest of the ulna and is the most important ligament preventing posterolateral rotatory instability. The RCL predominantly resists varus stress, while the annular ligament is a stabilizer of the proximal radioulnar joint and does not contribute to ulnohumeral stability.

PHYSICAL EXAMINATION

Physical examination can be difficult in acute trauma patients because of pain. In cases with extreme pain, examination under anesthesia is more reliable than the physical examination performed in the office setting. In delayed trauma cases, physical examination is more reliable. Patients may report mechanical-type symptoms (clicking, popping, and slipping) during elbow flexion and extension. The most sensitive test is the gravity-assisted varus stress test. The patient is asked to abduct the arm to 90° and, while in this position, the patient is asked to flex and extend the elbow. In patients with VPMRI, there will be a feeling of pain, grinding, or instability during range of motion because the glenohumeral joint is closed medially by the lack of the buttress from the medial coronoid facet.

IMAGING STUDIES

Standard anteroposterior (AP) and lateral view radiographs often indicate normal findings but may reveal small lateral epicondyle avulsion fractures and disruption of the coronoid architecture (**Fig. 1**). Stress AP and lateral view radiographs may show widening of the ulnohumeral joint. Coronoid factures may not always be evident in AP, and lateral views, and therefore, oblique views should be obtained in patients with possible coronoid fracture. The gold standard is a fluoroscopic examination under anesthesia because the dynamic instability can usually be revealed without patient guarding in this setting.

In the authors' institution, they consider computed tomography (CT) scanning with

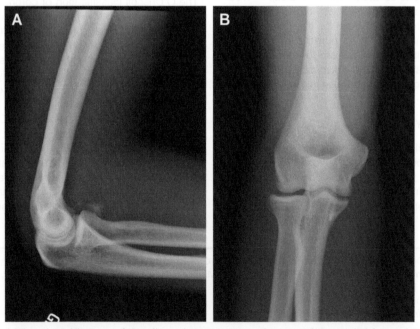

Fig. 1. Lateral (*A*) and AP (*B*) views of the elbow demonstrating a fracture of the medial facet of the coronoid.

3-dimensional (3D) reconstruction invaluable in treating these injuries. This modality can help identify the size and location of the medial facet of the coronoid fragment and may aid in preoperative planning (**Fig. 2**). MRI, especially arthrogram, although rarely required, might help identify injuries to the collateral ligaments and any osteochondral lesions that may have occurred as a result of trauma.

NONOPERATIVE VERSUS SURGICAL TREATMENT

The standard management of these injuries is surgical; studies have shown persistent varus instability and poor outcomes with nonsurgical treatment.[2,12] Therefore, in the authors' practice, the indications for treating these injuries nonoperatively are very few. These indications include elderly, inactive patients, and poor surgical candidates. If patients are treated nonoperatively, they are instructed to avoid shoulder abduction to avoid gravity varus stress across the elbow. It should be noted, however, that the understanding of this complex instability pattern is evolving and that further studies are required to accurately determine treatment indications.

SURGICAL MANAGEMENT
Preoperative Planning

Surgical planning begins in the office with careful review of the imaging studies. In particular, 3D CT

scan has been found to be invaluable because it gives an idea of the size of the coronoid fragment and helps in determining what hardware is required to fix the fracture and whether treatment will require lag screws, suture, or plate fixation. The authors have several systems available in case they need to change the fixation strategy intraoperatively, because CT scan does not adequately predict the quality of the available bone stock or the amount of comminution present. In cases of severe communution, internal fixation may not be possible, and the surgeon must be prepared to perform an anterior capsulodesis.

In the operating room, an examination of the elbow should be performed with the patient under general anesthesia and total paralysis.

The authors perform a pivot shift test, which is abnormal in most cases. If the test is negative, they typically also examine the elbow under fluoroscopy. Gapping of the lateral side of the ulnohumeral joint with varus stress usually indicates an incompetent LCL complex.

Patient Positioning

The patient is positioned supine on the operating room table. The authors prefer a radiolucent table with a hand table attachment (**Fig. 3**). They obtain fluoroscopic images before preparation and draping to make sure that adequate images are possible given the patient positioning and that the path of the fluoroscope does not interfere with the placement of the surgical team.

A nonsterile tourniquet is then applied and inflated to 225 mm Hg in most patients. The patient is prepared and draped in a sterile fashion, making sure that the arm is draped free.

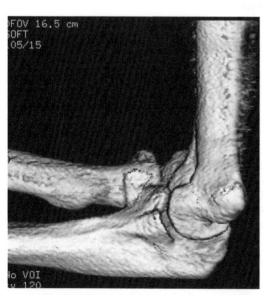

FOV 16.5 cm
SOFT
05/15

o VOI
v 120

Fig. 2. 3D CT scan of the elbow is obtained to further delineate the extent of the coronoid fragment and aid in preoperative planning.

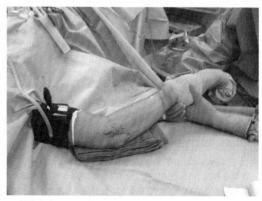

Fig. 3. Surgical setup. A radiolucent hand table is used with the arm draped free. A sterile tourniquet is applied.

Surgical Approach

Depending on surgeon preference, this injury can be approached through an extensile posterior approach or through medial and lateral approaches. The authors think that a single posterior skin incision with medial and lateral deep approaches allows the surgeon the required access to the entire elbow with few limitations. Alternatively, these injuries can also be treated arthroscopically assisted by addressing the coronoid fracture and repairing/reconstructing the LCL via a lateral mini-open approach.

Coronoid Fracture Fixation

The coronoid is approached via a medial approach through either a posterior incision or a separate medial incision as described above. The medial epicondyle is identified with the attachments of the flexor/pronator mass. At this point, the ulnar nerve can be identified and decompressed if indicated. The authors' typical approach is to decompress the nerve from the arcade of Struthers to the 2 heads of the flexor carpi ulnaris muscle. Once this is done, the anterior 50% of the flexor/pronator mass is detached from the medial epicondyle as described by Hotchkiss.[13] Care is taken to avoid the median nerve and brachial artery that lie just deep and anterior to these muscles. Once the flexor/pronator mass is elevated, the ulnar collateral ligament (UCL) is evaluated for integrity. The authors usually do not repair the ligament until the coronoid and LCL have been repaired. If instability persists, they typically repair this primarily with suture anchors as the last step of the case.

After the UCL is identified, the coronoid fracture is then exposed and evaluated. If the bone fragment is large, the authors typically opt to stabilize the fracture with an anterior mini-fragment plate with a combination of both locking and nonlocking screws. Alternatively, precontoured, low-profile plates are also available. The authors routinely provisionally stabilize the fracture with percutaneous posterior-to-anterior K-wires. Once they obtain adequate reduction under fluoroscopy, they apply the mini-fragment plate. Care is taken to avoid violating the ulnohumeral joint and the proximal radioulnar joint with screws. Several oblique fluoroscopic images are obtained to ensure that screws do not penetrate into the joint.

If the fracture pattern demands it, screw fixation can be used as shown in **Fig. 4**. If the fracture fragments are extensively comminuted and ORIF is not possible, the anterior capsule can be reattached to the ulna though bone tunnels.

Lateral Collateral Ligament Repair

Indications
Indications for LCL repair or reconstruction include symptomatic VPMRI in subacute/chronic injuries and persistent instability after coronoid fracture repair in acute cases (**Fig. 5**).

Surgical procedure
The authors use a utilitarian direct posterior skin incision with a combination of medial and lateral deep approaches as indicated. The advantages of a posterior approach are that it is extensile, allows for adequate exposure of the medial and lateral sides of the elbow, and does not preclude more extensive reconstruction is needed in the future.

Once the posterior approach is completed with thick subcutaneous flaps, the primary deep approach to the LCL is the Köcher interval between the anconeus and extensor carpi ulnaris muscles (see **Fig. 5**). The major caveat with this approach is that the posterior interosseus nerve can be injured with overzealous anterior retraction of the soft tissues.

The LCL is identified. In isolation with a coronoid fracture, the typical injury pattern is avulsion of the ligament from its attachment at the lateral epicondyle (**Fig. 6**). In this setting, a LCL repair is usually performed. In chronic injuries or situations where the ligament quality is poor, the ligament must be reconstructed. The integrity of the common extensor tendon is then evaluated. If the tendon is torn or avulsed, it is repaired back to the lateral epicondyle.

The authors' technique for LCL repair involves running a locked no. 2 nonabsorbable suture. Once this suture is passed, a decision is made as to lateral condyle fixation. Lateral condyle fixation can be done in a variety of ways, including suture anchors or anterior and posterior drill holes. The authors prefer to dock the ligament via bone tunnels. However, a good repair can be achieved with suture anchors.

Regardless of the procedure used to secure the ligament to the lateral epicondyle, it is imperative to place the ligament under appropriate tension in an isometric fashion. To accomplish this, the authors tighten the ligament with the elbow in pronation, 45° of flexion, and a small bump on the medial forearm to give a valgus stress. The elbow is then taken through a range of motion to confirm that the ligament remains isometric throughout the entire range of motion.

The muscular interval is then closed with a size 0 braided, nonabsorbable suture. The wound is subsequently closed, and the arm is placed in a

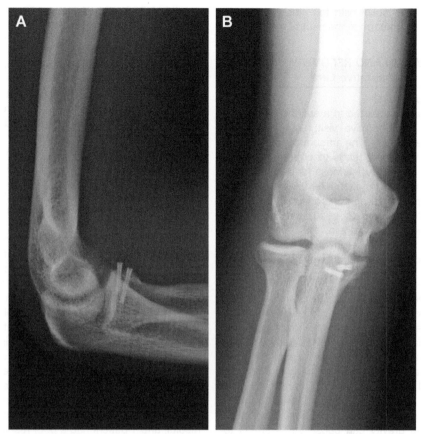

Fig. 4. Lateral (*A*) and AP (*B*) views of the elbow demonstrating the medial facet of the coronoid fracture fixed with 2.0-mm cannulated screws.

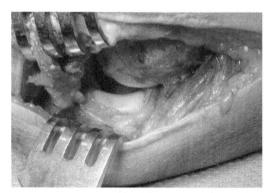

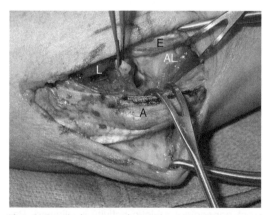

Fig. 5. Intraoperative stress test demonstrating persistent glenohumeral subluxation, an indication for LCL repair.

Fig. 6. Surgical approach to the LCL. The interval between the anconeus muscle (A) and extensor carpi ulnaris (E) is developed. The torn LCL ligament is identified. AL, annular ligament; L, lateral epicondyle.

posterior plaster splint with the elbow at 45° of flexion and the forearm in the neutral rotation.

REHABILITATION AND RECOVERY
Immediate Postoperative Care

Stage I (0–3 weeks)
The elbow is immobilized in a splint until the patient's first postoperative visit, usually at 7 to 10 days after surgery. The amount of surgery performed on the elbow tends to create significant scar tissue and elbow stiffness, and as a result, light active range of motion exercises are started early to help prevent postoperative stiffness. Patients are transitioned to a custom, removable splint at week 1 and are allowed to come out of the splint for gentle elbow, wrist, and hand range-of-motion exercises as well as bathing.

Stage II (3–6 weeks)
After 3 weeks, if desired, the patient can be advanced to a hinged elbow brace with limits set by the surgeon. Strict non-weight-bearing precautions are maintained during this phase. Occupational therapists may begin flexor–pronator isometrics and active-assisted range of motion from 0 to 120° of flexion with forearm pronated at all times. It is important to emphasize to therapists that patients need to avoid shoulder abduction because gravity can cause varus stress to the elbow and stress the repair.

Stage III (6–12 weeks)
At 12 weeks postoperatively, patients may discontinue brace immobilization if adequate healing is observed on follow-up radiographs. Passive range of motion and active-assisted range of motion are then instituted with specific attention to terminal stretching to tolerance. Therapists can begin unrestricted strengthening of flexor–pronators and extensors.

Stage IV (3–6 months)
The goals of this phase of postoperative care are to start transitioning to normal activities of daily living. By this point, the coronoid fracture and LCL are typically well healed. Patients typically have not regained full range of motion, but they usually regain most range of motion over the next 2 to 3 months. Strengthening is advanced, and therapists typically transition patients to a home/gym-based program at about 4.5 months. High-level athletics such as throwing or contact sports are prohibited until the 6-month time frame. Most noncontact athletic activity is allowed. Patients are allowed full unrestricted activity at 6 months as long as they have full motion and no evidence of persistent instability.

CLINICAL RESULTS IN THE LITERATURE

Data on outcomes after reconstruction for varus posteromedial instability are limited, and published results suggest relatively poor functional outcomes postoperatively.

Doornberg and Ring[9] studied 18 patients over a 6-year period. Fifteen patients were originally treated surgically, and 3 were treated nonoperatively. Patients were followed for an average of 26 months. Of the 18 patients, 4 patients required repeat surgery. One patient had a wound infection leading to osteomyelitis and subsequent fusion. Another patient had recurrent dislocation and infected hematoma requiring incision and drainage with external fixation. One patient had plate removal, and the fourth patient underwent elbow release secondary to heterotopic ossification and proximal radioulnar synostosis. Six patients were found to have varus malalignment of the anteromedial facet of the coronoid and varus subluxation, and all 6 developed radiographic arthritis and had fair or poor functional result according to the Broberg and Morrey score. Nine patients were reported to have secure fixation of the coronoid, and their outcomes were better. Average flexion-extension arc was 99° and forearm rotation was 149°. Based on the Broberg and Morrey score, 3 patients had excellent results, 5 had fair results, and 1 patient had a poor result.

A recent study by Park and colleagues[1] showed better patient outcomes compared with the previous series. In this retrospective series, 11 patients had an anteromedial facet fracture that was associated with an LCL injury in all patients and medial collateral ligament injury in 6 of 11 patients. At an average follow-up of 31 months, average range of motion was 128° with an average elbow flexion contracture of 6°. One patient had persistent ulnotrochlear incongruity, and 2 patients had ulnar nerve symptoms, one necessitating ulnar nerve transposition. Average Mayo performance score was 89, and results were reported as excellent in 4 patients, good in 6 patients, and fair in 1 patient.

SUMMARY

Varus posteromedial instability of the elbow is a result of traumatic injury to the medial facet of the coronoid and usually the LCL. Treatment of these fractures is usually surgical; poor outcomes have been described with nonoperative treatment. Surgical management consists of coronoid fracture fixation with plates, screws, or sutures, and RCL repair instead of reconstruction. Outcomes of these injuries are mixed, but most series report fair to good objective scores. The purpose of this article was to describe the pathophysiology of varus posteromedial instability, discuss the management of this injury, and report the outcomes of treatment.

REFERENCES

1. Park SM, Lee JS, Jung JY, et al. How should anteromedial coronoid facet fracture be managed? A surgical strategy based on O'Driscoll classification and ligament injury. J Shoulder Elbow Surg 2015; 24:74–82.

2. Ring D, Doornberg JN. Fracture of the anteromedial facet of the coronoid process. Surgical technique. J Bone Joint Surg Am 2007;89(Suppl 2 Pt.2):267–83.

3. Budoff JE. Coronoid fractures. J Hand Surg Am 2012;37:2418–23.

4. Closkey RF, Goode JR, Kirschenbaum D, et al. The role of the coronoid process in elbow stability. A biomechanical analysis of axial loading. J Bone Joint Surg Am 2000;82-A:1749–53.

5. Schneeberger AG, Sadowski MM, Jacob HA. Coronoid process and radial head as posterolateral rotatory stabilizers of the elbow. J Bone Joint Surg Am 2004;86-A:975–82.

6. Beingessner DM, Dunning CE, Stacpoole RA, et al. The effect of coronoid fractures on elbow kinematics and stability. Clin Biomech (Bristol, Avon) 2007;22: 183–90.

7. Steinmann SP. Coronoid process fracture. J Am Acad Orthop Surg 2008;16:519–29.

8. Doornberg JN, Ring D. Coronoid fracture patterns. J Hand Surg Am 2006;31:45–52.

9. Doornberg JN, Ring DC. Fracture of the anteromedial facet of the coronoid process. J Bone Joint Surg Am 2006;88:2216–24.

10. Pollock JW, Brownhill J, Ferreira L, et al. The effect of anteromedial facet fractures of the coronoid and lateral collateral ligament injury on elbow stability and kinematics. J Bone Joint Surg Am 2009;91: 1448–58.

11. Ring D, Jupiter JB, Zilberfarb J. Posterior dislocation of the elbow with fractures of the radial head and coronoid. J Bone Joint Surg Am 2002;84-A:547–51.

12. Tashjian RZ, Katarincic JA. Complex elbow instability. J Am Acad Orthop Surg 2006;14:278–86.

13. Hotchkiss RN. Elbow contracture. In: Green DP, Hotchkiss RN, Peterson WC, editors. Green's operative hand surgery. 4th edition. New York: Churchill Livingstone; 1999. p. 667–82.

Adult Monteggia and Olecranon Fracture Dislocations of the Elbow

Justin C. Wong, MD[a],*, Charles L. Getz, MD[b],
Joseph A. Abboud, MD[b]

KEYWORDS

- Monteggia • Transolecranon fracture dislocation • Elbow fracture dislocation • Adult
- Olecranon fracture

KEY POINTS

- Monteggia fractures in adults are most commonly posteriorly directed, may have associated radial head and coronoid fractures, and sometimes have lateral collateral ligament disruption.
- Olecranon fracture dislocations are fractures of the olecranon associated with ulnohumeral instability and may occur in anterior (transolecranon) or posterior directions.
- Optimal treatment of Monteggia fractures of the diaphysis is centered on restoration of ulnar alignment and length.
- Proximal ulnar fractures require stable anatomic reduction of the trochlear notch and coronoid process in relation to the ulnar diaphysis.

INTRODUCTION

The elbow is a complex joint formed by 3 articulations: ulnohumeral, radiocapitellar, and proximal radioulnar. These articulations allow for stable motion through an average arc of flexion-extension of 150° and pronation-supination of 160° to 170°.[1] During forearm rotation, the ulna remains fixed while the radius rotates around a longitudinal axis extending from the proximal radioulnar joint to the distal ulna. Because of this intimate relationship between the proximal radius and ulna, fractures involving the ulna can result in concomitant fracture of the radius and/or disruption of the proximal radioulnar or radiocapitellar joints. When an ulna fracture occurs in conjunction with proximal radioulnar joint dislocation this is termed a Monteggia fracture. The recognition that proximal radioulnar joint instability may occur anteriorly, posteriorly, or laterally, and may also include fracture of the proximal radius, led to an expanded definition of Monteggia fractures by Bado in 1967.[2] Monteggia fractures in adults can be difficult to treat and before the advent of stable internal fixation allowing earlier range of motion poor outcomes were common.[3–7] Improvements in radiographic imaging, which have allowed a better understanding of the injury patterns, combined with stable internal fixation have resulted in better surgical outcomes.[8–11] The purpose of this article is to review the relevant anatomy pertaining to Monteggia fractures and to describe the associated patterns of injury as well as treatment options.

Each author has contributed substantially to the research, preparation, and production of this article and approves of its submission to the journal.
[a] Department of Orthopaedic Surgery, Thomas Jefferson University Hospital, 1020 Walnut Street, College Building Room 516, Philadelphia, PA 19107, USA; [b] Department of Orthopaedic Surgery, The Rothman Institute, Thomas Jefferson University Hospital, 925 Chestnut Street, 5th Floor, Philadelphia, PA 19107, USA
* Corresponding author.
E-mail address: jcwong330@gmail.com

hand.theclinics.com

ANATOMY
Bony Structures

The 3 bony articulations of the elbow (ulnohumeral, radiocapitellar, and proximal radioulnar) allow for movement in the flexion-extension axis as well as forearm rotation (**Fig. 1**). The ulnohumeral joint is a highly congruent joint between the trochlea of the distal humerus and the trochlear notch, which is composed of the olecranon and coronoid processes of the proximal ulna. The trochlea is covered with a 300° arc of articular cartilage and has a sagittal depression that interdigitates with a corresponding sagittal ridge in the trochlear notch. The trochlear notch provides a nearly 180° arc of articulation with the trochlea but has a central transverse bare spot devoid of articular cartilage, which is important to consider when reconstructing the relationship between the coronoid and olecranon processes to prevent malreduction.[12] In profile, a line drawn from the tips of the coronoid and olecranon processes should form a 30° angle with the axis of the ulnar shaft (**Fig. 2**). The coronoid process itself is composed of a tip, body, anteromedial facet, anterolateral facet, and sublime tubercle. The sublime tubercle serves as the insertion point of the anterior bundle of the medial collateral ligament. Laterally, at the base of the proximal ulna is the

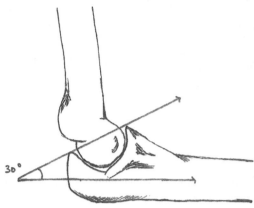

Fig. 2. Relationship of coronoid and olecranon processes. Lateral view of proximal ulna shows that a line drawn from the tips of the olecranon and coronoid processes should form an angle of 30° with a line drawn down the axis of the ulna diaphysis.

crista supinatoris, which serves as the insertion site for the lateral ulnar collateral ligament. As a whole, the coronoid serves as an anterior buttress for the ulnohumeral joint and because of the articular congruity with the trochlea and attachments of the ulnar collateral ligaments it provides varus, valgus, posteromedial, and posterolateral stability of the elbow.

The original Regan and Morrey[13] classification for coronoid fractures was based on lateral-view radiographs and the amount of coronoid involvement (type 1, tip avulsion; type 2, less than 50% of coronoid height; type 3, 50% of coronoid height). However, the use of computed tomography scans of the elbow has allowed for improved recognition of additional coronoid fracture patterns, including the anteromedial and anterolateral oblique coronoid fractures.[14] The O'Driscoll classification system takes into account coronoid fracture morphology and the fracture's relationship to capsular and ligamentous attachments.[15] The main categories of this classification are: transverse tip, anteromedial facet, and base of coronoid. Fractures involving the tip of the coronoid are more common in the valgus posterolateral rotatory instability patterns and the terrible triad, whereas anteromedial facet fractures occur with varus posteromedial elbow instability and generally large coronoid base fractures occur with Monteggia and olecranon fracture dislocations.[16]

The radial head is an elliptical dish that projects 15° obliquely from the radial shaft and is covered with articular cartilage proximally as well as along its margin. The margin of the radial head articulates with the ulna via the lesser sigmoid notch to

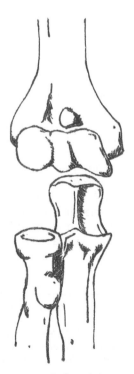

Fig. 1. Bony anatomy of elbow joint. Anterior view of distal humerus and proximal radius and ulna demonstrate highly congruous joint surfaces.

form the proximal radio-ulnar joint and proximally with the humerus via the radiocapitellar joint. The radial head serves as a secondary stabilizer to valgus forces.[17] Partial articular fractures of the radial head may lead to altered elbow kinematics especially in the setting of collateral ligament disruption.[18] Radial head fractures may be classified with the Mason[19] classification system in which type I fractures are nondisplaced or minimally displaced (<2 mm), type II fractures are displaced more than 2 mm and involve greater than 30% of the articular surface, and type III fractures are comminuted. Modifications of this system have been made to describe radial head fractures in association with elbow dislocation[20] or to more closely correlate classification type and treatment.[21]

Ligamentous Structures

Ligamentous structures on both the medial and lateral joint contribute significantly to stability of the elbow (**Fig. 3**). The medial collateral ligament complex is composed of an anterior bundle, posterior bundle, and transverse ligament. The anterior bundle of the medial collateral ligament is a primary stabilizer of the elbow and originates from the anterior-inferior aspect of the medial epicondyle and inserts on the sublime tubercle of the ulna, providing stability to valgus and posteromedial rotatory stresses. The fibers of the anterior bundle provide restraint against valgus force from full extension to 85° of flexion, whereas the posterior bundle is more important with greater degrees of elbow flexion.[17]

The lateral collateral ligament complex is composed of the radial collateral ligament, lateral ulnar collateral ligament, and the annular ligament. The radial collateral ligament takes its origin off of the lateral epicondyle at the isometric point of the flexion-extension axis of the elbow and extends to a broad insertion on the annular ligament.[17,22] The radial collateral ligament maintains a consistent level of tension throughout elbow flexion, provides restraint against varus forces and helps to stabilize the radial head. The lateral ulnar collateral ligament is considered a primary stabilizer of the elbow to varus and posterolateral rotatory stress and originates from the isometric point of the lateral epicondyle and inserts on the crista supinatoris of the lateral ulna. The annular ligament encircles the radial head. With an origin and insertion on the proximal ulna, it provides stability to the proximal radioulnar joint.

Elbow Stability

Elbow instability may occur with disruption of either bony or ligamentous stabilizers or oftentimes disruption of a combination of bony and ligamentous stabilizers. Biomechanical studies have helped to illustrate the relative contributions of bony and ligamentous structures to elbow stability.[18,23–29] In the absence of ligamentous or radial head injury, transverse fractures of the coronoid process involving greater than 50% to 60% of coronoid height can lead to axial and varus instability of the elbow.[25,28,29] However, with loss of the stabilizing effect of an intact radiocapitellar joint, posterolateral rotatory instability may be seen with coronoid fractures involving 30% of coronoid height.[26,27] These studies underscore that bony and ligamentous stabilizers work in concert to provide elbow stability, such that combined injuries may lead to instability in cases in which the individual components of an injury seen in isolation may not. When treating complex elbow instability cases, it is imperative to identify the bony and/or ligamentous stabilizers that require repair or reconstruction to restore joint stability and allow for early joint range of motion.

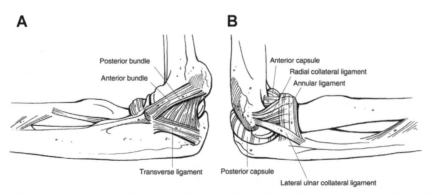

Fig. 3. Elbow ligamentous anatomy. Structure of the medial collateral ligament complex (*A*) and the lateral collateral ligament complex (*B*). (*From* Tashijian RZ, Katarinic JA. Complex elbow instability. J Am Acad Orthop Surg 2006;14(5):279; with permission.)

CLASSIFICATION

In the original description of the injury pattern that bears his name, Monteggia described the clinical scenario of a proximal ulnar fracture in conjunction with anterior dislocation of the radial head. In 1967, Bado[2] expanded the definition of Monteggia fractures by describing a 4-category classification system based on the location of ulna fracture, direction of radial head displacement, and presence or absence of concomitant proximal radius fracture, which he termed Monteggia lesion (**Fig. 4**).

Type I Monteggia lesions represent anterior dislocation of the radial head and apex anterior angulation of the ulnar fracture. Type II lesions represent posterior or posterolateral dislocation of the radial head and apex posterior angulation of the ulnar fracture. Type III lesions represent an anterolateral dislocation of the radial head in conjunction with a proximal ulnar metaphysis fracture. Type IV lesions represent an anterior dislocation of the radial head in conjunction with a proximal radial shaft fracture at the same level of the ulnar shaft fracture. From a practical standpoint, Monteggia fractures may be considered as either anterior or anterolateral (type I and type III) or posterior (type II) with type IV involvement of the radial shaft occurring with either anterior or posterior Monteggia fractures.[2,30]

The posterior Monteggia fractures (Bado type II) have been subdivided by Jupiter and colleagues[8] based on the ulnar fracture in relation to the coronoid (**Fig. 5**). Type IIA lesions represented ulnar fractures at the level of the coronoid with

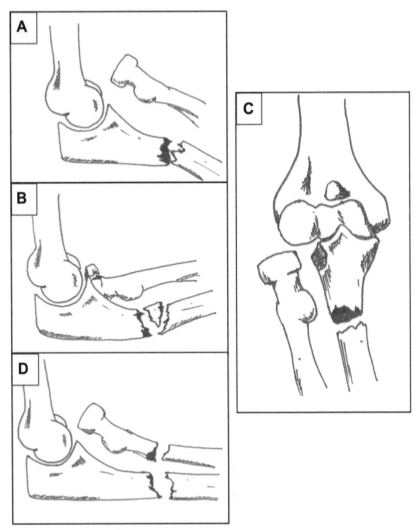

Fig. 4. Bado classification of monteggia fractures. (*A*) Type I, anterior monteggia. (*B*) Type II, posterior monteggia. (*C*) Type III, lateral monteggia. (*D*) Type IV, monteggia fracture with diaphyseal radial shaft fracture.

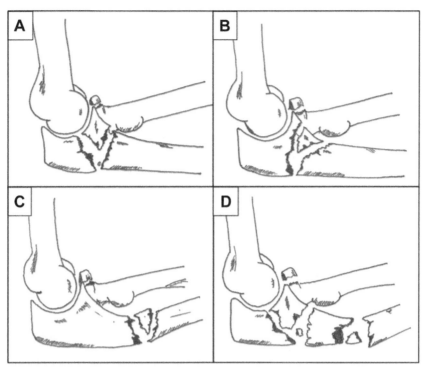

Fig. 5. Jupiter subclassification of posterior monteggia fractures (*A*): IIA, the ulnar fracture involves the distal olecranon and coronoid process. (*B*) IIB, the ulnar fracture is at the metaphyseal-diaphyseal junction distal to the coronoid. (*C*) IIC, the ulnar fracture is diaphyseal. (*D*) IID, ulnar fracture extends along proximal third to half of the ulna.

disruption of the greater sigmoid notch. Type IIB lesions represented ulnar fractures distal to the coronoid at the ulnar metaphysis with preservation of the greater sigmoid notch. Type IIC lesions have a diaphyseal ulna fracture and type IID lesions had comminuted involvement of the proximal ulna from the diaphysis to the greater sigmoid notch. One of the purposes for this subclassification was to highlight the varying complexity of ulnar fracture patterns and the need for anatomic alignment and stable fixation of the ulna, particularly with respect to reestablishing ulnar length and anatomically reducing the coronoid fracture.

When the ulna fracture occurs proximally in the olecranon and involves the trochlear notch, ulnohumeral joint instability may be compromised and these fractures may be termed olecranon fracture dislocations. The olecranon fracture dislocation is subdivided into 2 types: anterior and posterior, each of which has characteristic patterns of injury and outcomes. With anterior transolecranon fracture dislocation, the forearm translates anteriorly as a result of fracture through the olecranon and the proximal radioulnar joint remains stable.[31,32] This distinguishes these injuries from the anterior Monteggia fractures in which the proximal radioulnar joint is disrupted.

Posterior olecranon fracture dislocations are considered a type of posterior Monteggia lesion.[33,34] With posterior olecranon fracture dislocations, the radial head dislocates posteriorly and is often fractured, in conjunction with disruption of the proximal radioulnar joint and possible injury to the lateral ulnar collateral ligament. These injuries may be associated with more persistent instability despite restoration of bony alignment.

EPIDEMIOLOGY AND PATTERNS OF INJURY

In children, anterior Monteggia fracture (Bado type I) is the most common pattern seen; however, in adults, the anterior Monteggia is less common.[11,30,34] Proximal ulna fractures with anterior radiocapitellar dislocation can be misinterpreted as anterior Monteggia fractures when in fact they represent anterior transolecranon fracture dislocations with preservation of the proximal radioulnar joint.[32] The anterior transolecranon fracture dislocation often occurs as a result of a high-energy mechanism of injury. With the elbow in a flexed position, the trochlea is driven through the greater sigmoid notch, resulting in anterior translation of the forearm relative to the elbow. This pattern of injury was initially described by Biga and

Thomine[31] who noted that the olecranon fracture pattern may be simple but is more commonly associated with comminution of the sigmoid notch. The incidence of these injuries is unclear and several investigators suspect it may be under-reported because these injuries are often misdiagnosed as anterior Monteggia fractures.[9,35] In general, this injury pattern does not disrupt the proximal radioulnar joint or radial head nor does it result in disruption of the stabilizing ligaments of the ulnohumeral joint. Consequently, treatment aimed at restoration of the trochlear notch and olecranon generally confers ulnohumeral joint stability.

Anterior dislocation of the proximal radioulnar joint may occur in approximately 14.5% to 30% of Monteggia fractures.[9,11] These are often the result of high-energy mechanisms and can commonly be associated with polytrauma, open fractures, and peripheral nerve injury.[9,11] In one series, 4 of 7 subjects had Gustilo-Anderson type III open fracture and 3 of 7 had an ipsilateral diaphyseal humerus fracture resulting in a floating elbow.[9] Despite the severity of the injuries, concomitant radial head or coronoid fractures are generally uncommon with this injury.

Posterior Monteggia fractures (Bado type II) encompass a wide spectrum of injury from diaphyseal ulnar fractures with posterior radioulnar joint dislocation to posterior olecranon fracture-dislocations. In adults, these injuries can occur as a result of various mechanisms from seemingly innocuous ground-level falls to high-energy falls or motor vehicle accidents.[9] Injuries from a ground-level fall tend to occur in middle-to-older age women and can be associated with osteoporosis.[9] For younger patients, these injuries result from higher energy mechanisms of injury and may be associated with polytrauma, open fracture, and compartment syndrome. When using the Jupiter subclassification, most of these ulnar fractures occur at the metaphyseal level distal to the coronoid (type IIB), followed by fracture through the coronoid (type IIA), with diaphyseal (type IIC) and severely comminuted fracture of the proximal ulna being the least common.[9,11] In contrast to the anterior Monteggia, posterior Monteggia injuries are frequently associated with radial head or coronoid fractures and variable disruption of the lateral ulnar collateral ligament complex, which may impact ulnohumeral stability. Lateral ulnar collateral ligament injury may occur in half to two-thirds of posterior Monteggia fractures by some estimates,[30] although formal repair may only be required in the setting of persistent ulnohumeral instability despite stable anatomic fixation of the ulna and radial head.

Radial head fractures are most commonly seen with posterior Monteggia fractures, including the posterior olecranon fracture dislocation. Radial head involvement is rare with the anterior transolecranon fracture or anterior Monteggia. Concomitant radial head fracture may be seen with posterior Monteggia lesions in 35% to 100% of cases.[6–8,11] Using the Mason classification of radial head fractures, they are often Mason type II or III.[6–8,11,19] In a series of 7 patients, Penrose[7] observed that with the forearm placed in 30° of pronation, the radial head fracture plane faced anteriorly. He suggested a shearing mechanism of injury because the radial head dislocated past the capitellum.

Fractures involving the coronoid process are common with the posterior Monteggia and anterior or posterior transolecranon fracture dislocations but rare with anterior diaphyseal Monteggia. By definition, the coronoid is involved in the Jupiter IIA and IID subset of posterior Monteggia fractures. In a series of both anterior and posterior transolecranon fracture dislocation, coronoid involvement was seen in 50% of anterior and 100% of posterior fracture dislocations.[33] Using the Regan and Morrey classification system, the coronoid fractures are most often type III followed by type II.[9,11,13,33] Coronoid involvement requires special attention to reduction and fixation to restore stability to the ulnohumeral joint.

SURGICAL TECHNIQUE

These injury patterns are best treated through a posterior approach to the elbow and the subcutaneous border of the ulna. A posterior approach allows for potential subcutaneous flaps to be developed for direct medial or lateral approaches to the elbow if necessary.

Reduction and Fixation of the Ulna

For diaphyseal and metaphyseal Monteggia fractures (anterior Monteggia or posterior type IIB and IIC), restoration of ulnar length and alignment first leads to reduction of the proximal radio-ulnar joint. It is rare for the annular ligament or adjacent soft tissue structures to interpose and prevent radial head reduction when the appropriate ulnar length and alignment has been achieved. If the radiocapitellar joint does not reduce appropriately after ulna fixation, the ulna should be evaluated for possible malalignment of fracture fragments.

A posterior incision can be used to expose the fracture and the fracture fragments may be stabilized with a contoured 3.5 mm limited-contact dynamic compression plate. For true ulnar shaft fractures, the plate may be placed either on the medial or lateral aspect of the ulna. However, proximal fractures occurring through the metaphysis and olecranon process are best stabilized with a posterior plate that is contoured around the olecranon, which creates a stronger construct by allowing for additional fixation in the proximal fragment as well as screws in an orthogonal plane to the more distal screws[9,11,30,32] (**Fig. 6**). For complex fracture patterns, the use of tension band wiring or semitubular plates is not recommended because they may not provide sufficient fracture stability and can lead to loss of fracture alignment.[8,36,37] For posterior Monteggia fractures, there is frequently an anterior oblique fracture fragment of the ulna, which must be reduced and stabilized to help resist the tendency for recurrent posterior angulation of the fracture.[8]

When the ulna fracture involves the coronoid process and ulnohumeral joint (posterior Monteggia type IIA, IID), restoration of the alignment and stable fixation of the coronoid fragment is imperative for joint stability (**Fig. 7**). Exposure is again obtained through a posterior incision. Frequently, the coronoid fracture can be reduced through the fracture of the olecranon or if necessary can be exposed medially through a split in the flexor-pronator

mass or laterally if radial head comminution necessitates excision and prosthetic replacement. In general, these coronoid fragments are amenable to fixation with screws or transosseous suture directed from posterior to anterior or at times anterior to posterior. If required, the medial elbow can be approached through the posterior skin incision by raising a medial skin flap and splitting the flexor pronator mass. If plate fixation of the coronoid is intended, the ulnar nerve should be protected and controlled during exposure.

Complex ulna fractures with involvement of the trochlear notch or coronoid can be fixed either from proximal-to-distal[32] or distal-to-proximal.[38,39] In a series of anterior transolecranon fracture dislocations, Ring and colleagues[32] described a technique in which the proximal olecranon fragment is first temporarily stabilized to the trochlea with a smooth 0.062-in Kirschner wire. Using the trochlea as a reduction template, the trochlear notch can be reconstructed and the distal ulna can be realigned. These investigators also advocated using a temporary skeletal distractor to help in provisionally restoring length and alignment of the ulna. Alternatively, for fractures with significant comminution extending to the

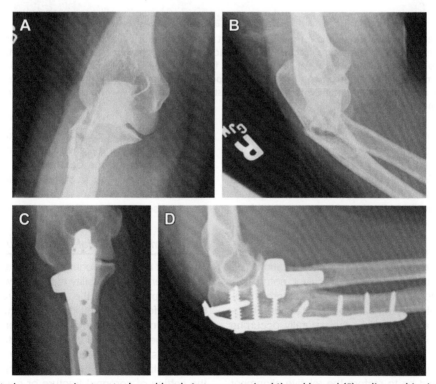

Fig. 6. Posterior monteggia at metaphyseal level. Anteroposterior (*A*) and lateral (*B*) radiographic views demonstrate posterior monteggia at metaphyseal level (Jupiter IIB) with associated radial head fracture. Postoperative anteroposterior (*C*) and lateral (*D*) radiographic views after stable fixation with posteriorly placed and contoured plate and metallic radial head arthroplasty.

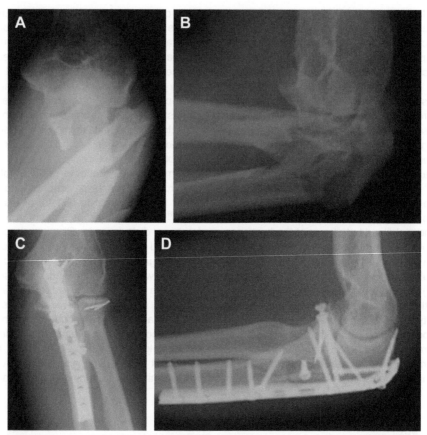

Fig. 7. Posterior monteggia with coronoid involvement anteroposterior (*A*) and lateral (*B*) radiographic views demonstrate a posterior monteggia fracture with characteristic large anterior quadrangular ulnar fragment extending into the coronoid process as well as radial head fracture. Anteroposterior (*C*) and lateral (*D*) radiographs after anatomic reduction and fixation of the ulna with posterior placed plate and screws. Supplemental fixation of the large anterior ulna fragment with anterior-to-posterior directed screws. The radial head fragment is fixed with Kirschner wires.

diaphysis of the ulna, fixation can proceed from distal-to-proximal with use of lag screws and mini-fragment plates.[39] Addressing the proximal olecranon fragment last allows the fracture plane to be used to view the reduction and allow placement of provisional fixation of the more distal fracture fragments. Provisional fixation with Kirschner wires and mini-plates allows the surgeon to confirm appropriate reduction of fracture fragments before placement of definitive fixation.

When reconstructing the trochlear notch it is important to remember the normal anatomic relationship between the coronoid process and olecranon process as well as the naturally occurring bare spot of the trochlear notch, which is devoid of articular cartilage, to prevent malreduction. The primary goal of reconstructing the trochlear notch should be to restore the relative alignment between the coronoid and olecranon processes. Residual articular incongruity in comminuted fractures may have less impact on outcomes than

trochlear notch alignment.[32] Stable fixation of the trochlear notch is imperative to allow for early joint range of motion in the postoperative period. For severely comminuted fractures, application of a static external fixator for a period of 4–6 weeks may be used to protect the construct stability.

Management of Radial Head Fractures

The intact radial head contributes to varus, valgus and posterolateral stability of the elbow as well as sharing up to 60% of the axial load transmission from the forearm to the distal humerus.[18,23,24,40] In isolation, fractures involving greater than one-third of the radial head can lead to altered elbow kinematics and subtle changes in varus-valgus joint stability.[24] These effects are compounded in the setting of coronoid fracture or collateral ligament injury. With this in mind, we believe Mason type II and some Mason type III radial head fractures should be treated with open reduction and internal fixation when possible to maximize the restoration of radiocapitellar joint congruency. However, some investigators have performed excision of small fragments of radial head or even complete radial head excision with no discernible effect on clinical outcome.[8,9,11] Additionally, it should be noted that attempts to fix Mason type III radial head fractures may lead to greater complications than radial head excision with radial head malunion leading to restriction in forearm pronation and supination.[9] The role of metallic radial head arthroplasty over radial head resection in these injuries is unclear as previous studies report on subjects treated before the use of metallic radial head implants.[8,9,11] However, because these injuries can occur in conjunction with complex instability patterns and the radiocapitellar joint contributes to elbow stability and load transmission it is prudent for the surgeon to consider the need for metallic radial head arthroplasty if the radial head fracture is deemed too comminuted to fix. In cases of ulnohumeral instability despite appropriate restoration of alignment of the ulna or longitudinal forearm instability, a radial head prosthesis may provide improved forearm and elbow stability.[41]

Residual and Late Instability

At the time of surgery, persistent elbow instability after fracture fixation may be the result of either[1] inadequate fracture reduction or[2] due to coronoid, radial head or capsuloligamentous deficiency.[37,42] It may also occur postoperatively, particularly in the case of posterior Monteggia fractures due to loss of fixation in osteoporotic bone.[37]

If radiocapitellar subluxation is detected intraoperatively, the first consideration should be to confirm adequate fracture alignment - inadvertent malalignment or shortening of the ulna fracture can result in failure to reduce the radiocapitellar joint. Similarly, ulnohumeral instability may occur if the ulna is inadequately reduced or stabilized. In particular, the coronoid fragment in posterior Monteggia fractures serves a prominent role as the anterior buttress to prevent ulnohumeral instability. If ulnohumeral instability persists despite appropriate reduction and fixation of the ulna fracture fragments, then attention should be turned to the lateral ulnar collateral ligament complex, which can be injured particularly with the posterior Monteggia injury patterns.[33,42]

Late malalignment of the radiocapitellar or ulnohumeral joint is often due to inadequate fixation of the ulna fracture.[8,37] Loss of fracture fixation has been most commonly observed when tension band wiring, semi-tubular or 1/3 tubular plates are used to stabilize complex fracture patterns.[8,9,37] As highlighted by Jupiter and colleagues,[8] in posterior Monteggia fractures, the fracture pattern often involves an anterior triangular or quadrangular fragment, which results in loss of a compression-resistant cortex and so more stout fixation is often required. Salvage of these injuries has been described with revision of the ulnar fixation and use of a posteriorly placed contoured 3.5 mm limited-contact dynamic compression plate with an external fixator.[8,9,11,30,37] In some cases of coronoid deficiency and radial head nonunion or malunion, the radial head may be replaced and a portion of the excised radial head can be used to reconstruct the coronoid.[43] This technique allows for reconstruction of deficiencies of 30% to 50% of the coronoid.

RESULTS AND COMPLICATIONS

Despite the challenges in management of these complex injuries, good outcomes may be achieved if attention is paid to understanding the full spectrum of the injury and a stable anatomic reduction of the fractures is obtained to allow for early elbow range of motion. In many cases, stable anatomic alignment of the fracture fragments alone imparts sufficient stability to the ulnohumeral joint, but in some cases, capsuloligamentous repair with or without external fixation is required. The Broberg and Morrey rating system[44] and the Disability of the Arm, Shoulder and Hand questionnaire[45] are 2 of the more commonly used instruments in the reporting of outcomes in the more contemporary reports of Monteggia and transolecranon fracture dislocations. Using the Broberg and Morrey scale, the outcomes of 70% to 80% of patients with these injury patterns can be considered good or excellent, although reoperation rates can be high. In general, worse outcomes are associated with the posterior Monteggia or posterior olecranon fracture dislocation patterns, concomitant radial head fracture, and ulna fractures with involvement of the coronoid process.[9,11,33,34] Complications of these injuries and their treatment include loss of fixation, elbow instability, posttraumatic arthrosis, heterotopic ossification, synostosis and symptomatic hardware.

Although the anterior transolecranon fracture dislocation injury pattern tends to occur as a result of high-energy mechanisms of injury and can often have associated open fractures, the fracture pattern spares involvement of the proximal radio-ulnar joint and ligamentous injury requiring repair is not commonly observed[32,35] (**Table 1**). Associated radial head fractures are uncommon with this injury pattern and although coronoid

Table 1
Outcomes of olecranon fracture dislocation

	Anterior Fracture Dislocation				Posterior Fracture Dislocation
Publication	Ring et al,[32] JOT 1997	Moushine et al,[35] JSES 2007	Mortazavi et al,[36] Injury 2006	Doornberg et al,[33] CORR 2004	Doornberg et al,[33] CORR 2004
Subjects	17	14	8	10	16
Average follow-up	25 mo (14–36)	42 mo (7–84)	37 mo (10–50)	7 y (3–10)	6 y (3–10)
Average age	38 (18–78)	54 (22–82)	35 (22–58)	42 (20–72)	53 (21–82)
Gender	14 male, 3 female	6 male, 8 female	7 male, 1 female	7 male, 3 female	8 male, 8 female
Ground-level fall	1 (6%)	2 (14%)	1 (12.5%)	2 (20%)	5 (31%)
High-energy fall	3 (18%)	3 (21%)	1 (12.5%)	2 (20%)	9 (56%)
MVA	11 (65%)	6 (43%)	4 (50%)	4 (40%)	1 (6%)
Other	2 (12%)	3 (21%)	2 (25%)	2 (20%)	—
Open fracture	5 (29%): 2 type II, 2 type IIIA, 1 type IIIB	6 (43%): 4 type II, 2 type IIIB	1 (13%): type I	3 (30%): 2 type II, 1 type IIIA	1 (6%): type IIIA
Radial head	2 (12%): 1 comminuted, 1 marginal fx	1 (7%)	2: 1 comminuted, 1 marginal fx	1 (10%)	13 (81%)
Coronoid	8 (47%)	5 (36%)	4	5 (50%)	16 (100%)
LCL	—	—	—	—	2 (20%)
Nerve injury	0	0	0	1 ulnar nerve palsy	—
Other injuries	7 segmental ulna fx	—	—	—	1 shoulder dislocation with brachial plexus palsy 2 distal radius fx

Method of fixation	2 tension band wire construct (simple pattern) 5 3.5 mm LC-DCP 4 3.5 mm DCP 2 3.5 mm recon plate 2 1/3 tubular plate 2 semitubular plate	7 tension band 2 3.5 mm 1/3 tubular plate 1 3.5 mm DCP 4 3.5 mm recon plate	1 tension band wiring 7 3.5 mm recon plate	2 tension band wiring 5 3.5 mm LC-DCP 1 3.5 mm DCP 1 stacked 1/3 tubular plate or tension band wiring	1 tension band wiring 11 3.5 mm LC-DCP 2 3.5 mm DCP 1 3.5 mm recon plate
F/E ROM	113 (14–127)	103 (22–125)	93 (22–115)	110 (20–130)	95 (30–125)
P/S ROM	Normal in all but 4	144 (68 pro, 76 sup)	158 (75 pro, 83 sup)	155 (80 pro, 75 sup)	115 (60 pro, 55sup)
Broberg-Morrey	Excellent 7 (41%) Good 8 (47%) Fair 2 (12%) Poor 0 (0%)	Excellent 4 (29%) Good 6 (43%) Fair 2 (14%) Poor 2 (14%)	Excellent 2 (25%) Good 5 (62.5%) Fair 1 (12.5%)	Excellent 4 (40%) Good 5 (50%) Fair 0 Poor 1 (10%)	Excellent 5 (31%) Good 7 (44%) Fair 1 (6%) Poor 3 (19%)
ASES score	—	—	89 (69–100)	89 (52–100)	78 (28.5–100)
DASH score	—	—	—	—	—
Reoperation	2 (12%) 1/3 tubular plates had loss of fixation	3 (21%) failed tension band wiring (43% of tension band constructs)	4: 1 (12.5%) failed tension band, 3 elective hardware removal	5 (50%): 1 failed tension band, 3 capsular release, 1 ulna nonunion	—
Arthrosis	2 (12%)	4 (29%)	0 (0%)	2 (20%)	9 (56%)
Heterotopic ossification or synostosis	1 (6%)	4 (29%) heterotopic ossification	1 (12.5%) heterotopic ossification	1 (10%) heterotopic ossification	4 (25%) synostosis

Abbreviations: DCP, dynamic compression plate; fx, fracture; LC-DCP, limited-contact dynamic compression plate; MVA, motor vehicle accident; pro, pronation; sup, supination.
Data from Refs.[32,33,35,36]

Table 2
Outcomes of adult monteggia fractures

	Anterior Monteggia			Posterior Monteggia	
Publication	Guitton et al,[10] JHS 2009	Ring et al,[9] JBJS 1998	Konrad et al,[11] JBJS Br 2007	Ring et al,[9] JBJS 1998	Konrad et al,[11] JBJS Br 2007
Subjects	11	7	15	38	37
Average follow-up	20 y (7–34)	6.5 (2–14) entire study	10 y (6–14)	6.5 (2–14) entire study	8 (5–11)
Average age	36 (14–50)	26 (18–41)	40 (22–70)	58 (27–88)	43 (21–72)
Gender	6 male, 5 female	5 male, 2 female	9 male, 6 female	15 male, 23 female	18 male, 9 female
Ground-level fall	—	—	—	—	—
High-energy fall	—	—	—	—	—
MVA	—	—	—	—	—
Other	—	7 (100%) high-energy fall	—	9 (24%) high-energy fall 29 (76%) low-energy fall	—
Open fx	—	4 (57%): 2 type IIIA, 2 type IIIC	2	3 (8%): 2 type I, 1 type IIIA	4
Radial head	0	1 nondisplaced	1	26 (68%): 7 type II, 19 type III	11
Coronoid	0	0	0	10 (26%)	11
LCL	—	—	—	—	—
Nerve injury	—	3: 1 radial, 1 ulnar, 1 median-ulnar	—	0 (0%)	—
Other injuries	1 distal humerus fx 1 medial epicondyle fx	3 floating elbow 3 compartment syndrome	—	3 distal radius fx 1 floating elbow 1 proximal humerus fx 1 shoulder dislocation	—

Method of fixation	10 3.5 mm DCP 1 external fixation	7 3.5 mm DCP	15 3.5 mm DCP or LC-DCP	3 tension band wiring 1 Steinmann pin 17 3.5 mm DCP 10 3.5 mm LC-DCP 2 3.5 mm recon plate 4 semitubular plate	11 tension band wiring 26 3.5 mm DCP or LC-DCP
F/E ROM	140 (0–140)	115 (80–140)	121 (90–130)	112 (65–140)	103 (50–130)
P/S ROM	160 (90–180)	135 (40–16)	144 (115–180)	126 (0–160)	128 (100–180)
Broberg-Morrey	Excellent 8 (73%) Good 2 (18%) Fair 1 (9%)	Excellent 3 (43%) Good 3 (43%) Fair 0 Poor 1 (14%)	Excellent 11 (73%) Good 3 (20%) Fair 1 (7%) Poor 0 (0%)	Excellent 14 (37%) Good 18 (47%) Fair 1 (3%) Poor 5 (13%)	Excellent 8 (30%) Good 9 (33%) Fair 6 (22%) Poor 4 (15%)
ASES score	—	—	—	—	—
DASH score	7 (0–34)	—	9 (0–31)	—	22 (0–70)
Reoperation	7: 2 (18%) nonunion, 5 elective hardware removal	0	12 subjects of entire study group (26%): 6 nonunion, 2 infection, 2 radial head loss of fixation, 2 synostosis	9 (24%): 6 (16%) loss of fixation, 3 (8%) for secondary radial head resection	12 subjects of entire study group (26%): 6 nonunion, 2 infection, 2 radial head loss of fixation, 2 synostosis
Arthrosis	3 (27%)	0	—	3 (8%)	—
Heterotopic ossification or synostosis	—	—	1 (7%) heterotopic ossification	2 (5%) synostosis	5 (14%) heterotopic ossification 2 (5%) synostosis

Abbreviations: DCP, dynamic compression plate; LC-DCP, limited-contact dynamic compression plate; MVA, motor vehicle accident; pro, pronation; sup, supination.
Data from Refs.[9-11]

involvement is common, coronoid fractures are frequently larger fragments that allow for stable reconstruction of the trochlear notch and restoration of ulnohumeral stability. Consequently, although flexion-extension motion may be affected, these injuries tend to cause less impairment of forearm rotation. Ring and colleagues[32] reported on a series of seventeen anterior transolecranon fracture dislocations treated with tension band wiring for simple fracture patterns and tubular/semitubular plates or 3.5 mm plates for more comminuted fractures. Failure of fixation was seen when tubular/semitubular plates were used to stabilize comminuted fractures. No ulnohumeral instability was observed after stable fixation of the fracture fragments. With an average follow-up period of 25 months, posttraumatic arthrosis was only observed in 12% of subjects. Although tension-band wiring was used with success in this subject series, other investigators have observed up to 50% failure rates of the tension band wiring constructs when used for these injuries.[33,35,36] The reported rates of posttraumatic arthrosis vary between 0% and 29% and may be due to differences in methods of grading joint arthrosis or length of follow-up.[32,33,35,36]

The posterior olecranon fracture dislocation is often considered as a subset of the posterior Monteggia fracture[33,34] and results of these injuries are often reported in conjunction with posterior Monteggia fractures.[9] In one study evaluating either anterior or posterior olecranon fracture dislocations, 62% were the posterior type and concomitant radial head and coronoid involvement was high.[33] Subjects with posterior olecranon fracture dislocation exhibited more limitations in flexion-extension as well as forearm rotation than subjects with anterior transolecranon fracture dislocation. Rates of radiographic arthrosis as well as radioulnar synostosis were also higher in these subjects, which contributed to worse outcomes.

The reported outcomes of anterior Monteggia fractures are generally more favorable than the posterior Monteggia fracture, which may be attributable to the lower incidence of radial head fracture and the lack of involvement of the coronoid process[9-11] (Table 2). Ring and colleagues[9] reported on a series of 7 anterior Monteggia fractures as part of a larger overall study of Monteggia fractures in adults and found a significantly lower need for reoperation in the anterior Monteggia fracture pattern. A later study from the same institution reported on eleven subjects with anterior Monteggia fracture at an average 20-year follow-up and found that subjects continued to improve their range of motion even after 1-year from surgery.[10] Similarly, the overall outcomes

according to the Broberg and Morrey elbow scale improved between early and late follow-up. Joint arthrosis was observed in 3 (27%) subjects although 2 of these subjects either had concomitant distal humerus fracture or long-standing ulnar nonunion. Konrad and colleagues[11] reported long-term outcomes on a group of adult subjects with Monteggia fracture and also found significantly improved outcomes according to Broberg and Morrey elbow scale and DASH questionnaire in anterior Monteggia as opposed to posterior Monteggia injuries.

SUMMARY

Monteggia fractures and olecranon fracture dislocations represent complex injuries with distinct patterns of bony and soft tissue involvement. Fractures of the proximal ulna and olecranon process may lead to disruption of the proximal radioulnar joint and/or ulnohumeral joint. The keys to treatment are recognition of the pattern of injury and formation of an algorithmic surgical plan to address all components of the injury process. Diaphyseal ulnar fractures require anatomic alignment and stable fixation of the ulnar shaft for restoration of proximal radioulnar joint stability. More proximal fractures extending into the coronoid and olecranon process require anatomic stable reconstruction of the trochlear notch with posteriorly placed and contoured plate and screws. When managing concomitant radial head fractures, open reduction and internal fixation or radial head arthroplasty may be preferable to radial head excision due to the relative contribution of an intact radiocapitellar joint to overall elbow and forearm stability. Lateral ulnar collateral ligament injuries may need to be repaired if ulnohumeral instability persists. In order to optimize outcomes, anatomic stable fixation must be achieved, which allows for earlier initiation of joint mobilization. Complications are common and may be related to the injury spectrum itself and/or inadequate fracture alignment/fixation.

REFERENCES

1. Wilkins KE, Morrey BF, Jobe FW, et al. The elbow. Instr Course Lect 1991;40:1–87.
2. Bado JL. The Monteggia lesion. Clin Orthop Relat Res 1967;50:71–86.
3. Watson-Jones R. Fractures and joint injuries. 3rd edition. Baltimore (MD): Williams and Wilkins; 1943. p. 520–35.
4. Speed JS, Boyd HB. Treatment of fractures of the ulna with dislocation of the head of the radius

(Monteggia fracture). J Am Med Assn 1940;115: 1699–705.

5. Bruce HE, Harvey JP Jr, Wilson JC Jr. Monteggia fractures. J Bone Joint Surg 1974;56-A:1563–76.

6. Pavel A, Pitman JM, Lance EM, et al. The posterior Monteggia fracture. A clinical study. J Trauma 1965;5:185–99.

7. Penrose JH. The Monteggia fracture with posterior dislocation of the radial head. J Bone Joint Surg Br 1951;33:65–73.

8. Jupiter JB, Leibovic SJ, Ribbans W, et al. The posterior Monteggia lesion. J Orthop Trauma 1991;5(4): 395–402.

9. Ring D, Jupiter JB, Simpson NS. Monteggia fractures in adults. J Bone Joint Surg Am 1998;80(12): 1733–44.

10. Guitton TG, Ring D, Kloen P. Long-term evaluation of surgically treated anterior Monteggia fractures in skeletally mature patients. J Hand Surg Am 2009; 34(9):1618–24.

11. Konrad GG, Kundel K, Kreuz PC, et al. Monteggia fractures in adults: long-term results and prognostic factors. J Bone Joint Surg Br 2007;89(3):354–60.

12. Tashijian RZ, Katarinic JA. Complex elbow instability. J Am Acad Orthop Surg 2006;14(5):278–86.

13. Regan W, Morrey B. Fractures of the coronoid process of the ulna. J Bone Joint Surg Am 1989;71(9): 1348–54.

14. Adams JE, Sanchez-Sotelo J, Kallina CF 4th, et al. Fractures of the coronoid: morphology based upon computed tomography scanning. J Shoulder Elbow Surg 2012;21(6):782–8.

15. O'Driscoll SW, Jupiter JB, Cohen MS, et al. Difficult elbow fractures: pearls and pitfalls. Instr Course Lect 2003;52:113–34.

16. Doornberg JN, Ring D. Coronoid fracture patterns. J Hand Surg Am 2006;31(1):45–52.

17. Regan WD, Korinek SL, Morrey BF, et al. Biomechanical study of ligaments around the elbow joint. Clin Orthop Relat Res 1991;271:170–9.

18. Beingessner DM, Dunning CE, Gordon KD, et al. The effect of radial head fracture size on elbow kinematics and stability. J Orthop Res 2005;23(1): 210–7.

19. Mason ML. Some observations on fractures of the head of the radius with a review of one hundred cases. Br J Surg 1954;42:123–32.

20. Broberg MA, Morrey BF. Results of treatment of fracture-dislocations of the elbow. Clin Orthop Relat Res 1987;216:109–19.

21. Hotchkiss RN. Displaced fractures of the radial head: internal fixation or excision? J Am Acad Orthop Surg 1997;5(1):1–10.

22. King GJ, Morrey BF, An KN. Stabilizers of the elbow. J Shoulder Elbow Surg 1993;2(3):165–74.

23. Beingessner DM, Dunning CE, Gordon KD, et al. The effect of radial head excision on elbow kinematics and stability. J Bone Joint Surg Am 2004;86-A(8):1730–9.

24. Johnson JA, Beingessner DM, Gordon KD, et al. Kinematics and stability of the fractured and implant-reconstructed radial head. J Shoulder Elbow Surg 2005;14(1 Suppl S):195S–201S.

25. Closkey RF, Goode JR, Kirschenbaum D, et al. The role of the coronoid process in elbow stability. A biomechanical analysis of axial loading. J Bone Joint Surg Am 2000;82-A(12):1749–53.

26. Deutch SR, Jensen SL, Tyrdal S, et al. Elbow joint stability following experimental osteoligamentous injury and reconstruction. J Shoulder Elbow Surg 2003;12(5):466–71.

27. Schneeberger AG, Sadowski MM, Jacob HA. Coronoid process and radial head as posterolateral rotatory stabilizers of the elbow. J Bone Joint Surg Am 2004;86-A(5):975–82.

28. Hull JR, Owen JR, Fern SE, et al. Role of the coronoid process in varus osteoarticular stability of the elbow. J Shoulder Elbow Surg 2005;14(4):441–6.

29. Jeon IH, Sanchez-Sotelo J, Zhao K, et al. The contribution of the coronoid and radial head to the stability of the elbow. J Bone Joint Surg Br 2012;94(1):86–92.

30. Ring D. Monteggia fractures. Orthop Clin North Am 2013;44(1):59–66.

31. Biga N, Thomine JM. La luxation trans-olecranienne du coude. Rev Chir Orthop 1974;60:557–67.

32. Ring D, Jupiter JB, Sanders RW, et al. Transolecranon fracture-dislocation of the elbow. J Orthop Trauma 1997;11(8):545–50.

33. Doornberg J, Ring D, Jupiter JB. Effective treatment of fracture-dislocations of the olecranon requires a stable trochlear notch. Clin Orthop Relat Res 2004; 429:292–300.

34. Ring D, Jupiter JB. Fracture-dislocation of the elbow. J Bone Joint Surg Am 1998;80(4):566–80.

35. Moushine E, Akiki A, Castagna A, et al. Transolecranon anterior fracture dislocation. J Shoulder Elbow Surg 2007;16(3):352–7.

36. Mortazavi SM, Asadollahi S, Tahririan MA. Functional outcome following treatment of transolecranon fracture-dislocation of the elbow. Injury 2006;37(3): 284–8.

37. Ring D, Tavakolian J, Kloen P, et al. Loss of alignment after surgical treatment of posterior Monteggia fractures: salvage with dorsal contoured plating. J Hand Surg Am 2004;29(4):694–702.

38. Athwal GS, Ramsey ML, Steinmann SP, et al. Fractures and dislocations of the elbow: a return to the basics. Instr Course Lect 2011;60:199–214.

39. Beingessner DM, Nork SE, Agel J, et al. A fragment-specific approach to Type IID Monteggia elbow fracture-dislocations. J Orthop Trauma 2011;25(7):414–9.

40. Lanting BA, Ferreira LM, Johnson JA, et al. The effect of excision of the radial head and metallic radial

head replacement on the tension in the interosseous membrane. Bone Joint J 2013;95-B(10):1383–7.

41. Harrington IJ, Sekyi-Out A, Barrington TW, et al. The functional outcome with metallic radial head implants in the treatment of unstable elbow fractures: a long-term review. J Trauma 2001;50(1):46–52.

42. Ring D, Hannouche D, Jupiter JB. Surgical treatment of persistent dislocation or subluxation of the ulnohumeral joint after fracture-dislocation of the elbow. J Hand Surg Am 2004;29(3):470–80.

43. Ring D, Guss D, Jupiter JB. Reconstruction of the coronoid process using a fragment of discarded radial head. J Hand Surg Am 2012;37(3):570–4.

44. Broberg MA, Morrey BF. Results of delayed excision of the radial head after fracture. J Bone Joint Surg Am 1986;68A:669–74.

45. Jester A, Harth A, Germann G. Measuring levels of upper-extremity disability in employed adults using the DASH Questionnaire. J Hand Surg 2005;30A: 1074.e1–10.

Olecranon Fractures

Tyler J. Brolin, MD, Thomas Throckmorton, MD*

KEYWORDS

- Olecranon fracture • Review • Outcomes • Locking plate • Tension band • Intramedullary nail

KEY POINTS

- A majority of olecranon fractures occur from a low-energy mechanism, such as a fall from standing height in a middle-aged patient, and result in a displaced yet noncomminuted fracture.
- Goals of olecranon fracture fixation are to restore joint stability, articular congruity, and the triceps extensor mechanism with stable fixation to allow for early range of motion.
- Tension band wiring (TBW) acts essentially only as a static compression device and not a dynamic compression device. Recent trends have seen an increased use of locking plate and intramedullary nail fixation.
- A majority of olecranon fractures heal uneventfully with good/excellent results with a small loss of motion to be expected. Due to the subcutaneous nature of the olecranon hardware, irritation continues to be a potential postoperative issue.

INTRODUCTION

Olecranon fractures are common upper extremity injuries that are usually the result of a direct blow onto the elbow after a fall from standing height. Less commonly they result from an indirect tension injury from the triceps attachment. Although a majority are treated surgically, there still is some debate regarding the optimal surgical fixation technique. This has led to a shift from TBW to locking plate fixation and, more recently, intramedullary fixation. Although most patients can expect a good outcome, there are some well-known complications, including loss of motion, hardware irritation, and wound healing problems. This article reviews the available evidence and current understanding of olecranon fractures.

ANATOMY

The elbow is a trochoid joint with various contributions to stability from osseous and soft tissue structures. The olecranon and coronoid processes compose the greater sigmoid notch and are separated by an area of the articular surface devoid of hyaline cartilage, commonly referred to as the "bare spot." More recently there has been better understanding of the unique anatomy of the proximal ulna. The sagittal anatomy of proximal ulna is variable but 96% of patients have dorsal angulation, known as the proximal ulnar dorsal angulation, which averages 5.7°.[1–3] The proximal ulna also has on average 14° of varus angulation.[4] This is important because it pertains to implant selection, especially with precontoured locking plates.[4]

EPIDEMIOLOGY

Olecranon fractures represent approximately 10% of all upper extremity fractures. From retrospective data collected through a trauma database in Edinburgh, Scotland, fractures of the olecranon

Disclosures: None (Dr T.J. Brolin). Consultant – Biomet, Zimmer; Speakers bureau – Biomet; Research support – Biomet; Royalties – Saunders/Mosby-Elsevier; Editorial Board – *Instructional Course Lectures*, *Techniques in Shoulder & Elbow Surgery*, *Journal of Orthopaedic Trauma*, and *American Journal of Orthopaedics*; Board/Committee appointments – AAOS and MAOA; Stock – Gilead (Dr T. Throckmorton).
Department of Orthopaedic Surgery & Biomedical Engineering, University of Tennessee-Campbell Clinic, 1211 Union Avenue, Suite 510, Memphis, TN 38104, USA
* Corresponding author.
E-mail address: tthrockmorton@campbellclinic.com

Hand Clin 31 (2015) 581–590
http://dx.doi.org/10.1016/j.hcl.2015.07.003
0749-0712/15/$ – see front matter © 2015 Elsevier Inc. All rights reserved.

accounted from 0.9% of all fractures and 18% of all proximal forearm fractures and have an overall incidence of 12 per 100,000 people. By far the most common mechanism was a fall from standing height, representing 70% of all olecranon fractures. Less commonly, high-energy mechanisms, such as those resulting from sporting event or motor vehicle accidents, result in direct trauma whereas an indirect avulsion fracture can result due to the triceps attachment; 22% of all olecranon fractures resulted in an associated ipsilateral upper extremity injury, with fractures of the radial head and neck the most common. The mean age of all olecranon fractures was 50 years for men and 63 years for women.

The most common fracture seen was a simple, displaced fracture representing 73.5% of all such injuries.[5]

CLASSIFICATION

Three main classification schemes exist for olecranon fractures. The Mayo classification was described by Morrey[6] and is based on several factors, including displacement, comminution, and elbow stability. Type I is nondisplaced, type II is displaced but the elbow is stable, and type III is displaced with elbow instability. Groups are further subclassified into groups A and B based on the presence of comminution[6] (**Fig. 1**).

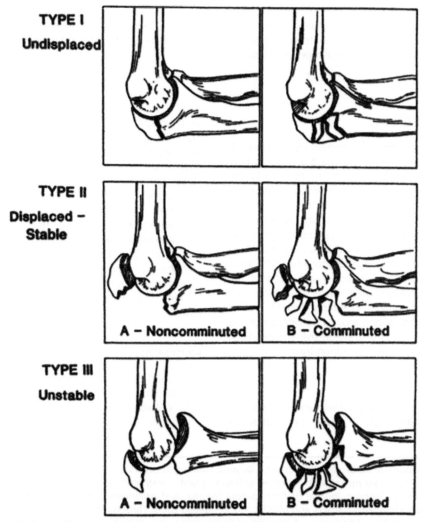

Fig. 1. Mayo classification of olecranon fractures as described by Morrey. Type I fractures are nondisplaced, type II fractures are displaced, and type III fractures represent elbow instability. Fractures are further subclassified into types A and B, indicating the presence or absence of comminution. (*Modified from* Cabanela ME, Morrey BF. Fractures of the olecranon. In: Morrey BF, editor. The elbow and its disorders. 3rd edition. Philadelphia: WB Saunders; 2000. p. 400; with permission.)

The Schatzker classification delineates olecranon fractures into 6 groups based on fracture orientation, articular surface impaction, comminution, and associated injuries[7] (**Fig. 2**).

The AO classification is usually reserved for research purposes and gives the proximal forearm the designation of 21. From there each fracture is classified into A for exta-articular, B if 1 bone has an intra-articular fracture, and C if both bones have intra-articular fractures. These are further subclassified depending whether both bones are involved and on degree of comminution.

NONOPERATIVE TREATMENT

The first decision in the treatment algorithm is nonoperative versus operative treatment. Because olecranon fractures not only are articular injuries but also are essential for the extensor mechanism through the attached triceps, typically only truly nondisplaced fractures are considered nonoperative. Furthermore, to avoid late fracture displacement and prolonged immobilization, patients may reasonably elect for surgical stabilization even in those situations.

Recent evidence by Duckworth and colleagues,[8] however, has suggested reasonable outcomes after nonoperative treatment in low-demand elderly patients. All were Mayo type II fractures with a mean age of 78 years. In short-term follow-up, 72% had excellent results even with 78% of these patients going on to nonunion. Long-term results showed 91% of patients were satisfied; however, 17% had weakness or an inability to push themselves up from a chair. Nevertheless, most authorities reserve nonoperative treatment to extremely low-demand or infirm patients, those with soft tissues that preclude surgical management, and those with significant medical contraindications to surgery.

OPERATIVE TREATMENT

The goals of operative treatment include restoration of joint stability, articular congruity, and the extensor mechanism with stable fixation to allow early pain-free range of motion. These can be accomplished with various techniques, including TBW, standard plate fixation, locked plate fixation, intramedullary fixation, and fragment excision with triceps advancement.

Preoperative planning consists of fracture characterization and thorough inspection of the posterior soft tissue envelope. The presence and location of comminution are key to understanding the fracture morphology and appropriate treatment. A recent study found that 52 of 80 patients had an intermediate fragment present and the investigators recommended CT for routine evaluation[9] (**Fig. 3**). The authors rely on plain radiographs alone for most fracture patterns but obtain a CT scan if there is a high suspicion for unrecognized articular impaction or comminution.[10]

There has been a shift recently in treatment from TBW to plate fixation. TBW is based on the premise that distraction forces at the outer cortex are converted to compressive forces at the articular surface. This dynamic compression mechanism has been called into question by studies showing there is negligible compression of the articular surface during active extension with a maximum occurring at 75° of flexion. This also was significantly less compression compared with compression plating techniques.[11,12] Using an

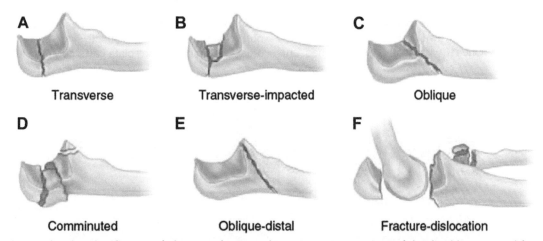

A	B	C
Transverse	Transverse-impacted	Oblique
D	E	F
Comminuted	Oblique-distal	Fracture-dislocation

Fig. 2. Schatzker classification of olecranon fractures. (*From* Perez EA. Fractures of the shoulder, arm, and forearm. In: Canale ST, Beaty JH, editors. Campbell's operative orthopaedics. 12th edition. Philadelphia: Mosby Elsevier; 2013. Fig. 57–70. p. 2879; with permission.)

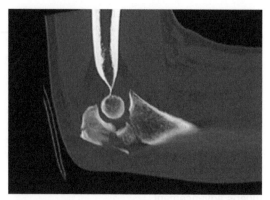

Fig. 3. Sagittal reconstruction view of CT scan demonstrating an intermediate fragment. It is important to recognize and reduce such fragments to obtain articular congruence.

intramedullary screw with associated TBW is another option that has been found to have significantly less gap formation compared with Kirschner (K)-wires.[13]

An ideal indication for traditional TBW is a simple transverse fracture with no comminution. The patient is positioned according to surgeon preference, either supine or lateral decubitus. A standard posterior approach that curves laterally around the olecranon tip is made with attention to soft tissue handling. Dissection is carried to bone to facilitate hardware insertion and joint visualization through medial and lateral windows.

Two smooth K-wires are inserted taking care to engage the second cortex and travel through the subchondral bone. These 2 steps have been shown to lessen wire instability and failure with the possibility of decreasing wound irritation and development of osteoarthrosis.[14,15] Anterior cortical perforation of the ulna has been found safe with the median nerve and ulnar artery found greater than 10 mm away from the proposed perforation ite.[16] Once K-wire insertion is performed, an

18-gauge wire is passed in a figure-of-eight pattern through a predrilled hole in the dorsal cortex of the ulna distal to fracture line. Small longitudinal incisions are made in the triceps to bury the K-wire and the tension band construct is tensioned in unison and excess wire cut and buried (**Fig. 4**).

Precontoured locking plate fixation has also emerged in the treatment of olecranon fractures (**Fig. 5**). It allows for significantly more compression at fracture site than does TBW as well as the ability to manage more complex and comminuted fracture patterns.[12] The approach to the olecranon is the same as TBW and again a longitudinal split can be made in the triceps to help decrease plate prominence. As fracture complexity increases, the surgeon must be aware of the normal proximal ulna anatomy (described previously). A radiograph of the contralateral elbow may serve as a control or template. Even with the advent of "anatomic" precontoured proximal ulna plates, there are many times when there is a need for recontouring to prevent malreduction. Surgeons must also be aware of the significant variability within plate manufacturers.[4]

A couple of specific considerations must be taken into account with these complex fractures. The first is to recognize the presence of an intermediate fragment and articular impaction. A Freer elevator can disengage the impacted fragment from either the lateral or medial window. Also, a K-wire can be inserted into the dorsal cortex just opposite of the impaction. The K-wire can be removed and the blunt side reinserted into the previously made hole and used as a tamp to gently elevate the impacted articular fragment. The home run screw can then aid in stabilization if it is placed in the subchondral bone to support the impacted fragment (**Fig. 6**).

The second consideration is to be aware of the width of the greater sigmoid notch and take care not to over-compress, and effectively narrow, the articular surface. A small plate can nicely augment

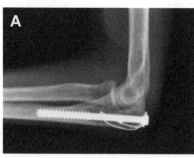
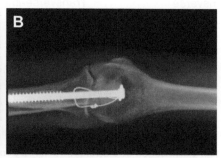

Fig. 4. Anteroposterior (A) and lateral (B) radiographs showing a TBW construct using an intramedullary screw for fixation.

A B

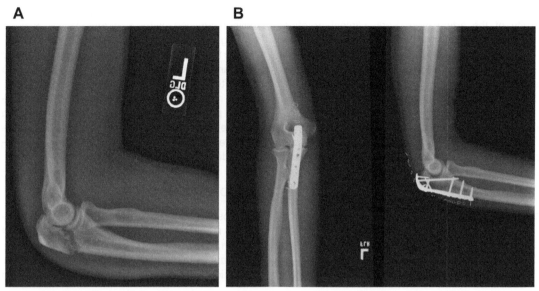

Fig. 5. (A) Preoperative radiograph of a short oblique olecranon fracture. (B) Final anteroposterior and lateral views showing good reduction and stable fixation.

fixation when the medial or lateral cortical surface is comminuted. With a small proximal fragment, it is strongly encouraged to aim a retrograde screw to add additional fixation. A recent study examined 5 different plates and all ultimately had catastrophic failure when the proximal segment pulled away from the implant in an osteoporotic model. The average force to failure was 4.4 kg, which is less than the 6.6 kg the investigators proposed would be the force of a patient rising from a chair. There was no difference between locking, non-locking, stainless steel, and titanium devices.[17] To help protect fracture fixation, augmentation with suture into the triceps has been described. This involves placing a no. 2 FiberWire-type suture in a running-locking pattern within the triceps and

securing this to the plate through suture holes. In a biomechanical cadaver model, plate fixation with suture augmentation significantly increased the strength of repair with ultimate strength greater than 200 N above the 500 N it takes to rise from a chair.[18] Appropriate tension was described as advancing the triceps distally 5 mm, and furthermore, the investigators were confident in starting motion 10 to 14 days after fixation.[19]

Unfortunately, there are situations where significant comminution precludes anatomic fixation and a technique has been described that involves excision of the intercalary fragments with advancement of the proximal segment using fixation with 2 lag screws.[20] A rongeur can be used to contour the fracture surface and use the distal

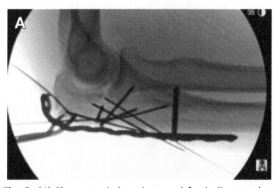 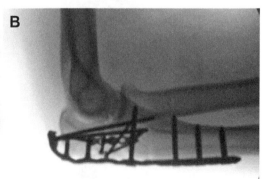

Fig. 6. (A) Fluoroscopic imaging used for indirect reduction of the intermediate fragment. A K-wire is inserted into the dorsal cortex and then withdrawn. The blunt end is then replaced and used as a tamp to elevate the intermediate fragment. (B) Final construct with subchondral screws supporting the intermediate fragment. Because of extensive comminution, a separate medial plate was used.

humeral articular surface as a guide for the congruity of the articulation. Early clinical practice accepted excision of as much as 80% of the olecranon; however, more recently this has been challenged.[21,22] A recent biomechanical model has shown that removal of as little as 12.5% of the olecranon alters joint stability.[23]

When excision is the only option in highly comminuted fractures or in instances of failed fixation, the triceps must be advanced. Previous reports have recommended anterior attachment; this has been contradicted recently with posterior attachment leading to increased strength of the triceps mechanism, albeit decreased strength compared with the contralateral extremity[24] (**Fig. 7**).

Multiplanar locked intramedullary nailing is another option and may be beneficial in certain clinical situations, such as elderly patients who rely on a walker or polytrauma patients[25] (**Fig. 8**).

A biomechanical study showed intramedullary nailing survived with a higher failure weight, 14.4 kg versus 8.7 kg, and a higher number of cycles to failure. Another cadaveric study compared TBW and intramedullary nail fixation and showed that after 300 cycles the TBW group had significantly more displacement.[26] These studies have shown promise but cost remains a concern, which may be offset if the number of symptomatic hardware removals is significantly decreased with intramedullary fixation.[25,27]

POSTOPERATIVE COURSE

The postoperative course depends on several variables, including soft tissue status, the stability of fixation, and the type of implant used. In most circumstances the elbow is immobilized in 30° to 45° of flexion with an anterior slab splint for 7 to

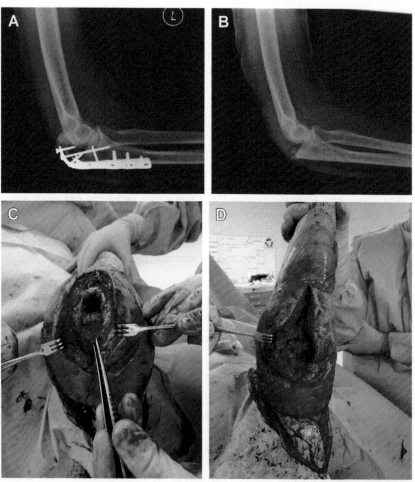

Fig. 7. (*A*) Failed attempt at fixation of a small olecranon tip fragment. (*B*) After excision of the olecranon tip with triceps advancement. (*C, D*) Intraoperative photographs show triceps advancement to the remaining olecranon segment after excision of the olecranon tip.

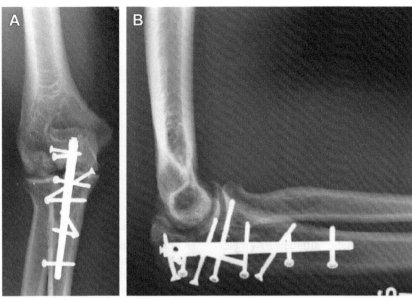

Fig. 8. Anteroposterior (*A*) and lateral (*B*) radiographs of a comminuted olecranon fracture with intramedullary nail fixation.

10 days to allow for soft tissue healing and to unload the triceps. With stable fixation and adequate soft tissues, this immobilization can be shortened and range of motion begun almost immediately. Active range-of-motion exercises can be initiated after splint removal with strengthening delayed until osseous healing has occurred.

OUTCOMES

Outcomes after olecranon fracture fixation are generally predictable with the majority achieving good or excellent results. A study out of Sweden examined 73 patients with 15- to 25-year follow-up and showed that 96% achieved good/excellent results.[28] Only 12% of patients had occasional pain and 4% had daily pain. Radiographic analysis showed 6% with osteoarthritic changes and 50% had degenerative changes compared with 0% and 11% in the contralateral extremity, respectively. Patients lost on average of 3° of flexion and 4° of extension. Radiographic arthrosis is common after elbow trauma but is relatively rare after olecranon fractures. At an average of 19.5 years after a traumatic elbow injury, only 5 of 54 patients with olecranon fractures developed moderate to severe arthrosis, which did not always correlate with function.[29]

Even though outcomes have been historically good, these are articular injuries requiring anatomic reduction and restoration of the dimension and contour of the sigmoid notch. A retrospective review of 58 patients found that suboptimal fixation and fracture pattern correlated with arthrosis.[30] Looking specifically at plate fixation, multiple studies have shown good to excellent outcomes. One study found 22 of 25 patients achieved good to excellent Mayo Elbow Performance Index scores and satisfaction was 9.7 out of 10.[31] Another retrospective review of 18 patients treated with locking plate fixation for comminuted olecranon fractures found 12 of 18 patients had very good to good results and all achieved union at an average of 4.4 months with an average flexion/extension arc of 116°.[32] There are few head-to-head comparisons of fixation; however, locked compression plating (LCP) outperformed TBW in 1 study, with 92% of LCP and 77% of TBW having good/excellent results. The plating group had increased operating room time and cost but less hardware irritation. There was no difference in motion of Disabilities of the Arm, Shoulder and Hand score.[33]

Olecranon fractures treated with multiplanar locked intramedullary nail fixation have shared similar results in the literature. In a series from Germany, 68 of 73 patients had good to excellent results with a combination of simple and comminuted olecranon fractures.[34] After 1 year of follow-up, 28 patients treated with intramedullary nails showed range of motion within 10° of contralateral elbow with no pain and full return to activities.[27]

COMPLICATIONS

The most commonly seen complications after olecranon fractures include loss of motion, malunion, nonunion, symptomatic hardware, wound

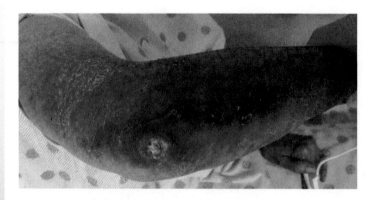

Fig. 9. Wound dehiscence with an exposed olecranon plate. This is a common complication after fixation of high-energy olecranon fractures.

dehiscence, heterotopic ossification, ulnar neuritis, and posttraumatic arthrosis. A minor loss of terminal flexion and extension is expected after olecranon fracture fixation and patients should be counseled appropriately. The average arc of motion ranged from near normal in some studies to 111° in others.[27,32,35]

Symptomatic hardware is a common complication due to the subcutaneous nature of the olecranon process. The rates of hardware removal vary in the literature and according to fixation technique. Up to 75% of TBW constructs are symptomatic.[36] Plate fixation also has a significant rate of symptomatic hardware, with some reports exceeding 50%.[10,21,32,37] In a matched cohort study, Amini and colleagues (Amini MH, et al, unpublished data, 2015) found TBW to have more hardware-related symptoms than plate fixation, which trended toward significance. Multiple studies have shown an increase in flexion arc after removal of hardware, including both TBW and LCP.[37] It also seems that intramedullary nail fixation may decrease the rate of these symptoms with no painful hardware reported in 1 study.[27]

Ulnar neuritis occurs in up to 12% of olecranon fractures and up to 25% of fracture/dislocations. Usually observation is sufficient. One case series, however, examined ulnar nerve palsy after surgical treatment of olecranon fractures and found medial fracture displacement can lead to ulnar nerve compression within the cubital tunnel. With careful attention to the anteroposterior radiograph, this medical displacement can be seen and addressed.[38]

Heterotopic ossification (HO) is common after elbow trauma but is less prevalent with olecranon fractures. In fractures of the proximal ulna and radius, there is a 7% to 37% risk of heterotopic ossification, with 20% reaching clinical significance. Heterotopic bone formation is more often associated with transolecranon fracture/dislocations, distal humerus fractures, and terrible

triad injuries.[39,40] There is some debate regarding HO prophylaxis, but the role of radiation therapy has been curtailed. Patients receiving prophylaxis with 1 dose of 700 mCGy (microgray - absorbed radiation dose of ionizing radiation, usually written μGy) had a nonunion rate of 38% compared with 4% in the control group in a randomized controlled study of elbow fractures.[41]

Nonunions are rare after olecranon fracture fixation and approach 1%. These are seen more frequently with higher-energy injuries.[42,43] Careful attention to all fracture fragments and the proximal ulnar geometry can guard against both intraarticular and extra-articular malunions. Special consideration must be given to the so-called intermediate fragment, both to recognize it and then reduce anatomically. Intra-articular malunions can lead to rapid joint destruction and posttraumatic arthritis. Prudent rehabilitation must be carried out with tenuous fixation constructs to guard against fixation failure.

Wound healing problems are typically seen in patients with higher-energy injury mechanisms (**Fig. 9**). Such elbows warrant vigilant and meticulous handling of the soft tissues to avoid dehiscence and infection. Specifically, suture techniques with no tension on the soft tissues and judicious anterior splint immobilization are helpful.

SUMMARY

Olecranon fractures are common fractures of the upper extremity and most frequently result from a fall from standing height. Most fractures are displaced and require surgical fixation. Although TBW may be indicated for simple transverse fractures, there has been a shift toward locked plating and intramedullary nail fixation. With the evidence currently available, both locking plate fixation and intramedullary nail fixation provide greater construct stability and less symptomatic hardware with similar clinical outcomes. Good to excellent outcomes can be expected in a majority of patients, with the most common complications symptomatic hardware, loss of motion, ulnar neuritis, and posttraumatic arthrosis.

REFERENCES

1. Rouleau DM, Faber KJ, Athwal GS. The proximal ulnar dorsal angulation: a radiographic study. J Shoulder Elbow Surg 2010;19:26–30.
2. Rouleau DM, Canet F, Chapleau J, et al. The influence of proximal ulnar morphology on elbow range of motion. J Shoulder Elbow Surg 2012; 21:384–8.
3. Beser CG, Demiryürek D, Ozsoy H, et al. Redefining the proximal ulna anatomy. Surg Radiol Anat 2014; 36:1023–31.
4. Puchwein P, Schildhauer TA, Schöffman S, et al. Three-dimensional morphometry of the proximal ulna: a comparison to currently used anatomically preshaped ulna plates. J Shoulder Elbow Surg 2012;21:1018–23.
5. Duckworth AD, Clement ND, Aitken SA, et al. The epidemiology of fractures of the proximal ulna. Injury 2012;43:343–6.
6. Morrey BF. Current concepts in the treatment of fractures of the radial head, the olecranon, and the coronoid. Instr Course Lect 1995;44:175–85.
7. Hak DJ, Golladay GJ. Olecranon fractures: treatment options. J Am Acad Orthop Surg 2000;8: 266–75.
8. Duckworth AD, Bugler KE, Clement ND, et al. Nonoperative management of displaced olecranon fractures in low-demand elderly patients. J Bone Joint Surg Am 2014;96:67–72.
9. von Rüden C, Woltmann A, Hierholzer C, et al. The pivotal role of the intermediate fragment in initial operative treatment of olecranon fractures. J Orthop Surg Res 2011;6:9.
10. Wellman DS, Lazaro LE, Cymerman RM, et al. Treatment of olecranon fractures with 2.4- and 2.7-mm plating techniques. J Orthop Trauma 2015;29:36–43.
11. Brink PR, Windolf M, de Boer P, et al. Tension band wiring of the olecranon: is it really a dynamic principle of osteosynthesis? Injury 2013;44:518–22.
12. Wilson J, Bajwa A, Kamath V, et al. Biomechanical comparison of interfragmentary compression in transverse fractures of the olecranon. J Bone Joint Surg Br 2011;93:245–50.
13. Hutchinson DT, Horwitz DS, Ha G, et al. Cyclic loading of olecranon fracture fixation constructs. J Bone Joint Surg Am 2003;85:831–7.
14. van der Linden SC, van Kampen A, Jaarsma RL. K-wire position in tension-band wiring technique affects stability of wires and long-term outcome in surgical treatment of olecranon fractures. J Shoulder Elbow Surg 2012;21:405–11.
15. Saeed ZM, Trickett RS, Yewlett AD, et al. Factors influencing K-wire migration in tension-band wiring of olecranon fractures. J Shoulder Elbow Surg 2014;23:1181–6.
16. Prayson MJ, Iossi MF, Buchalter D, et al. Safe zone for anterior cortical perforation of the ulna during tension-band wire fixation: a magnetic resonance imaging analysis. J Shoulder Elbow Surg 2008;17:121–5.
17. Edwards SG, Martin BD, Fu RD, et al. Comparison of olecranon plate fixation in osteoporotic bone: do current technologies and designs make a difference? J Orthop Trauma 2011;25:306–11.
18. Wild JR, Askam BM, Margolis DS, et al. Biomechanical evaluation of suture-augmented locking plate fixation for proximal third fractures of the olecranon. J Orthop Trauma 2012;26:533–8.
19. Izzi J, Athwal GS. An off-loading triceps suture for augmentation of plate fixation in comminuted osteoporotic fractures of the olecranon. J Orthop Trauma 2012;26:59–61.
20. Iannuzzi N, Dahners L. Excision and advancement in the treatment of comminuted olecranon fractures. J Orthop Trauma 2009;23:226–8.
21. Gartsman GM, Sculco TP, Otis JC. Operative treatment of olecranon fractures. Excision or open reduction with internal fixation. J Bone Joint Surg Am 1981;63:718–21.
22. An KN, Morrey BF, Chao EY. The effect of partial removal of proximal ulna on elbow constraint. Clin Orthop Relat Res 1986;(209):270–9.
23. Bell TH, Ferreira LM, McDonald CP, et al. Contribution of the olecranon to elbow stability: an in vitro biomechanical study. J Bone Joint Surg Am 2010; 92:949–57.
24. Didonna M, Fernandez JJ, Lim TH, et al. Partial olecranon excision: the relationship between triceps insertion site and extension strength of the elbow. J Hand Surg Am 2003;28:117–22.
25. Argintar E, Martin BD, Singer A, et al. A biomechanical comparison of multidirectional nail and locking plate fixation in unstable olecranon fractures. J Shoulder Elbow Surg 2012;21:1398–405.
26. Nowak TE, Burkhart KJ, Mueller LP, et al. New intramedullary locking nail for olecranon fracture fixation—an in vitro biomechanical comparison with tension band wiring. J Trauma 2010;69:E56–61.
27. Argintar E, Cohen M, Eglseder A, et al. Clinical results of olecranon fractures treated with multiplanar locked intramedullary nailing. J Orthop Trauma 2013;27:140–4.
28. Karlsson MK, Hasserius R, Karlsson C, et al. Fractures of the olecranon: a 15- to 25-year followup of 73 patients. Clin Orthop Relat Res 2002;(403):205–12.
29. Guitton TG, Zurakowski D, van Dijk NC, et al. Incidence and risk factors for the development of radiographic arthrosis after traumatic elbow injuries. J Hand Surg Am 2010;35:1976–80.

30. Rommens PM, Küchle R, Schneider RU, et al. Olecranon fractures in adults: factors influencing outcome. Injury 2004;35:1149–57.

31. Bailey CS, MacDermid J, Patterson SD, et al. Outcome of plate fixation of olecranon fractures. J Orthop Trauma 2001;15:542–8.

32. Erturer RE, Sever C, Sonmez MM, et al. Results of open reduction and plate osteosynthesis in comminuted fracture of the olecranon. J Shoulder Elbow Surg 2011;20:449–54.

33. Schliemann B, Raschke MJ, Groene P, et al. Comparison of tension band wiring and precontoured locking compression fixation in Mayo type IIA olecranon fractures. Acta Orthop Belg 2014;80:106–11.

34. Gehr J, Friedl W. Intramedullary locking compression nail for the treatment of an olecranon fracture. Oper Orthop Traumatol 2006;18:199–213.

35. Wang YH, Tao R, Xu H, et al. Mid-term outcomes of contoured plating for comminuted fractures of the olecranon. Orthop Surg 2011;3:176–80.

36. Macko D, Szabo RM. Complications of tension-band wiring of olecranon fractures. J Bone Joint Surg Am 1985;67:1396–401.

37. Buijze G, Kloen P. Clinical evaluation of locking compression plate fixation for comminuted olecranon fractures. J Bone Joint Surg Am 2009;91:2416–20.

38. Ishigaki N, Uchiyama S, Nakagawa H, et al. Ulnar nerve palsy at the elbow after surgical treatment for fractures of the olecranon. J Shoulder Elbow Surg 2004;13:60–5.

39. Foruria AM, Augustin S, Morrey BF, et al. Heterotopic ossification after surgery for fractures and fracture-dislocations involving the proximal aspect of the radius or ulna. J Bone Joint Surg Am 2013;95:e66.

40. Koh KH, Lim TK, Lee HI, et al. Surgical treatment of elbow stiffness caused by post-traumatic heterotopic ossification. J Shoulder Elbow Surg 2013;22:1128–34.

41. Hamid N, Ashraf N, Bosse MJ, et al. Radiation therapy for heterotopic ossification prophylaxis acutely after elbow trauma: a prospective randomized study. J Bone Joint Surg Am 2010;92:2032–8.

42. Papagelopoulos PJ, Morrey BF. Treatment of nonunion of olecranon fractures. J Bone Joint Surg Br 1994;76:627–35.

43. Baecher N, Edwards S. Olecranon fractures. J Hand Surg Am 2013;38:593–604.

Distal Humerus Fractures
Open Reduction Internal Fixation

Mark A. Mighell, MD[a,b,c,d],*, Brent Stephens, MD[c], Geoffrey P. Stone, MD[c],
Benjamin J. Cottrell, BS[e]

KEYWORDS

- Distal humerus fracture • Fracture fixation • Open reduction internal fixation • Plate fixation
- Orthogonal plates • Parallel plates

KEY POINTS

- The treatment should be selected according to the type of fracture. Type A, type B1, and type B2 fractures can be treated without extensive exposure of the joint. Type B3 and type C fracture should be treated after the joint has been exposed.
- The goal of treatment is to restore the two columns and articular surface, restoring the "triangle." The different types of distal humerus fracture are thought of as descriptions on how this triangle is disrupted.
- Screw-only constructs do not provide adequate restoration. These constructs lack the buttressing offered by plates to maintain the reconstruction and have a higher chance of failure.
- When possible, plates should be applied only after reduction of the columns and articular surface has been achieved. However, plate reduction may be required in highly comminuted fractures.

INTRODUCTION

Fractures of the distal humerus have traditionally been a significant challenge to treat for the orthopedic surgeon. The anatomic complexity, limited bone stock of the distal segment, frequent fracture comminution, and the close proximity of neurovascular structures add to the difficulty of fracture treatment.[1,2] In the 1960s and 1970s, nonoperative treatment was considered a practical option. This included bag of bones, skeletal traction, and closed reduction and immobilization.[3] The last several decades have seen the evolution of innovative techniques to fix these fractures. These techniques were first described by the Arbeitsgemeinschaft für Osteosynthesefragen, and with modern implant designs, improved patient outcomes have been reported.[4–8]

This article presents surgical strategies to reconstruct complex injuries to the distal humerus based on fracture classification. The authors' preferred method of approach and fixation is described in detail. The article concludes with a description of the most common treatment-related complications and the appropriate manner in which to handle them.

Disclosure: Dr M.A. Mighell receives royalties, speakers bureau payments, consultancy fees, and research support from DJO Surgical. In addition, he receives research support as an investigator from Biomet. Dr B. Stephens and Dr G.P. Stone have nothing to disclose.
[a] The American Board of Orthopaedic Surgery, 400 Silver Cedar Court, Chapel Hill, NC 27514, USA; [b] Department of Orthopaedic Surgery, University of South Florida, 13220 USF Laurel Drive, Tampa, FL 33612, USA; [c] Florida Orthopaedic Institute, 13020 Telecom Parkway North, Tampa, FL 33637, USA; [d] Uniformed Services University of the Health Sciences, F. Edward Hébert School of Medicine, 4301 Jones Bridge Road, Bethesda, MD 20814, USA; [e] Foundation for Orthopaedic Research and Education, 13020 Telecom Parkway North, Tampa, FL 33637, USA
* Corresponding author. Florida Orthopaedic Institute, 13020 Telecom Parkway North, Tampa, FL 33637.
E-mail address: saskiavm@aol.com

hand.theclinics.com

Anatomy

Stable anatomic fixation is the most important treatment goal when fixing these complex fractures. To accomplish this requires a thorough understanding of the three-dimensional anatomy of the elbow.

It is helpful to think of the distal humerus as a triangle. The sides of the triangle are defined by the bony medial and lateral columns, which are then linked by the articular segment. The articular segment represents the horizontal limb of the triangle (**Fig. 1**). Applying the triangular concept allows for systematic reconstruction of the distal humerus.[9]

It is important to recognize that the distal articular surface is in 5 to 7° of internal rotation, 5 to 8° of valgus, and projects 30° anterior to the humeral diaphysis (**Fig. 2**). The radial and coronoid fossae allow for flexion, whereas the olecranon fossa allows for extension. Malposition or overreduction of these restricts postoperative range of

motion.[4] The more prominent medial epicondyle serves as the attachment of the ulnar collateral ligament and the flexor-pronator group. The lateral collateral ligament and supinator-extensor muscle group attach to the lateral epicondyle. These structures must be protected during the surgical approach because they provide dynamic stability to the elbow after fixation.

Classification

There are several classifications described for distal humerus fractures; however, the most commonly referenced classification system is the Orthopedic Trauma Association Classification (**Fig. 3**). Fractures are separated into three categories: (1) extra-articular (type A), (2) partial articular (type B), and (3) complete articular (type C). Further division is based on the degree of comminution and position or orientation of the fracture pattern.[4] The goals of a classification system are to guide treatment for surgeons and to provide an efficient way for researchers to communicate with each other.

Indications and Contraindications

Nonoperative treatment has a limited role in distal humerus fractures. This only remains appropriate for very low-demand patients and those unable to undergo surgery. Before the introduction of Arbeitsgemeinschaft für Osteosynthesefragen plating techniques, outcomes were unpredictable. The advent of newer plating techniques and implants has dramatically improved results.[5–7,10–14] Controversy still remains regarding the optimal surgical approach and plate position. The surgical approach should be tailored to the personality of the fracture (types A, B, or C).

SURGICAL TECHNIQUE
Preoperative Planning

Distal humerus fractures are often the result of a high-energy injury, which can mask damage to other body parts. Therefore, the surgeon should perform a thorough examination of the patient to evaluate for other injuries. The elbow should be carefully inspected for breaks in the skin and any blisters noted. A complete neurovascular assessment should be completed, with specific documentation regarding each neurovascular element.

Good quality radiographs are often difficult to achieve because of patient discomfort, but effort should be made to obtain a true anteroposterior and lateral radiograph. Traction views can aid in understanding fracture displacement and required reduction maneuvers. Although not always

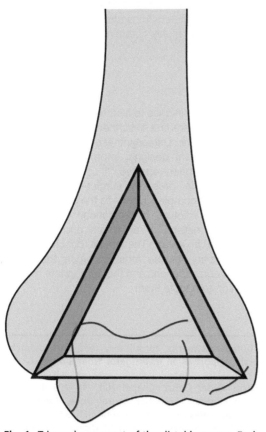

Fig. 1. Triangular concept of the distal humerus. Each column represents a limb of the triangle. The articular surface is represented by the horizontal limb. The concept requires that the articular bridge and each column be reconstructed for stability. (Printed with permission from F. O. R. E., Tampa, FL.)

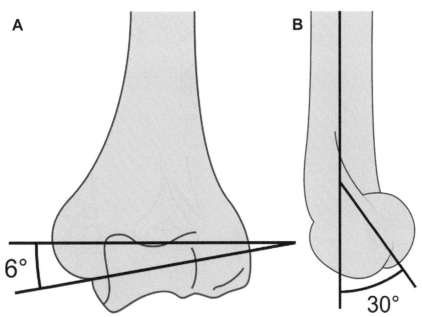

Fig. 2. (A) Anteroposterior and (B) lateral drawing of the distal humerus depicting the anterior projection and valgus angulation of the distal humerus. (Printed with permission from F. O. R. E., Tampa, FL.)

necessary, a computed tomography scan with three-dimensional reconstruction should be considered for poorly defined fractures or those involving the articular surface.

Preparation and Patient Positioning

After intubation, all patients are positioned in the lateral decubitus position with the arm draped over a post (**Fig. 4**). Time is taken to ensure that all bony prominences are well padded and the nonoperative arm is comfortably positioned. The C-arm is brought in from the head, allowing it to be brought in and out of the surgical field. Before draping several fluoroscopic images are taken to ensure adequate intraoperative visualization of the fracture. Our selected surgical approach directly relates to involvement of the articular surface.

Surgical Approach

Types A, B1, and B2: paratricipital approach, joint exposure not required

There is limited involvement of the articular surface in type A, B1, and B2 fractures. The paratricipital approach allows the surgeon to create windows to expose both columns by working on either side of the triceps mechanism. The triceps attachment to the olecranon is not compromised. If greater articular exposure is required, this can be converted to an olecranon osteotomy.[15]

The upper extremity is exsanguinated and a sterile tourniquet is inflated. A midline posterior incision is then made beginning proximal to the level of the fracture. The incision can be curved lateral around the olecranon tip to minimize the possibility of painful scar formation. Full-thickness medial and lateral flaps are created. The ulnar nerve is identified proximally in the wound along the medial border of the triceps muscle. The nerve is carefully dissected from proximal to distal, which allows for complete mobilization (**Fig. 5**). The decision to transpose the nerve is made by the surgeon intraoperatively.

The interval between the triceps and medial intermuscular septum is developed, followed by elevation of the triceps off the posterior and lateral aspects of the humerus. The triceps can be mobilized as a unit in either direction to allow optimal visualization and fixation of the fracture. If the dissection is extended proximally, the radial nerve is encountered along the lateral border of the triceps and should be identified.[15]

This approach does not provide complete articular visualization. However, it offers several benefits. First, the triceps mechanism is not disrupted allowing early active range of motion. Second, it preserves the innervation and blood supply of the anconeus, allowing maximal postoperative stability. Finally, this approach can safely be converted to a transolecranon approach if further exposure is required.[16]

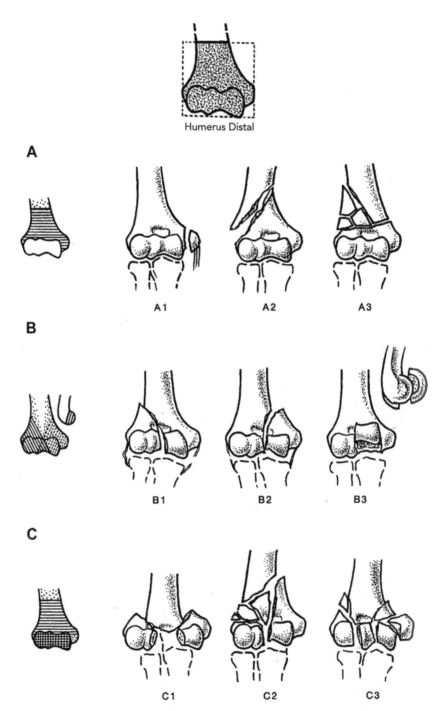

Fig. 3. Orthopedic Trauma Association Classification of distal humerus fractures. (*A*) Extra-articular, articular limb intact. (*B*) Partial articular, one column intact. (*C*) Complete articular, complete disruption of both columns and the articular segment. (*From* Williams GR, Yamaguchi K, Ramsey ML, et al. Shoulder and elbow arthroplasty. Philadelphia: Lippincott Williams & Wilkins; 2005; with permission.)

Types B3 and C: olecranon osteotomy, joint exposure required

We use the olecranon osteotomy when treating distal humerus fractures requiring complete articular visualization (types B3 and C). The initial approach is the same as the triceps-sparing approach. A capsulotomy is performed on either side of the olecranon. The "bare area," a nonarticular portion of the ulna between the olecranon articular facet and coronoid articular facet,

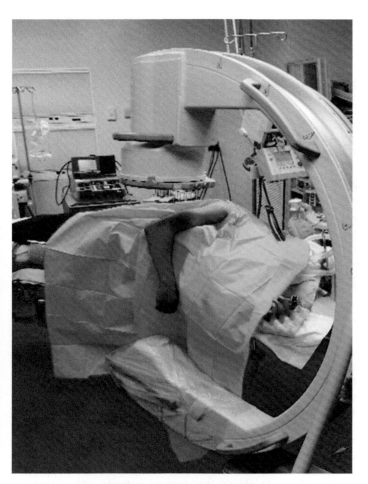

Fig. 4. The patient is positioned beanbag lateral, with the entire arm draped free. Note the C-arm is positioned to allow it to roll in and out of the surgical field. (Printed with permission from F. O. R. E., Tampa, FL.)

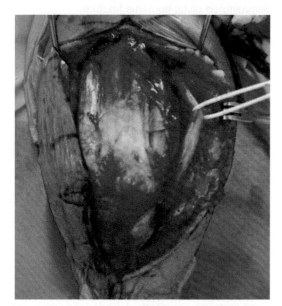

Fig. 5. The ulnar nerve should be mobilized to allow for hardware placement. A vessel loop is used to manipulate the nerve during release to minimize trauma. (Printed with permission from F. O. R. E., Tampa, FL.)

is identified.[15] A vessel loop can be placed across the joint as a visual guide to determine this location. The olecranon is predrilled and tapped before creation of the osteotomy to facilitate extensor mechanism repair at the completion of the case. A chevron-shaped intra-articular osteotomy is then created with the apex pointing distally. The osteotomy is initiated with an oscillating saw and completed with an osteotome. This creates irregularities along the cut surface that allows for interdigitation. The olecranon osteotomy provides the greatest exposure of the articular surface (**Fig. 6**).[17]

Historically, the disadvantages have been hardware irritation after repair. Recent literature has shown that two lag screws across the osteotomy site results in a high rate of union and low rate of hardware irritation. The disadvantages are increased rates of malunion, nonunion, and hardware irritation after repair. Although postoperative osteotomy complications are not completely avoidable, there are several tricks to minimize these problems.

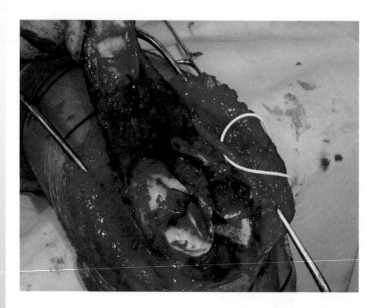

Fig. 6. The olecranon osteotomy allows the greatest visualization of the articular segment. (Printed with permission from F. O. R. E., Tampa, FL.)

The first is to predrill the olecranon before performing the osteotomy. This facilitates anatomic restoration of olecranon position. Another is to use tenaculum clamps on either side of the osteotomy to create compression across the osteotomy site. We prefer the use of two parallel screws instead of K-wires for repair of the olecranon. This can be supplemented with a cerclage if the surgeon believes it is necessary. Although K-wires provide adequate strength they have an increased incidence of hardware irritation, requiring additional surgery for hardware removal.[18,19]

Severely comminuted fractures

Severely comminuted fractures of the distal humerus are particularly challenging. In most instances, it is possible to find a fracture key from which the distal humerus can be reconstituted. Minifragment screws can be used to reassemble the small fracture fragments. Articular fragments that are too small to reliably lag together serve as templates to reduce the risk of overreduction of the trochlea. Most distal humeral nonunions occur in the supracondylar region.[20] In cases with extensive comminution, it may only be possible to achieve stable fixation by removing the comminuted fragments and shortening the distal humerus. The comminuted segments can then be morselized and used as bone graft. Although this surgical technique achieves a more stable construct, distal humerus shortening comes at a cost. Hughes and colleagues[21] found that shortening the distal humerus by 1 cm reduced extension strength by 11%, whereas 3 cm of shortening resulted in a 21% loss at 90° of flexion.

Our approach is different in elderly patients with extensive comminution. The unacceptably high complication rates seen with severely comminuted fractures[8] makes total elbow arthroplasty an attractive alternative. Cobb and Morrey[22] reviewed 21 patients treated with primary total elbow arthroplasty for distal humerus fractures. At 2-year follow-up, they had 15 excellent and 5 good results, with an average range of motion of 130 to 25°.[22] This has now become our approach to elderly low-demand patients with a severely comminuted distal humerus fracture.

Surgical Procedure

Reduction and fixation of intra-articular fractures

The strategy for reduction must take into account the restoration of the articular surface. This requires understanding of the three-dimensional structure of the distal humerus. The missing fragments often encountered in these fractures must be taken into account to avoid overreduction of the trochlea. A shortened trochlea does not allow proper seating of the olecranon, causing an incongruous fit.

Fixation goals include anatomic restoration of the articular surface and secure fixation of the joint to the humeral shaft in a compressive mode. The orientation and anatomic position of any small free fragments are noted if they are to be temporarily removed before reconstruction. The fractured surfaces are gently debrided. The articular surface is first reduced and temporarily held with K-wires. Of note, K-wires should be used for this step rather than small drill bits because of their increased risk of breakage. The K-wires are replaced with a subchondral screw that can provide compression in cases where comminution is not present. Subchondral screws should generally be of smaller diameter (2.0 or 2.7). These smaller screws leave sufficient room for additional screws through the fracture plates. In addition, it eliminates the need to work around K-wires during plate placement.

The next step in reconstruction of the distal humerus requires compression of the articular surface to the humeral shaft. To accomplish this, the columns are assessed to determine which keys in better. This column is then reduced and secured with 2.7-mm screws, followed by reduction of the remaining column. When significant comminution exists in both columns, humeral shortening is used to achieve secure fixation.

Although beginning with reduction of the articular surface is ideal, it is not always feasible. Many C3 fractures have a severely comminuted articular surface making the initial reduction challenging. When encountered with these fractures, we prefer to start by securing one column to the humeral shaft with 2.0- or 2.7-mm screws (**Fig. 7**). We then reduce pieces of the articular surface to the stable column with 2.0 screws and a long column screw. The remaining column is then reduced to the articular surface with a column screw (**Fig. 8**). The use of K-wires is minimized to allow better C-arm visualization of the fragments and prevent difficulty with plate placement.

Plate placement
Ideally, the plates should only be applied after the fracture is adequately reduced. In no circumstance should the surgeon rely on screw fixation alone to stabilize type C fractures (**Figs. 9** and **10**).

In type C fractures, anatomic reduction is often difficult to achieve without using indirect reduction techniques with the plates. Plate application provides the rigidity required to optimize fracture union. The two constructs that provide the greatest stability are parallel plating (**Figs. 11** and **12**) and orthogonal ("90 to 90") plating (**Figs. 13** and **14**). Traditional 90 to 90 plating has been shown to have superior mechanical strength compared with screws or Y-plate fixation.[23]

In certain fractures, such as low transverse and severely comminuted fractures, orthogonal plating has been less than ideal. In this fracture pattern, parallel plating allows a greater number of screws to capture the articular fragments, increasing the stability of the construct (see **Fig. 12**). Although biomechanical studies have shown mixed results when comparing these two plating methods, most seem to favor parallel plating for low transverse fractures.[13,24,25]

The senior author prefers to evaluate the fracture pattern and the soft tissues when deciding which plate construct to use. Fractures with severe comminution are provisionally fixed as described in the previous section and plated in a parallel fashion, providing maximum intra-articular stability (see **Figs. 10** and **11**). Close attention should be given to the trochlea to ensure that it is not overreduced. We continue to use orthogonal plating with B3 fractures to capture the coronal fracture of the capitellum with the posterolateral plate.

The final step in fracture fixation is the repair of the olecranon osteotomy. Reduction of the

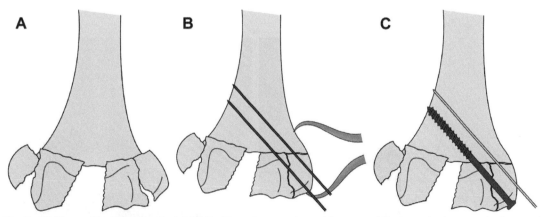

Fig. 7. (*A*) Illustration depicting the initial fixation of a comminuted fracture of the lateral column to the humeral shaft with a 2.7-mm screw. (*B*) The lateral segment is first reduced with a tenaculum and two 2-mm K-wires. (*C*) The distal K-wire is removed, and the fragment is fixated with a 2.7-mm screw. (Printed with permission from F. O. R. E., Tampa, FL.)

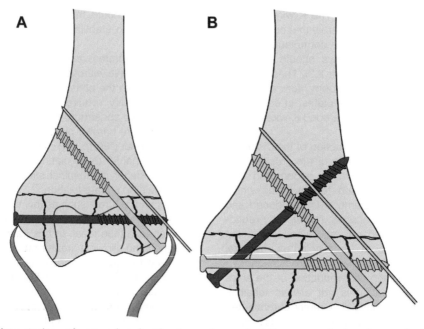

Fig. 8. (*A*) The articular surface is reduced with a tenaculum and a 2.7-mm screw is placed across the joint. (*B*) The medial column is now fixed in the same fashion to the humeral shaft as **Fig. 7**. (Printed with permission from F. O. R. E., Tampa, FL.)

predrilled osteotomy is achieved under direct visualization with pointed reduction clamps placed medial and lateral (see **Fig. 12**).

K-wires are placed in the predrilled holes to ensure proper angle and replaced with 2.7- or 3.5-mm screws, depending on the size of the olecranon. Both screws should engage the anterior cortex of the proximal ulna to ensure maximal purchase. After radiographs confirm reduction of the osteotomy, the elbow is taken through a full range of motion to make certain that there is no mechanical block. Before skin closure, the wound

should be copiously irrigated. We routinely place vancomycin powder in the wound before final closure. A drain should be used in most fracture cases.

Ulnar nerve

Ulnar nerve neuropathy following open reduction of distal humerus fractures is a common complication, ranging from 0% to 51%.[26–29] The ulnar nerve is susceptible to injury with fracture because of its fixed position within the cubital tunnel. The nerve may also be injured because of manipulation

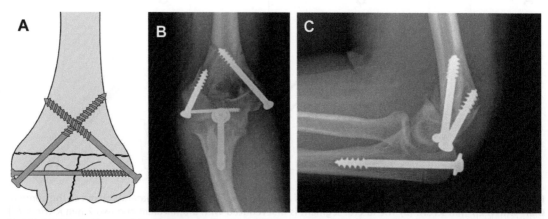

Fig. 9. (*A*) Illustration and (*B*, *C*) radiographs depicting a screw-only construct. Isolated screw fixation without plates is unacceptable when treating these fractures. (Printed with permission from F. O. R. E., Tampa, FL.)

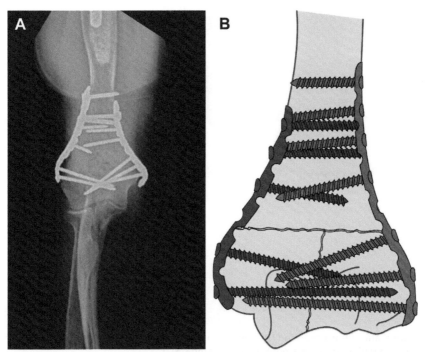

Fig. 10. (*A*) Intraoperative image and (*B*) drawing showing parallel plating after provisional fixation of the distal humerus. Note that parallel plating allows the greatest number of screws into the distal articular piece. These screws often interdigitate, further enhancing the strength of the construct. (Printed with permission from F. O. R. E., Tampa, FL.)

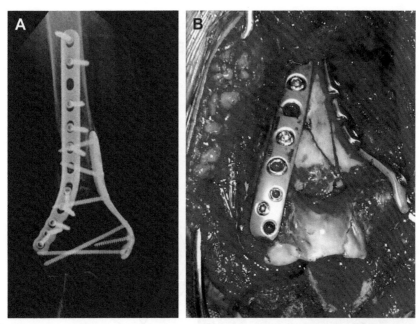

Fig. 11. (*A*) Radiograph and (*B*) intraoperative image of a C2 fracture depicting orthogonal plating technique. (*B*) In this case posterolateral plating allowed for capture of the intact capitellar fragment. (Printed with permission from F. O. R. E., Tampa, FL.)

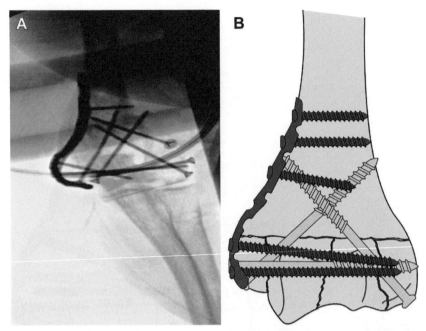

Fig. 12. (*A*) Intraoperative fluoroscopy and (*B*) illustration depicting placement of medial plate after reduction of the fracture. (Printed with permission from F. O. R. E., Tampa, FL.)

during fracture fixation. In most cases, we prefer subcutaneous transposition. When transposition is performed, it is important to completely release the nerve proximally and distally to ensure minimal tension.

Immediate Postoperative Care

The patient receives antibiotics for 24 hours after surgery. Although shoulder, hand, and wrist motion is encouraged, the elbow is splinted in 60° of flexion and immobilized for 10 to 14 days to allow

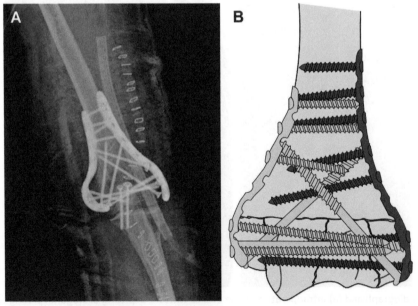

Fig. 13. (*A*) Radiograph and (*B*) illustration depicting final construct with column screws and parallel plating. (Printed with permission from F. O. R. E., Tampa, FL.)

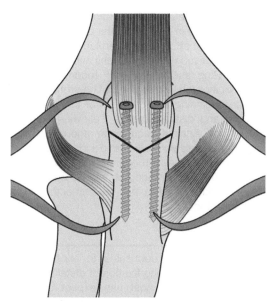

Fig. 14. Reduction of osteotomy with dual tenaculums allows for maximum compression before final lag screw placement. (Printed with permission from F. O. R. E., Tampa, FL.)

for skin healing. The splint is then removed, and the patient is encouraged to perform active and active-assisted elbow range of motions exercises. Light resistance is permitted at 6 weeks, with increasing levels of resistance allowed once the fracture has healed. Radiographs are taken at 1, 6, and 12 weeks.

CLINICAL RESULTS IN THE LITERATURE

Distal humerus fractures are difficult injuries to treat, requiring a thorough understanding of elbow anatomy. Outcomes should be interpreted with the type of fracture and patient's age in mind. Younger patients typically suffer high-energy trauma, possibly resulting in multiple injuries. In his study looking at results for open reduction, Henley and colleagues[30] had a younger patient population, with an average age of 32 years. Although 92% reported an excellent outcome, there was a 45% complication rate. Half of these were related to the olecranon osteotomy. Huang and colleagues[8] evaluated the functional outcome after fixation in patients older than 65 years. Although all fractures united, only 43% reported excellent outcomes. Given the inconsistent results with complex intra-articular patients in this age group, some have advocated for primary total elbow arthroplasty.[22,31] Unfortunately, this restricts patients to a lifelong 10-lb lifting restriction. Regardless of the patient's age, the keys to successful union must include an anatomic restoration of the articular surface, rigid fixation, and early mobilization.

Ulnar Neuropathy

Ulnar neuropathy following distal humerus fractures has reported rates ranging from 0% to 51%.[26–29,32] This can be caused by the initial injury, during intraoperative manipulation, by scar tissue, or hardware irritation. There is not a clear consensus regarding optimal intraoperative handling of the ulnar nerve. Vazquez and colleagues[29] looked at 69 patients with surgically treated distal humerus fractures, without preoperative ulnar nerve findings. They found that 10.1% had ulnar nerve symptoms immediately following surgery, whereas 16% had ulnar symptoms after 12 months. Interestingly, 64% of the patients who had ulnar nerve symptoms after 1 year did not present with immediate postoperative symptoms. Worden and Ilyas[28] found a 38% incidence of ulnar nerve symptoms following surgical treatment of distal humerus fractures. All patients with preoperative findings continued to have late ulnar nerve symptoms, with no benefit of anterior transposition.

Ulnar nerve neurolysis in patients with postoperative neuropathy seems to be an effective treatment. McKee and colleagues[33] evaluated the outcome of 21 elbows that developed neuropathy after primary treatment of elbow fracture, requiring subsequent neurolysis. They found that 17 of those patients had good or excellent results with return of intrinsic power and high patient satisfaction.

Nonunion

The rate of nonunion has been reported between 2% and 10% in the literature, with many cases involving the supracondylar region.[20] Although nonunion may not be a common complication, when present patients can experience significant compromise to quality of life. Therefore, nonunions typically require a return to the operating room for a repeat procedure.

Helfet and colleagues[34] analyzed the results of 52 surgically treated nonunions over a 26-year period. They found that 51 of the 52 patients had healing of the nonunion after the index procedure, with an average time to union of 6 months. Patients had mild improvement in the preoperative range of motion. Of note, they suggested the elbow stiffness that frequently accompanies nonunions be addressed during the revision surgery. Failure to release the elbow contracture results in increased forces across the nonunion site and eventual failure of the construct.

Ring and colleagues[20] reported the results of 15 patients treated for an unstable nonunion of the distal humerus. They also found success with repeat revision surgery, joint contracture release, and bone grafting. Patients had an average arc of ulnohumeral motion of 95° with most reporting only mild pain. In reporting his 30-year experience dealing with distal humerus malunions, Jupiter[35] reported that ulnar nerve dysfunction can be significant with the ulnar nerve encased in scar. He recommends ulnar nerve exploration and transposition be done under loupe magnification.[35]

Although repeat rigid internal fixation and elbow contracture release is ideal for young active patients, some patients may benefit from a total elbow arthroplasty. Ramsey and colleagues[36] reported on 16 patients treated with a semiconstrained total elbow arthroplasty for an unstable distal humeral nonunion. They recommended this treatment be considered for patients older than 60 years and select younger patients with significant bone loss.

Infection

Infection rates are low when treating distal humerus fractures. However, it should be suspected in any patient with a delayed union or nonunion. Persistent drainage or difficulty healing the incision often indicates postoperative infection. There are few papers dealing with management of this difficult complication.[37] Treatment options must strike a balance between stabilizing the fracture and eradicating the infection. Serial debridements with maintenance of implants are an effective treatment of acute nonaggressive infections. This allows minimal disruption of the stable construct, maximizing potential for healing.

If multiple debridements and systemic antibiotics fail to treat the infection, implants should be removed to allow for a more thorough debridement of the distal humerus.

Heterotopic Ossification

The incidence of heterotopic ossification after surgically treated distal humerus fractures varies widely in the literature. Risk factors include concomitant head injury, delayed internal fixation, use of bone graft, extended postoperative immobilization, and method of fracture fixation.[38,39] Abrams and colleagues[40] found that in patients who ultimately developed heterotopic ossification, it was visible on radiographs obtained 2 weeks after surgery 86% of the time, suggesting a more positive outcome with absence of early radiographic findings.

Excision of heterotopic ossification should be considered within 6 to 9 months of injury, limiting degeneration of articular cartilage. Maturation can be assessed with bone scans and serial radiographs. Ring and colleagues[5] recommended a posterior incision with removal of heterotopic ossification beginning at the margin of the olecranon process and distal humerus. Following surgery, prophylaxis against recurrence should include continuous passive motion and indomethacin or low-dose radiation. Although preventative measures before initial fixation should be considered in select patients, it is not recommended as a routine protocol.

Stiffness

Patients should be counseled to expect some loss of motion following fixation of distal humerus fractures; however, most can expect good to excellent results.[2,3,14] The key to preserving motion is early postoperative mobilization. Stiffness resulting from either heterotopic ossification or capsular contraction can effectively be treated with surgical intervention.[41]

Failure of Olecranon Osteotomy

Although the olecranon osteotomy provides the best view of the articular surface, it requires additional hardware for secure fixation. Symptomatic implant prominence and nonunion are the most common sited complications in the literature. Woods and colleagues[18] reported an 11.9% overall nonunion rate, whereas Henley and coworkers[30] reported a 10.3% nonunion rate. Both studies recognized a significant increase in complications in the K-wire/tension band construct.[39,41] Coles and colleagues[19] looked at 70 olecranon osteotomies fixed with either a screw/tension band construct or plate stabilization and found 0 nonunions, although 8% required an isolated implant removal for symptomatic irritation. Olecranon osteotomy complications are rare, regardless of the fixation method used.

SUMMARY

Open reduction internal fixation offers good results in distal humerus fractures. The surgeon should base treatment around the "personality" of the fracture pattern, including the degree of comminution and the feasibility of reduction. To simplify this concept for the multitude of different fractures seen in patients, surgeons should internalize the concept of restoring the triangular construct formed by the articular surface and the two columns. The focus of this approach is to attain reconstruction of each disrupted limb of the triangle using a combination of screws and plates. Achieving this allows the surgeon to restore anatomic structure, promoting positive outcomes.

REFERENCES

1. Throckmorton TW, Zarkadas PC, Steinmann SP. Distal humerus fractures. Hand Clin 2007;23(4): 457–69.

2. Pollock JW, Faber KJ, Athwal GS. Distal humerus fractures. Orthop Clin North Am 2008;39(2):187–200.

3. Ramsey ML, Bratic AK, Getz CL, et al. Open reduction and internal fixation of distal humerus fractures. Tech Shoulder Elbow Surg 2006;7(1):44–51.

4. Webb L. Fractures of the distal humerus. In: Rockwood CA Jr, Gree DP, Bucholz RW, et al, editors. Fractures in adults. Philadelphia: Lippincott-Raven; 2001. p. 953–72.

5. Ring D, Jupiter J. Complex fracture of the distal humerus and their complications. J Shoulder Elbow Surg 1999;8:85–97.

6. Doornberg JN, van Duijn PJ, Linzel D, et al. Surgical treatment of intra-articular fractures of the distal part of the humerus. Functional outcome after twelve to thirty years. J Bone Joint Surg Am 2007;89(7): 1524–32.

7. Kozánek M, Bartonicek J, Chase SM, et al. Treatment of distal humerus fractures in adults: a historical perspective. J Hand Surg Am 2014;39(12):2481–5.

8. Huang JI, Paczas M, Hoyen HA, et al. Functional outcome after open reduction internal fixation of intra-articular fractures of the distal humerus in the elderly. J Orthop Trauma 2011;25(5):259–65.

9. Bonczar M, Rikli D, Ring D. Distal humerus fractures. AO Surg Ref. 2007.

10. Risenborough EJ, Radin EL. Intercondylar T fractures of the humerus in the adult. A comparison of operative and non-operative treatment in twenty-nine cases. J Bone Joint Surg Am 1969;51:130–41.

11. Ring D, Jupiter JB, Gulotta L. Articular fractures of the distal part of the humerus. J Bone Joint Surg Am 2003;85A:232–8.

12. Sotelo-Sanchez J, Barwood S, Blaine T. Current concepts in elbow fracture care. Curr Opin Orthop 2004;15:300–10.

13. Babhulkar S, Babhulkar S. Controversies in the management of intra-articular fractures of distal humerus in adults. Indian J Orthop 2011;45(3):216–25.

14. McCarty LP, Ring D, Jupiter JB. Management of distal humerus fractures. Am J Orthop 2005;34(9): 430–8.

15. Pollock JW, Athwal GS, Steinmann SP. Surgical exposures for distal humerus fractures: a review. Cliin Anat 2008;21(8):757–68.

16. Schildhauer TA, Nork SE, Mills WJ, et al. Extensor mechanism-sparing paratricipital posterior approach to the distal humerus. J Orthop Trauma 2003;17(5): 374–8.

17. Wilkinson JM, Stanley DJ. Posterior surgical approaches to the elbow: a comparative anatomic study. Shoulder Elbow Surg 2001;10(4):380–2.

18. Woods BI, Rosario BL, Siska PA, et al. Determining the efficacy of screw and washer fixation as a method for securing olecranon osteotomies used in the surgical management of intraarticular distal humerus fractures. J Orthop Trauma 2015;29(1): 44–9.

19. Coles CP, Barei DP, Nork SE, et al. The olecranon osteotomy: a six-year experience in the treatment of intraarticular fractures of the distal humerus. J Orthop Trauma 2006;20(3):164–71.

20. Ring D, Gulotta L, Jupiter JB. Unstable nonunions of the distal part of the humerus. J Bone Joint Surg Am 2003;85-A(6):1040–6.

21. Hughes RE, Schneeberger AG, An KN, et al. Reduction of triceps muscle force after shortening of the distal humerus: a computational model. J Shoulder Elbow Surg 1997;6(5):444–8.

22. Cobb TK, Morrey BF. Total elbow arthroplasty as primary treatment for distal humeral fractures in elderly patients. J Bone Joint Surg Am 1997;79(6):826–32.

23. Helfet DL, Hotchkiss RN. Internal fixation of the distal humerus: a biomechanical comparison of methods. J Orthop Trauma 1990;4(3):260–4.

24. Shin SJ, Sohn HS, Do NH. A clinical comparison of two different double plating methods for intraarticular distal humerus fractures. J Shoulder Elbow Surg 2010;19(1):2–9.

25. Scolaro JA, Hsu JE, Svach DJ, et al. Plate selection for fixation of extra-articular distal humerus fractures: A biomechanical comparison of three different implants. Injury 2014;45(12):2040–4.

26. Ruan HJ, Liu JJ, Fan CY, et al. Incidence, management, and prognosis of early ulnar nerve dysfunction in type C fractures of distal humerus. J Trauma 2009; 67(6):1397–401.

27. Chen RC, Harris DJ, Leduc S, et al. Is ulnar nerve transposition beneficial during open reduction internal fixation of distal humerus fractures? J Orthop Trauma 2010;24(7):391–4.

28. Worden A, Ilyas AM. Ulnar neuropathy following distal humerus fracture fixation. Orthop Clin North Am 2012;43(4):509–14.

29. Vazquez O, Rutgers M, Ring DC, et al. Fate of the ulnar nerve after operative fixation of distal humerus fractures. J Orthop Trauma 2010;24(7):395–9.

30. Henley MB, Bone LB, Parker B. Operative management of intra-articular fractures of the distal humerus. J Orthop Trauma 1987;1(1):24–35.

31. Frankle MA, Herscovici D Jr, DiPasquale TG, et al. A comparison of open reduction and internal fixation and primary total elbow arthroplasty in the treatment of intraarticular distal humerus fractures

in women older than age 65. J Orthop Trauma 2003;17(7):473–80.

32. McKee MD, Wilson TL, Winston L, et al. Functional outcome following surgical treatment of intra-articular distal humeral fractures through a posterior approach. J Bone Joint Surg Am 2000;82-A(12):1701–7.

33. McKee MD, Jupiter JB, Bosse G, et al. Outcome of ulnar neurolysis during post-traumatic reconstruction of the elbow. J Bone Joint Surg Br 1998;80(1):100–5.

34. Helfet DL, Kloen P, Anand N, et al. Open reduction and internal fixation of delayed unions and non-unions of fractures of the distal part of the humerus. J Bone Joint Surg Am 2003;85-A(1):33–40.

35. Jupiter JB. The management of nonunion and mal-union of the distal humerus: a 30-year experience. J Orthop Trauma 2008;22(10):742–50.

36. Ramsey ML, Adams RA, Morrey BF. Instability of the elbow treated with semiconstrained total elbow arthroplasty. J Bone Joint Surg Am 1999;81(1):38–47.

37. Brinker MR, O'Connor DP, Crouch CC, et al. Ilizarov treatment of infected nonunions of the distal humerus after failure of internal fixation: an outcomes study. J Orthop Trauma 2007;21(3):178–84.

38. Foruria AM, Lawrence TM, Augustin S, et al. Heterotopic ossification after surgery for distal humeral fractures. Bone Joint J 2014;96-B(12):1681–7.

39. Bauer AS, Lawson BK, Bliss RL, et al. Risk factors for posttraumatic heterotopic ossification of the elbow: case-control study. J Hand Surg Am 2012;37(7):1422–9.e1–6.

40. Abrams GD, Bellino MJ, Cheung EV. Risk factors for development of heterotopic ossification of the elbow after fracture fixation. J Shoulder Elbow Surg 2012;21(11):1550–4.

41. Lindenhovius AL, Linzel DS, Doornberg JN, et al. Comparison of elbow contracture release in elbows with and without heterotopic ossification restricting motion. J Shoulder Elbow Surg 2007;16(5):621–5.

Total Elbow Arthroplasty for Distal Humerus Fractures

Luke S. Harmer, MD, MPH, FRCSC, Joaquin Sanchez-Sotelo, MD, PhD*

KEYWORDS

- Elbow • Arthroplasty • Distal humerus fractures • Treatment • Technique

KEY POINTS

- Total elbow arthroplasty (TEA) provides a successful treatment alternative for selected distal humerus fractures.
- Elbow arthroplasty is selected over internal fixation for elderly patients with low anticipated physical demands on the elbow as well as fractures with severe osteopenia and/or comminution or too low to be amenable to internal fixation.
- Elbow arthroplasty for fractures is best performed by exposing the joint on both sides of the triceps and resecting the fractured fragments, which provides a reasonable working space for canal preparation and component implantation.
- Although elbow arthroplasty for fractures provide a high rate of satisfactory short to midterm outcomes, several patients experience implant failure over time, and some complications may be catastrophic and difficult to solve.
- Do not underestimate the rate of persistent sensory and/or motor ulnar neuropathy as a complicating factor leading to a worse clinical outcome when this complication does occur.

INTRODUCTION

Complex distal humerus fractures continue to present a challenge for orthopedic surgeons. These injuries occur commonly; a recent study in the Scottish population reported an incidence of 5.7/ 100000 individuals.[1] Like many other injuries, distal humerus fractures occur in a bimodal distribution, with a majority occurring in elderly osteopenic patients and a smaller peak occurring among younger patients.[1] The complex osseous, articular, ligamentous, musculotendinous, and neurologic anatomy involved in these injuries and the often osteopenic bone in which they often occur make surgical treatment of any kind challenging.[2] Internal fixation remains the treatment of choice for most patients with distal humerus fractures; however, elbow arthroplasty has emerged as an attractive solution for selected patients.

RATIONALE

Intra-articular distal humerus fractures have been a challenge to orthopedic surgeons from the advent of surgical fracture care. In 1969, Riseborough and Radin[3] reported outcomes on operative and nonoperative care of these patients and concluded that operative treatment was rarely indicated due to the difficulty and morbidity of open reduction and internal fixation (ORIF). With the advent of modern fracture fixation principles in the 1980s, fixation of these injuries was again advocated but with limited expectations for excellent outcomes.[4]

Department of Orthopedic Surgery, Mayo Clinic, 200 First Street SW, Rochester, MN 55905, USA
* Corresponding author.
E-mail address: sanchezsotelo.joaquin@mayo.edu

Hand Clin 31 (2015) 605–614
http://dx.doi.org/10.1016/j.hcl.2015.06.008

In 1997, Cobb and Morrey[5] first reported on a series of patients treated with a TEA for an acute distal humerus fracture. This cohort of patients did reasonably well, and the use of arthroplasty for acute fracture in the elderly and osteoporotic population gained in popularity. **Table 1** summarizes the chief benefits and potential disadvantages of elbow arthroplasty for distal humerus fracture.

Third-generation fixation principles along with the widespread use of precountoured periarticular plates have improved substantially the reliability and outcome of internal fixation compared with what was available historically.[3–5] Sanchez-Sotelo[6] described in detail the use of parallel periarticular plates for these difficult fractures and reported excellent outcomes in a selected group of particularly complex injuries, with a Mayo Elbow Performance Score (MEPS) of 85 and a low complication rate. This outcome has been replicated in other recent series using various fixation constructs.[7,8]

When selecting internal fixation or arthroplasty for a patient presenting with a distal humerus fracture, factors related to be fracture itself, the patient, and the surgeon or system used must all be weighed, as reflected in **Table 2**.

TECHNIQUE

Implants used for elbow arthroplasty are generally divided in 2 broad categories: linked and unlinked. Unlinked designs require competent humeral condyles and collateral ligaments to render the elbow stable.[9] Linked designs, in contrast, allow the ligaments and even the humeral condyles to be sacrificed when needed, because joint stability is maintained by the linked nature of the prosthesis.[9] Although use of an unlinked implant with internal fixation of the columns has been reported by some investigators, especially when using a humeral hemiarthroplasty,[10–12] the authors' preference has been to resect the fractured fragments and use a linked implant (described later).

Approach

There are several approaches that have been advocated for exposing the elbow to perform a TEA. In 1982, Bryan and Morrey[13] pioneered elbow arthroplasty and advocated a triceps-sparing approach that nonetheless did lift the insertion of the triceps off the olecranon in continuity with the fascia of the common extensor origin and anconeus creating in effect a digastric sleeve.[13] Wolfe and Ranawat[14] modified this technique to leave a sliver of bone attached to the triceps insertion to allow for a healthy cancellous bony bed to repair and allow bony healing. Multiple variations of so called triceps-off approaches have been reported over time (split, tongue, and others), but the emphasis more recently is on triceps-on exposures, which are particularly appropriate and useful when replacement is considered for a distal humerus fracture.

Table 2
Relative indications for total elbow arthroplasty for acute fracture

Fracture factors	• Irreducible comminution • End segment is unable to fit a screw • Cartilage sheer fracture • Osteoporotic bone
Patient factors	• Need use of arm for activities of daily living • Elderly physiologic age • Unable to comply with immobilization for 6–12 wk
Surgeon/system factors	• Ability to achieve anatomic reduction and stable fixation • Relative cost of implants and rehabilitation pathway

---

Table 1
The relative advantages and disadvantages of total elbow arthroplasty for management of acute distal fractures

Advantages of Total Elbow Arthroplasty for Acute Fracture	Disadvantages of Total Elbow Arthroplasty for Acute Fracture
Early range of motion and rehabilitation	Loss of bone stock
No need for bony union	Mechanical wear with time
No need for screw purchase in osteoporotic bone	Activity restriction
No risk of posttraumatic osteoarthritis	Infection risk
Early return to activities of daily living	

Adapted from Sanchez-Sotelo J. Distal humeral fractures: role of internal fixation and elbow arthroplasty. J Bone Joint Surg Am 2012;94:559; with permission.

Pierce and Herndon[15] first described adapting the classic Alonso-Llames bilaterotricipital approach for elbow arthroplasty, where windows on both the medial and lateral sides of the triceps are developed after removing the fractured portions of the distal humerus while leaving the central portion of the triceps attached to the olectanon. The distal humerus can be delivered to either side of the triceps and the ulna can be delivered by rotating the forearm[15] (**Fig. 1**).

The Pierce and Herndon approach is particularly suited to acute trauma situations where the fracture provides space at the elbow joint in which to work and negates the need to release the triceps to create working space.[15,16] This approach may result in shorter operative time, avoids triceps-related complications, and allows early unprotected range of motion.[16] McKee and colleagues[17] showed that resecting the humeral condyles did not affect range of motion, strength, or MEPS when using a semiconstrained implant and a triceps-preserving approach. Most TEAs for acute trauma now use this triceps-preserving approach along with condyle resection.

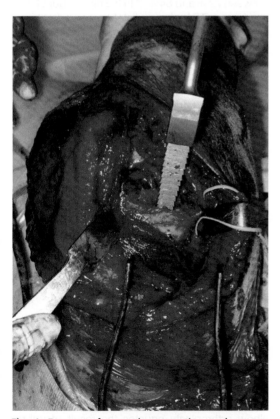

Fig. 1. Exposure for canal preparation and component implantation can be successfully achieved working on both sides of the triceps using the space created by the resected fragments.

Implants

Each implant system has specific instrumentation that should be well known to the surgeon. The position of the humeral component can be difficult to judge due to the distorted anatomic landmarks after trauma. When judging length, the proximal olecranon fossa is a reliable landmark but soft tissue tension should be used as well.[18] With the trial implants in place and the arm held in 90° of flexion, the forearm can pulled distally with moderate force and the humeral component position noted.[18] The elbow should extend but not hyperextend with the implant in this position.[18] The elbow should be able to be flexed so that the hand comes to the mouth. With regard to rotation, the flexion extension axis is 13° and 16° internally rotated relative to the posterior humeral axis in men and women, respectively.[19] The humeral component should be implanted in this correct rotation.

Not uncommonly, exposing the proximal ulna to instrument the canal and implant the ulnar component is difficult given the bulk of the common extensor origin. It is important to remember that the triceps insertion can be partially peeled from the lateral or medial side of the olecranon to improve exposure without compromising the insertion strength.[20] The position of the ulnar component is important as well; the component should be positioned so that the center of rotation is equidistant between the tip of the coronoid and the olecranon.[18] The ulnar component should be positioned so that the component is perpendicular to the dorsal surface of the ulna[18] (**Fig. 2**).

Cement restrictors should be used for the humeral and ulnar components when possible. When commercially available cement restrictors are too large, which is particularly common on the ulnar side, an osseous cement restrictor can often be fashioned. The senior author routinely mixes vancomycin powder (1g) and methylene blue (1 mL) in each package of polymethylmetacrylate cement. The blue color demarcates the border between cortical bone and cement to facilitate cement removal at a later date, if needed.

OUTCOMES

There are many studies that report outcomes after TEA performed specifically for distal humerus fractures.[5,16,21–33] These studies are summarized in **Table 3**. These studies were conducted at a wide variety of centers around the world and the results are fairly tightly clustered. The mean

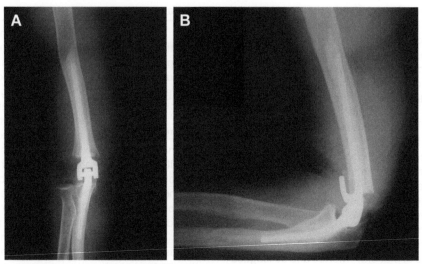

Fig. 2. (*A*) Anterolateral and (*B*) lateral radiographs after implantation of an elbow arthroplasty for a distal humerus fracture. Note the absence of distal humerus after resection of the fractured fragments.

MEPS scores are between 73 and 96, representing good and excellent results. The ranges of motion vary between 10° and 33° for flexion contracture and 116° to 137° for flexion.

There has only been 1 randomized trial comparing TEA for acute fracture with any other treatment modality. McKee and colleagues[32] randomized 40 patients who met their inclusion criteria of age greater than 65, Arbeitsgemeinschaft für Osteosynthesefragen/Orthopedic Trauma Association (AO/OTA) C-type distal humerus fracture, closed or type 1 open fracture treated within 12 hours, and surgeon recommendation for surgical treatment; 21 patients were randomized to each group and 1 patient in each group died prior to follow-up, leaving 20 patients in each group. Importantly, 5 patients in the ORIF group crossed over to the TEA group intraoperatively when the surgeon decided the fracture was not amenable to ORIF. The intension-to-treat analysis showed the MEPS was statistically and clinically significantly better at all time points, including the final follow-up at 2 years. The Disabilities of the Arm, Shoulder and Hand questionnaire outcome showed the TEA group statistically better only at the 6-week and 6-month marks, with no difference at the final 2-year assessment. The reoperation rates and complication rates were similar. This study demonstrates that in a carefully selected population the outcome of TEA is slightly better than ORIF. One important caution in applying this study is that the ORIF group was managed with a now outdated strategy of nonlocking hardware and in many cases non– precontoured plates.

COMPLICATIONS

TEA for all indications has a 5-year survival rate of between 72% and 84%.[34] In the elderly population receiving a TEA after a distal humerus fractures, medical complications may be more likely to happen in patients with severe comorbidities, and wound complications may be more likely to happen in the presence of skin fragility, especially when the soft tissue injury associated with the fracture is substantial. Complications after TEA for trauma are listed in **Table 4**.

A recent retrospective study reviewed the outcome of 719 patients who had undergone TEA for trauma in New York State between 1997 and 2006.[35] There was a 9.5% overall complication rate and 10.6% of patients were readmitted to hospital after TEA.[35] Mechanical complications were most common (4.6%), followed by infection (2.5%); only 1.7% underwent revision TEA.[35] In this study, the 5-year survival was better than in inflammatory arthritis or osteoarthritis.[35]

ARTHROPLASTY AFTER FAILED OPEN REDUCTION AND INTERNAL FIXATION

Advocates of fracture fixation for most distal humerus fractures argue that fixation should always been attempted, and if fixation fails it can then be salvaged with an elbow arthroplasty. The question then becomes whether the result of a primary elbow arthroplasty equates the result of arthroplasty as a salvage of early failure of fixation.

Prasad and Dent[36] compared a cohort of patients who underwent TEA for an acute distal

Table 3
Outcomes of cohort studies reporting outcomes of total elbow arthroplasty used for acute fracture

	n	Female:Male	Inclusion	Fractures Treated with Open Reduction and Internal Fixation During Enrollment	Fracture Classification	Implant	Follow-up (y) (%)	Mayo Elbow Performance Score	Range of Motion E-F/S-P Arc	Complications
Ducrot et al,[24] 2013	20	18:2	Age: >65	80	A: 2, B: 2 C:15, ?: 1	CM	3.4 (1.7–5.5) (75%)	83 (60–100)	33–130/ 152	Ulnar nerve: 2 (1 nonop improved, 1 needed surgery HO: 6 (no surg)
Mansat et al,[31] 2013	87	80:7	Age: >65 Isolated #	—	A: 9 B: 8 C: 70	CM: 85 Lat: 1 Discovery: 1	37.5 (6–106) (100%)	86 (45–100)	29– 125/—	Hematoma: 5 CRPS: 2 Skin necrosis: 1 Neuro injury: 7 Deep infection: 1 Stem #: 1 Stem loosening: 2 Elbow stiffness: 2 Peripros #: 1 Total reop: 8
Antuna et al,[21] 2012	16	1–15	?	—	B3:2 C2: 2 C3: 12	CM	57(24–91)	73 (30–100)	28–117/ 153	Infection: 3 Loosening: 3
Egol et al,[25] 2011	9	0:9	Age >60, female, records available, unilateral injury Intra-articular	11	C: 9	CM: 4 Solar: 5	14.8 (6–38)	79 (<60–100)	24–116/ 169	Death: 2 Loosening: 4 (2 ORs) Infection: 1 (OR but included previously with loosening)

(continued on next page)

Table 3
(continued)

	n	Female:Male	Inclusion	Fractures Treated with Open Reduction and Internal Fixation During Enrollment	Fracture Classification	Implant	Follow-up (y) (%)	Mayo Elbow Performance Score	Range of Motion E-F/S-P Arc	Complications
Baksi et al,[22] 2010	21	17:24 (In larger cohort, including nonunion)	?	—	C2: 12 C3: 9	Baksi sloppy hinge	55.5 (12–88)	96 (<60–100)	25–130/125	—
Chalidis et al,[23] 2009	11	2:9	Age: >75	—	C2: 3 C3: 8	Discovery: 11	2.8 (1–5)	90 (80–95)	10–117/121	Ulnar nn: 1 Peripros hum #: 1
McKee et al,[32] 2009	25	23:2	Age: >65, C type	15	C: 25	CM: 25	2 y (100%)	86 (82–89)	26–133/172	Ulnar nn: 3 (1 operation) Wound prob/hematoma: 4 Stiffness: 3 (2 ORs)
Kamineni et al,[30] 2004	43	31:12	All patients treated with elbow arthroplasty	182	A: 6 B: 5 C1: 5 C2: 8 C3: 25	CM: 43 (different generations, however)	7 (2–15)	93 (75–100)	24–131/—	17 Complications Stroke: 1, MI: 1, PE: 1, ulnar nn: 2 (no OR), CRPS: 1, ulnar PP #: 1 (nonop), hematoma: 3 (OR), wound dehiscence: 2 (OR), K wire removal: 1, deep infection: 1
Frankle et al,[26] 2003	12	0:12	Women, age >65	12	C3: 4 C?: 8	CM	45 mo (2–6 y)	95 (85–100)	15–125/160	Ulnar nn: 2 (no surg), uncoupling: 1, hematoma: 1, sup inf: 1

Study	N	Indication	Age	Fracture	Implant	Follow-up	MEPS	ROM	Complications
Garcia et al,[28] 2002	16 4:12	Age >50, osteopenia, comminution	—	A: 2 B: 2 C: 11 ?: 4	CM	3 (1–5.5)	93 (80–100)	24–125/160	MI: 1 Sup inf: 1 nonop Neuropraxia: 1 (preop) HO: 1 (nonop) Loosening: 1 (nonop)
Gambirasio et al,[27] 2001	10 0:10	Surgeon deemed # unfixable	43	B: 2 C: 8	CM	17.8 (12–34)	94 (80–100)	23.5–125/153.5	HO: 1 Loosening: 2 (nonop) CRPS: (1)
Hildebrand et al,[29] 2000	7 0:7	Surgeon deemed needs a TEA	—	—	CM	46.4 (±20.2)	78 ±18	30–137/158	Loosening: 4/18 Intraop #: 2/7 Neuropraxia: ? Infection: ?
Hall & McKee,[16] 2000	10 —	Age: >65	—	—	—	—	"…evaluation with [MEPS] found all patient with excellent or good results"	—	Radial nn palsy: 1 (resolved)
Ray et al,[33] 2000	7 0:7	Comminuted distal humerus #	—	C2: 1 C3: 3 ?: 3	CM	2.6 (2–4)	92 (85–100)	20–130/—	Sup inf: 1
Cobb & Morrey,[5] 1997	21 6:15	Comminuted distal humerus fracture with RA or comminuted distal humerus fracture age >65	108	A: 1 B: 7 C2: 5 C3: 6 Prox ulna: 2	CM (various iterations)	3.3 (2–5 Excluding 3 deceased patients)	95	25–130/147	MI: 1 Stroke: 1 PE: 1 Superficial infection: 1 (nonop) Ulnar nn: 3 Ulnar component #: 1 CRPS: 1 Osteotomy nonunion: 1

Abbreviations: CM, Coonrad-Morrey; E-F, extension-flexion; K, Kirschner; S-P, supination-pronation.
Data from Refs.[5,16,21–33]

Table 4 Complications reported in outcomes studies	
Major (requires reoperation)	• Deep infection • Ulnar nerve symptoms requiring surgery • CRPS • Olecranon fracture or nonunion • Symptomatic loosening • Hematoma requiring evacuation • Wound dehiscence • Implant fracture • Periprosthetic fracture • Elbow stiffness
Minor (no reoperation)	• Superficial infection • Neuropraxia • Radiographic loosening • Intraoperative fracture • HO
Medical	• Death • MI • Stoke • PE

Abbreviations: CRPS, chronic regional pain syndrome; HO, heterotopic ossification; MI, myocardial infarction; PE, pulmonary embolus.
Data from Refs.[5,16,21–33]

humerus fracture with a second cohort who underwent a TEA at an average of 56 weeks after initial nonoperative or ORIF treatment. The early TEA group had an MEPS of 85 whereas the delayed TEA group has an MEPS of 80.[36] The range of motion was also similar with an arc of 27° to 120° in the early group and 30° to 120° in the delayed group.[36] Although these functional outcomes were similar between the groups, survival for the early group was 93% at 88 months whereas the delayed group was 76% at 84 months.[36] Although this may indicate a trend, this difference was not statistically significant.[36]

Unpublished data from the authors' institution seem to suggest that when elbow arthroplasty is performed within 1 year of failed internal fixation for a distal humerus fracture, pain and function are improved, but the rate of implant revision or removal is high. The authors reviewed the outcome of 21 linked semiconstrained TEAs with an average timeframe between ORIF and TEA of 8 months. At most recent follow-up, 6 elbows had required a reoperation, including implant revision or removal in 4 elbows (19%). These 6 patients required a total of 14 reoperations, 9 of which involved revision or removal of implants. For patients with surviving implants, the mean MEPS score was 85.5 points, 89% reported no or mild pain, and 78% considered their elbow much better. Flexion increased from 94° to 138° and extension increased from 43° to 18°. The overall infection rate was 5%.

These studies seem to indicate that although failed internal fixation can be salvaged with an elbow arthroplasty, some price is paid in terms of a higher implant failure rate than typically reported when the arthroplasty is performed as the primary procedure (**Fig. 3**).

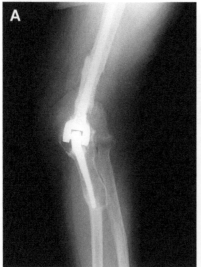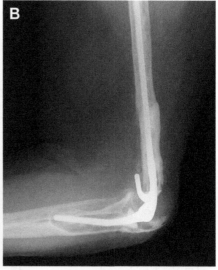

Fig. 3. Catastrophic implant failure may happen at mid- to long term after elbow arthroplasty for fracture. Ulnar loosening with severe bone loss, as seen on this example, represents a phenomenal treatment challenge. (*A*) Anterolateral view. (*B*) Lateral view.

SUMMARY

TEA is a good treatment alternative for selected patients with distal humerus fractures. Its attractiveness is related to several factors, including the possibility of performing the procedure leaving the extensor mechanism intact; the faster, easier rehabilitation compared with internal fixation; and the overall good outcomes reported in terms of both pain relief and function. Implant failure leading to revision surgery does happen, however, and patients must comply with certain limitations to extend the longevity of their implant. Development of high-performance implants may allow expanding the indications of elbow arthroplasty for fractures, but currently this procedure should be considered only if internal fixation is doomed to failure secondary to comminution, preexisting arthritis elbow pathology, or severe osteopenia, typically in older patients.

REFERENCES

1. Robinson CM, Hill RMF, Jacobs N, et al. Adult distal humeral metaphyseal fractures: epidemiology and results of treatment. J Orthop Trauma 2003;17:38–47.
2. Axelrod TS. Exposures of the Elbow. Hand Clin 2014;30:415–25.
3. Riseborough EJ, Radin EL. Intercondylar T fractures of the humerus in the adult. A comparison of operative and non-operative treatment in twenty-nine cases. J Bone Joint Surg Am 1969;51:130–41.
4. Jupiter JB, Neff U, Holzach P, et al. Intercondylar fractures of the humerus. An operative approach. J Bone Joint Surg Am 1985;67:226–39.
5. Cobb TK, Morrey BF. Total elbow arthroplasty as primary treatment for distal humeral fractures in elderly patients. J Bone Joint Surg Am 1997;79:826–32.
6. Sanchez-Sotelo J. Complex distal humeral fractures: internal fixation with a principle-based parallel-plate technique. J Bone Joint Surg Am 2007;89:961.
7. Kaiser T, Brunner A, Hohendorff B, et al. Treatment of supra- and intra-articular fractures of the distal humerus with the LCP Distal Humerus Plate: a 2-year follow-up. J Shoulder Elbow Surg 2011;20:206–12.
8. Shin S-J, Sohn H-S, Do N-H. A clinical comparison of two different double plating methods for intraarticular distal humerus fractures. J Shoulder Elbow Surg 2010;19:2–9.
9. Wright TW, Wong AM, Jaffe R. Functional outcome comparison of semiconstrained and unconstrained total elbow arthroplasties. J Shoulder Elbow Surg 2000;9:524–31.
10. Argintar E, Berry M, Narvy SJ, et al. Hemiarthroplasty for the treatment of distal humerus fractures: short-term clinical results. Orthopedics 2012;35:1042–5.
11. Burkhart KJ, Nijs S, Mattyasovszky SG, et al. Distal humerus hemiarthroplasty of the elbow for comminuted distal humeral fractures in the elderly patient. J Trauma 2011;71:635–42.
12. Hohman DW, Nodzo SR, Qvick LM, et al. Hemiarthroplasty of the distal humerus for acute and chronic complex intra-articular injuries. J Shoulder Elbow Surg 2014;23:265–72.
13. Bryan RS, Morrey BF. Extensive posterior exposure of the elbow. A triceps-sparing approach. Clin Orthop Relat Res 1982;(166):188–92.
14. Wolfe SW, Ranawat CS. The osteo-anconeus flap. An approach for total elbow arthroplasty. J Bone Joint Surg Am 1990;72:684–8.
15. Pierce TD, Herndon JH. The triceps preserving approach to total elbow arthroplasty. Clin Orthop Relat Res 1998;(354):144–52.
16. Hall JA, McKee MD. Total elbow arthroplasty for intra-articular fractures of the distal humerus. Tech Orthop 2000;15(2):120–7.
17. McKee MD, Pugh DMW, Richards RR, et al. Effect of humeral condylar resection on strength and functional outcome after semiconstrained total elbow arthroplasty. J Bone Joint Surg Am 2003;85-A:802–7.
18. Sanchez-Sotelo J, Ramsey M, King G, et al. Elbow arthroplasty: Lessons learned from the past and directions for the future. Instr Course Lect 2011;60:157–69.
19. Sabo MT, Athwal GS, King GJW. Landmarks for rotational alignment of the humeral component during elbow arthroplasty. J Bone Joint Surg Am 2012;94:1794–800.
20. Grogan B, Blair J, Blease R, et al. Exposure of the distal humerus using a triceps hemi-peel approach. Orthopedics 2014;37:e455–459.
21. Antuna SA, Laakso RB, Barrera JL, et al. Linked total elbow arthroplasty as treatment of distal humerus fractures. Acta Orthop Belg 2012;78:465–72.
22. Baksi DP, Pal AK, Baksi D. Prosthetic replacement of elbow for intercondylar fractures (recent or ununited) of humerus in the elderly. Int Orthop 2010;35:1171–7.
23. Chalidis B, Dimitriou C, Papadopoulos P, et al. Total elbow arthroplasty for the treatment of insufficient distal humeral fractures. A retrospective clinical study and review of the literature. Injury 2009;40:582–90.
24. Ducrot G, Ehlinger M, Adam P, et al. Complex fractures of the distal humerus in the elderly: Is primary total elbow arthroplasty a valid treatment alternative? A series of 20 cases. Orthop Traumatol Surg Res 2013;99:10–20.
25. Egol KA, Tsai P, Vazques O, et al. Comparison of functional outcomes of total elbow arthroplasty vs plate fixation for distal humerus fractures in

osteoporotic elbows. Am J Orthop (Belle Mead NJ) 2011;40:67–71.

26. Frankle MA, Herscovici D, DiPasquale TG, et al. A comparison of open reduction and internal fixation and primary total elbow arthroplasty in the treatment of intraarticular distal humerus fractures in women older than age 65. J Orthop Trauma 2003;17:473–80.

27. Gambirasio R, Riand N, Stern R, et al. Total elbow replacement for complex fractures of the distal humerus. An option for the elderly patient. J Bone Joint Surg Br 2001;83:974–8.

28. Garcia JA, Mykula R, Stanley D. Complex fractures of the distal humerus in the elderly. The role of total elbow replacement as primary treatment. J Bone Joint Surg Br 2002;84:812–6.

29. Hildebrand KA, Patterson SD, Regan WD, et al. Functional outcome of semiconstrained total elbow arthroplasty. J Bone Joint Surg Am 2000;82-A: 1379–86.

30. Kamineni S, Morrey BF. Distal humeral fractures treated with noncustom total elbow replacement. J Bone Joint Surg Am 2004;86-A:940–7.

31. Mansat P, Degorce HN, Bonnevialle N, et al. Total elbow arthroplasty for acute distal humeral fractures in patients over 65 years old – Results of a multi-center study in 87 patients. Orthop Traumatol Surg Res 2013;99:779–84.

32. McKee MD, Veillette CJH, Hall JA, et al. A multicenter, prospective, randomized, controlled trial of open reduction–internal fixation versus total elbow arthroplasty for displaced intra-articular distal humeral fractures in elderly patients. J Shoulder Elbow Surg 2009;18:3–12.

33. Ray PS, Kakarlapudi K, Rajsekhar C, et al. Total elbow arthroplasty as primary treatment for distal humeral fractures in elderly patients. Injury 2000; 31:687–92.

34. Kim JM, Mudgal CS, Konopka JF, et al. Complications of total elbow arthroplasty. J Am Acad Orthop Surg 2011;19:328–39.

35. Gay DM, Lyman S, Do H, et al. Indications and reoperation rates for total elbow arthroplasty: an analysis of trends in New York State. J Bone Joint Surg Am 2012;94(2):110–7.

36. Prasad N, Dent C. Outcome of total elbow replacement for distal humeral fractures in the elderly: a comparison of primary surgery and surgery after failed internal fixation or conservative treatment. J Bone Joint Surg Br 2008;90:343–8.

Capitellar and Trochlear Fractures

Michael J. Carroll, MD, FRCSC, George S. Athwal, MD, FRCSC,
Graham J.W. King, MD, MSc, FRCSC, Kenneth J. Faber, MD, MPHE, FRCSC*

KEYWORDS

- Capitellum • Trochlea • Coronal shear • Fracture • Distal humerus

KEY POINTS

- Capitellum and trochlea fractures are commonly associated with concomitant injuries, such as radial head fracture and lateral ligament instability.
- Computed tomography is recommended as plain radiographs often underestimate fracture displacement and comminution.
- A single posterior skin incision is preferred as it can be used to for surgical exposure of both the lateral and medial aspects of the elbow.
- Anatomic reduction and stable fixation are required for early range of motion. This technique may be accomplished with cannulated standard or headless compression screws, fine-threaded Kirschner wire, bone graft, and/or posterolateral locking plate fixation.
- Restricted range of motion or a protective, ligament-specific protocol is used for rehabilitation if stable fixation or joint stability is not achievable.

INTRODUCTION

Coronal shear fractures of the distal humerus may involve the capitellum alone; however, most extend medially to include a portion of the trochlea. Isolated fractures of the trochlea have been described but are especially rare.[1] Fractures of the capitellum compose 6% of distal humerus fractures and 1% of all elbow fractures, making them relatively uncommon.[2] Associated bone and soft tissue injuries to the elbow are common[3–9]; however, clinicians need to be vigilant in their assessment. Lateral collateral ligament (LCL) injury or radial head fracture may be seen in up to approximately 60% of patients with this type of fracture.[3]

Open reduction and internal fixation (ORIF) is the favored treatment of most displaced coronal shear fractures of the distal humerus. The evidence to support this, however, is limited to small case series.[3–7,9–15] In addition to ORIF, several other treatment options have been described and include closed reduction,[16–18] fragment excision, excision,[8,19,20] and arthroscopic-assisted reduction and internal fixation (AARIF).[21–23] Arthroplasty is indicated when stable internal fixation cannot be achieved for intra-articular distal humerus fractures in the elderly[24,25]; however, its application to coronal shear fractures of the distal humerus is not well studied. The ideal management of these fractures is uncertain as no comparative studies exist and available studies use varying rating

Disclosures: Dr G.J.W. King is a consultant for Wright Medical Technologies and receives royalties for implant development. Wright Medical Technologies had no input into this research in any manner. All other authors, their immediate families, or any research foundation with which they are affiliated have not received any financial payment or other benefits from any commercial entity related to the subject of this article.
Division of Orthopedic Surgery, Roth|McFarlane Hand & Upper Limb Centre, St. Joseph's Health Center, Western University, 268 Grosvenor Street, London, Ontario N6A 4L6, Canada
* Corresponding author.
E-mail address: kjfaber@uwo.ca

Hand Clin 31 (2015) 615–630
http://dx.doi.org/10.1016/j.hcl.2015.07.001

instruments to report clinical outcomes. The details of selected clinical studies are summarized in **Table 1**.

This article reviews the preoperative evaluation and classification, surgical technique, rehabilitation and recovery, clinical outcomes, and complications of coronal shear fractures of the distal humerus.

SURGICAL TECHNIQUE
Preoperative Planning

Most capitellum fractures are the result of a low-energy injury, such as a fall on the outstretched hand (FOOSH), with varying degrees of elbow flexion. Biomechanical studies have yet to demonstrate the mechanisms that cause coronal shear fractures of the distal humerus. In the instance when patients recall a FOOSH injury, we may infer 2 mechanisms resulting in fracture. In the first instance, the fracture may occur following direct transfer of energy to the capitellum through axial loading of the radius. Alternatively, the fracture may occur after an episode of elbow instability and/or LCL injury. In this scenario, the capitellum and trochlea may be sheared off by the radial head and coronoid following the reduction of a posterolateral subluxation or dislocation of the elbow.

A thorough physical examination of patients is essential as associated injuries are common.[3–6,9,11] An LCL injury or radial head fracture was noted in 60% of patients in one study[3]; Brouwer and colleagues[4] reported that 33% of patients in their study sustained an elbow dislocation and/or a radial head fracture; a collateral ligament injury or radial head fracture was reported in 57% of patients by Dubberley and colleagues.[9] Inspection may demonstrate generalized swelling of the elbow and/or ecchymosis along the lateral aspect of the joint. Careful palpation of bony prominences about the elbow should be performed; tenderness over the medial epicondyle, lateral epicondyle, or radial head should raise suspicion for injury to collateral ligaments or fracture of the radial head or epicondyles. Elbow flexion-extension and forearm rotation should be compared with the uninjured side and deficits or blocks to motion noted. The ipsilateral shoulder and wrist, including the interosseous membrane, should be evaluated for concomitant injury. Neurologic or vascular injuries have not been commonly reported in the literature; however, a detailed examination of the distal function should be performed.

A full series of plain radiographs including anteroposterior, lateral, oblique, and radiocapitellar views of the elbow should be obtained and is helpful in making the diagnosis of a coronal shear fracture as well as identifying concomitant injuries. Plain radiographs often cannot identify subtle fracture planes and underestimate the extent of comminution; the authors prefer to use computed tomography (CT) with 3-dimensional reconstruction. The use of CT has been shown to improve intrarater and interrater reliability in identifying the specifics of distal humerus fractures.[26] The additional information can influence the management strategy and helps with preoperative planning.

Fracture Classification

Several classification systems for coronal shear fractures of the distal humerus have been described. Bryan and Morrey[2] proposed a classification based on 3 types of capitellum fractures. A type 1 (Hahn-Steinthal) lesion involves a fracture isolated to the capitellum with attached subchondral bone; type 2 fractures (Kocher-Lorenz) are those involving primarily the articular cartilage overlying the capitellum; type 3 (Broberg-Morrey) lesions are defined as comminuted capitellum fractures. A type 4 lesion (McKee) was later added to the classification scheme and involves a capitellum fracture that extends medially into the trochlea.[15]

The Orthopedic Trauma Association (OTA) classification[27] defines partial articular fractures of the distal humerus as type 13-B. A partial articular fracture in the coronal plane is subclassified as 13-B3. Fractures involving the capitellum are further subdivided as involving only the capitellum (13-B3.1), the trochlea (13-B3.2), or both (13-B3.3).

Dubberley and colleagues[9] developed another classification following the review of 28 patients who underwent ORIF (**Fig. 1**). The benefit of their classification system over others is that it helps direct surgical management and provides prognostic information based on fracture types. The type 1 fracture involves the capitellum with or without extension to the lateral trochlear ridge and may be treated with ORIF through a muscle-splitting approach. The type 2 fracture involves disruption of the capitellum and trochlea as a single fragment. Visualization and access to the medial portion of the joint in a type 2 fracture may require a more extensile approach. The type 3 fracture involves the capitellum and trochlea as 2 independent fragments and may require an olecranon osteotomy to accurately assess and treat the injury. Fractures demonstrating posterior condylar comminution are denoted with a B modifier. Recognizing and treating posterior comminution by bone grafting the defect and applying a

Table 1
Selected clinical studies in the treatment of coronal shear fractures of the distal humerus

Author	Study	Follow-up	Fracture Classification	Outcomes	Complications	Associated Injuries
ORIF						
Bilsel et al,[10] 2013	Case series: 18 patients, ORIF (different types of screws) using extensile lateral approach	44 mo (16–70)	B&M Type 1–7 Type 2–0 Type 3–5 Type 4–6	MEPI 86.7 DASH 15.3 Flex 8.9 Ext 132.8 Pro 90 Sup 90	1 of 18 HO 0 AVN	None
Heck et al,[3] 2012	Case series: 15 patients, ORIF (fine-thread k-wire) using Kocher approach	58.5 (12–167)	B&M Type 1–7 Type 2–3 Type 3–2 Type 4–3 Dubberley 1A–9 2A–2 2B–1 3A–2 3B–1	MEPI 90 DASH 10.8 ASES 91.5 B-M score 90.8 Morrey score 87.3 Flex-ext arc 124 Pro-sup arc 174	All healed No instability	5 complex ligament injury 3 radial head fracture 1 ulnar nerve
Brouwer et al,[4] 2011	Case series: 30 patients, ORIF (HCS, plate/screw/wire)	Min 1 y	Dubberley 2A–6 2B–6 3B–18	8 of 8 Dubberley type 3B had nonunion	Nonunion Infection Loose implants Posttrauma arthritis	6 elbow dislocations 2 dislocations + radial head fracture 2 radial head fracture 6 polytrauma
Mighell et al,[11] 2010	Case series: 18 patients, ORIF (HCS) using Kaplan approach	25.5 mo (12–64)	Dubberley 1A–11 2A–7	ASES 83.1 B-M 93.3 Flex-ext arc 128 Pro-sup arc 176	100% union No instability 3 AVN 3 HO 5 arthrosis 1 stitch abscess 1 persistent stiffness	3 LCL (all in the class 2)

(continued on next page)

Table 1
(continued)

Author	Study	Follow-up	Fracture Classification	Outcomes	Complications	Associated Injuries
Giannicola et al,[5] 2010	Case series: 15 patients, ORIF using lateral or combined approach, external fixator for 6 wk	29 mo (12–49)	Dubberley 1A–3 1B–3 2A–5 3A–2 3B–2 B&M Type 1–6 Type 4–9	MEPS 98 Flex 140 Ext 13 Pro-sup arc full	2 arthritis 2 loose screws 1 intra-articular hardware and pin site infection	4 elbow dislocations + MCL and LCL injury 3 lateral epicondyle fracture 1 medial epicondyle fracture 5 MCL
Singh et al,[12] 2010	Case series: 14 patients (3 delayed union), ORIF using extensile Kocher approach	4.8 y (3–7 y)	B&M Type 1–7 Type 2–1 Type 4–3	MEPS (10 excellent, 4 good) Flex 7.5 Ext 132 Pro-sup arc full	3 nonunions No AVN Good stability No pain	None
Ruchelsman,[6] 2008	Case series: 16 patients, ORIF using extensile lateral approach	27 mo (13–69)	B&M Type 1–6 Type 3–2 Type 4–8 OTA B3.1–8 B3.3–8	MEPI 92 Ext 10 Flex 133 Pro-sup arc full Stability = all Union = all	No AVN No instability 6 HO (no functional implication) 1 malreduction	5 rad head fracture 1 elbow dislocation + LCL
Mahirogullari et al,[13] 2006	Case series: 11 patients, ORIF using Kocher approach	23.4 mo (12–60)	B&M Type 1–11	MEPI 93.6 Flex-ext arc 117 Pro-sup arc 117	No AVN No instability No infection	None
Dubberley et al,[9] 2006	Case series: 28 patients, ORIF using Boyd, Kaplan, Kocher approach; 14 had olecranon osteotomy	56 mo (14–121)	Dubberley 1A–9 1B–2 2A–1 2B–3 3A–3 3B–8	MEPI 91 ASES 29 PREE 16 Flex 138 Ext 19 Sup 74 Pro 82	3 AVN 4 HO 9 arthritis 1 screw in PRUJ 1 malreduction 6 painful hardware from olecranon osteotomy 7 elbow contracture 3 nonunion	11 LCL 3 radial head fracture 2 MCL 1 scaphoid fracture 1 distal radius fracture 1 triceps rupture

Study	Design/Intervention	Follow-up	Outcome Measure	Results	AVN/Instability	Other Complications
Sano et al,[14] 2005	Case series: 6 patients, ORIF using Kocher or olecranon osteotomy	5.6 y (2.5–9.3)	Grantham	Grantham criteria (3 excellent, 3 good) Ext 7.5 Flex 139.2 Pro-sup arc full	No AVN No instability	None
Mckee et al,[15] 1996	Case series: 6 patients, ORIF using extensile Kocher	22 mo (18–26)	B&M Type 4–6	B-M (3 excellent, 3 good) Flex 141 Ext 15 5 of 6 had full pro-sup	No AVN No instability No arthritis	None
Ring et al,[7] 2003	Case series: 21 patients, ORIF using extensile lateral approach or olecranon osteotomy	40 mo (24–90)	Ring	MEPI (4 excellent, 12 good, 5 fair) Flex 123 Ext 27 Pro-sup arc full	No instability No nonunion 10 of 21 required reoperation (6 stiff w contracture release, 2 ulnar neuropathy, 1 painful hardware, 1 loss fixation)	3 ulnohumeral subluxation 3 radial head fracture 1 olecranon fracture
Fragment Excision						
Dushuttle et al,[20] 1985	Case series: 5 patients (3 of 5 had concomitant medial-sided injury)	1–14 y	B&M Type 1–5	Flex-ext arc 114 Flex 129 Ext 15	2 valgus instability (both with medial-side injury)	2 MCL 1 medial condyle fracture
Grantham et al,[8] 1981	Case series: 20 patients (11 have follow-up)	1–15 y	B&M Type 2–8 Type 3–3	Mostly fair to poor Avg 40° loss of ROM	—	6 of 27 with radial head fracture
Feldman,[19] 1997	Report of 2 cases	17 and 15 mo	B&M Type 2–2	Case 1 had full ROM Case 2 flex-ext arc of 0–125	None	2 of 2 had radial head impression fracture
Closed Reduction						
Ochner et al,[16] 1996	Case series: 9 patients (6 have follow-up)	32.3 mo (5–108)	Not stated	<15° ext loss and otherwise complete ROM	No AVN	—
Cutbush et al,[18] 2014	Case series: 7 patients	41.6 mo (18–77)	B&M Type 1–7	DASH 4.36 97% flex and 83% ext of contra side	None	None
Ma et al,[17] 1984	Case series: 8 of 9 patients had closed reduction assisted by percutaneous pin	48.4 mo (19–80)	Not stated	6 excellent 2 good (loss of rom <30°, mild pain)	1 of 9 failed closed reduction No AVN	—

(continued on next page)

Table 1
(continued)

Author	Study	Follow-up	Fracture Classification	Outcomes	Complications	Associated Injuries
Puloski et al,[36] 2012	Case series: 7 patients, immobilized 14 d	18 mo (12–46)	B&M Type 1–7	DASH 9.1 Flex-ext arc 126 Pro-sup arc normal	No loss of reduction No AVN 6 of 7 reductions were anatomic	None
Dushuttle et al,[20] 1985	Case series: 4 patients, immobilized 21 d	1–14 y	B&M Type 1–4	Flex 145 Ext 5	—	—
AARIF						
Kuriyama et al,[21] 2010	Report of 2 cases, AARIF (percutaneous HCS)	Pt 1–20 mo Pt 2–17 mo	Dubberley 1A & 3A	Flex-ext arc 5–125 Pro-sup arc 85–90	None	None
Mitani et al,[22] 2009	Case report of AARIF (percutaneous HCS)	1 y	Dubberley 1A	Full ROM	United at 2 mo	No radial head, trochlea injury seen during arthroscopy
Hardy et al,[23] 2002	Case report of AARIF (percutaneous 3.5-mm cannulated screws)	—	B&M Type 1	Full ROM	United at 2 mo	No radial head, trochlea injuyi seen during arthroscopy

Abbreviations: ASES, American Shoulder and Elbow Scores; Avg, average; AVN, avascular necrosis; B-M, broberg and morrey scale; B&M, bryan & morrey; DASH, Disabilities of the Arm, Shoulder, and Hand; Ext, extension; Flex, flexion; k-wire, Kirschner wire; MEPI, Mayo Elbow Performance Index; PREE, patient rated elbow evaluation; Pro, pronation; Pro-sup, pronation-supination; PRUJ, proximal radioulnar joint; ROM, range of motion; Sup, supination.
Data from Refs.[3–23,36]

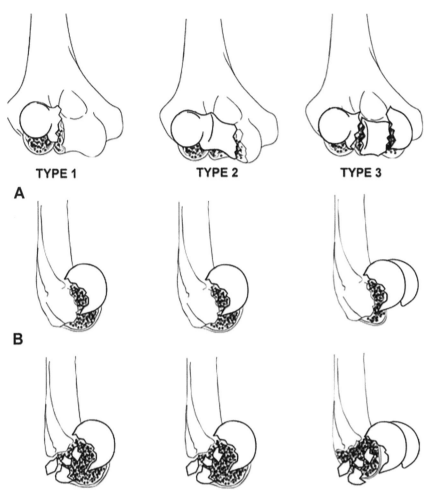

Fig. 1. Dubberley classification of capitellar and trochlear fractures. (*From* Dubberley JH, Faber KJ, Macdermid JC, et al. Outcome after open reduction and internal fixation of capitellar and trochlear fractures. J Bone Joint Surg Am 2006;88(1):47; with permission.)

column plate may help maintain reduction of the articular surface.

Patient Positioning

Patients are initially placed supine; following general or regional anesthesia, an image intensifier is used to evaluate for associated varus, valgus, or posterolateral rotatory instability. The integrity of the collateral ligaments is examined with the elbow in full extension as well as at 15° to 30° of flexion. With the shoulder in full external rotation, valgus stability of the elbow is evaluated by applying a valgus force to the forearm. The shoulder is then placed in internal rotation, and a varus force is applied about the elbow. The lateral pivot shift test is used to evaluate for posterolateral rotatory instability.[28]

The patients' position during the operative procedure depends on the fracture type, surgical approach, and surgeon preference. Some investigators prefer the lateral decubitus position, whereas others place patients supine with the arm across the chest. When positioned laterally, the elbow is propped up using rolled linen placed between the patients' arm and body. This technique avoids having to drape the arm over a bolster, avoiding the risk of compression of the anterior neurovascular structures; the linen can be easily removed allowing the arm to be positioned for intraoperative fluoroscopy. For simple fractures or those extending medially, one investigator prefers patients supine with the arm across the chest. In this position, the lateral elbow can be hinged open on the intact medial structures facilitating access to the trochlea. In all instances, a sterile tourniquet is applied after standard sterile prep and draping.

Surgical Approach

Several surgical exposures may be used; the optimal choice depends on fracture characteristics, associated periarticular injuries, and surgeon familiarity. The authors prefer a posterior skin incision for coronal shear fractures of the distal humerus. Superficial dissection for isolated capitellum fractures begins by elevating a laterally based full-thickness skin flap off the deep fascia. If access to the medial aspect of the elbow is required to address a trochlear fracture or soft tissue injury, a medial flap is raised using the same posterior skin incision.

The deep exposure to the lateral elbow is simplified in situations whereby the LCL has been disrupted or the lateral epicondyle has been fractured. Access to the capitellum is gained by reflecting the fractured epicondyle distally or the elbow may be hinged open when the LCL is incompetent.

If the LCL complex remains intact, the authors prefer to work through the intermuscular plane of the anconeus and extensor carpi ulnaris (ECU [Kocher interval[29]]). The dissection is carried anteriorly beneath the ECU, and an arthrotomy is created along the midaxis of the epicondyle to avoid iatrogenic disruption of the lateral ulnar collateral ligament (LUCL). To improve visualization of the anterior compartment, a Kocher interval may be extended proximally to release an inferior portion of the common extensor mass. In performing this extensile maneuver, the forearm should be maintained in pronation to avoid injury to the posterior interosseous nerve and the proximal dissection should avoid the radial nerve.

Access to the posterior aspect of the capitellum may be required to mobilize impacted fragments or for placement of plates and screws. When this is required, the authors prefer to release the LUCL from it origin on the epicondyle. Following fracture fixation, a meticulous LUCL repair must be performed to avoid iatrogenic posterolateral rotatory instability. Alternatively, the posterior capitellum can be exposed using the proximal extent of the approach described by Boyd,[30] whereby the ECU is elevated from the subcutaneous border of the ulna.

Capitellum fractures extending into the trochlea may not be adequately accessed using laterally based extensile maneuvers. If medial fracture visualization is not satisfactory, the flexor-pronator mass may be split and elevated anteriorly off the medial epicondyle as described by Hotchkiss[31] or an olecranon osteotomy may be used. To facilitate early motion, the authors prefer fixation of the olecranon osteotomy with a plate and screw construct (**Fig. 2**); alternatively, tension-band fixation may be used.

Fracture Fixation

Once the fracture is adequately exposed, the hematoma is carefully removed and the morphology of the fracture, the degree of displacement and the presence of comminution are determined. To minimize risk of avascular necrosis, the fracture fragments are gently manipulated into a reduced position taking care to preserve remaining soft tissue attachments (**Fig. 3**). Flexion of the elbow and pronation of the forearm assists in maintaining the reduction while internal fixation is placed.

Several methods of fixation have been used in the treatment of coronal shear fractures of the distal humerus and include fine-threaded Kirschner wires (k-wires), biodegradable pins, headless compression screws, small fragment cancellous screws, and plates.[3–7,9–15,21–23] In vitro biomechanical testing of these methods of fixation exists only for partially threaded cancellous and headless compression screws. Elkowitz and colleagues[32] simulated capitellar fractures and made the following observations: (1) Load to failure was equivalent when the partially threaded cancellous screws were introduced in a posterior-anterior direction. (2) Headless compression screws provided superior resistance to cyclic loading. If the cancellous screws were directed anterior to posterior, they had inferior resistance to pull out, less load to failure, and increased the risk of splitting the fracture fragment.

For a large capitellum fracture with sufficient subchondral bone, the authors prefer to use cannulated partially threaded screws (**Fig. 4**). The k-wire is inserted into the fragment from a posteroanterior direction and perpendicular to the fracture plane. The trajectory is assessed with fluoroscopy, and the screws are advanced over the k-wire to compress the fracture. Alternatively, the fracture may be compressed manually and fully threaded cannulated screws may be used. The fully threaded screws may prevent the fracture from shearing.

Stable fixation with posteroanterior screws cannot be reliably achieved when the capitellum fracture lacks sufficient subchondral bone. Those fractures with only a thin shell of subchondral bone are fixed with anteroposteriorly directed cannulated headless compression screw.

Comminuted coronal shear fractures with associated bone defects should be recognized and

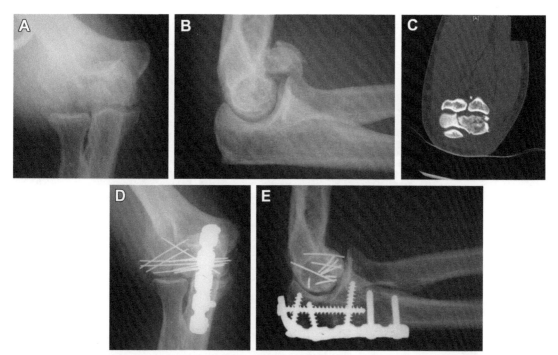

Fig. 2. Olecranon osteotomy. (*A*) Anteroposterior and (*B*) lateral radiographs with (*C*) axial CT demonstrating a comminuted coronal shear fracture involving the capitellum and trochlea. (*D, E*) An olecranon osteotomy was required for visualization and postoperative anteroposterior and lateral radiographs the osteotomy repaired with a plate and screw construct.

addressed. When extensive comminution of the fracture exists, small fragment fixation may be achieved with the use of countersunk fine-threaded k-wires (**Fig. 5**). Nonthreaded k-wires can migrate and should be avoided. Bone defects may result from comminution or are often seen following the reduction of larger impacted fracture fragments. To improve stability and maintain anatomic reduction of the articular surface, these defects are reinforced with bone graft and/or augmented with locking posterolateral plate fixation (**Fig. 6**). When possible, the authors prefer to use iliac crest autograft or, alternatively, synthetic bone graft substitute.

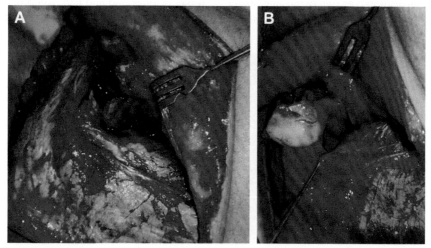

Fig. 3. (*A, B*) To minimize the risk of avascular necrosis, care is taken to preserve remaining soft tissue attachments to displaced fragments.

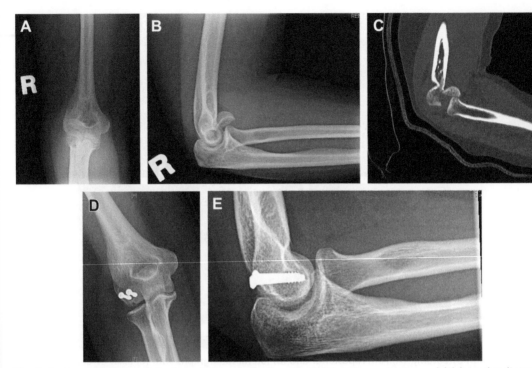

Fig. 4. Posteroanterior, partially threaded screw fixation. (*A–C*) (*A*) Anteroposterior and (*B*) lateral radiographs with (*C*) sagittal CT scan. (*D, E*) Postoperative image showing the use of posteroanterior-directed partially threaded screw fixation.

The final fracture reduction and internal fixation are evaluated both clinically and radiographically. The full arc of elbow flexion-extension and pronation-supination is examined while examining for a mechanical block or crepitation. Intraoperative fluoroscopy is used to evaluate the reduction of the articular surfaces, joint congruity, and hardware position.

The LCL is repaired before closure (**Fig. 7**). It may have been disrupted as part of the initial injury or released from its origin on the lateral epicondyle to enhance visualization of the fracture. A strong repair is essential to avoid instability. The tissue is captured using a running, locked technique with a heavy nonabsorbable. Two divergent transosseous tunnels originating at the isometric point on the lateral epicondyle and exiting posterior to the supracondylar ridge are created with a 2-mm drill. After the suture ends are retrieved posteriorly, the elbow is placed in pronation/flexion and the repair is tensioned and tied over a bony bridge. A bone button or cortical augment may be

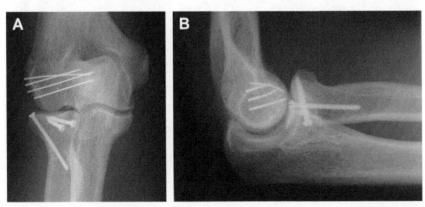

Fig. 5. (*A, B*) Postoperative anteroposterior and lateral radiographs of a comminuted capitellum fracture extending into the trochlear, which was treated with ORIF fine-threaded k-wire.

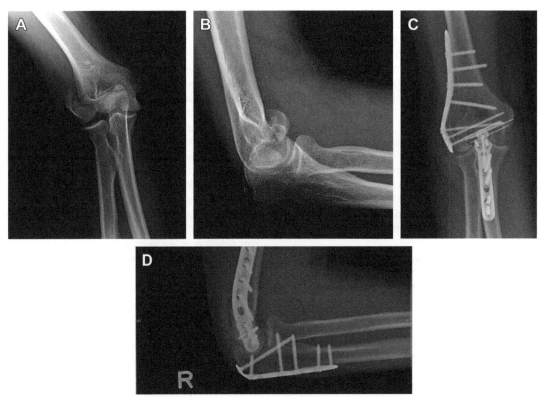

Fig. 6. Posterolateral plate fixation. (*A*) Anteroposterior and (*B*) lateral radiographs demonstrating a coronal shear fracture of the distal humerus with comminution and extension into the lateral epicondyle. (*C, D*) Postoperative (*A*) anteroposterior and (*B*) lateral radiographs of fracture fixation using fine-threaded k-wires and a posterolateral plate.

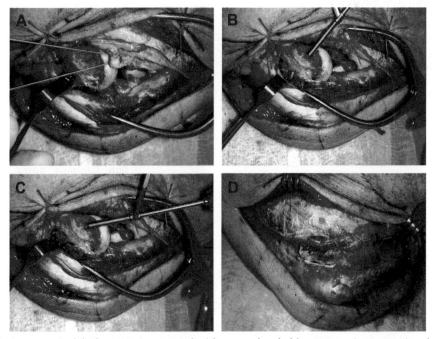

Fig. 7. Soft tissue repair. (*A*) The LUCL is captured with a nonabsorbable suture using a running, locked technique. (*B, C*) Two divergent tunnels originate at the isometric point on the lateral epicondyle and exit posterior to the supracondylar ridge. (*D*) The fascia overlying the intermuscular planes is closed with interrupted figure-of-eights using an braided absorbable suture.

necessary if bone comminution is present posteriorly. If the medial collateral ligament (MCL) is disrupted, the elbow should be carefully evaluated for residual instability. In most cases, the MCL does not require repair; but if the fixation is tenuous or residual elbow instability is present, then transosseous MCL repair should be performed.

The fascia overlying the intermuscular planes is closed to augment elbow stability. Interrupted figure-of-eight stitches using a heavy, braided absorbable suture is used to achieve this. The subcutaneous layer is closed with a 3-0 braided suture in a simple, inverted pattern. A 3-0 monofilament suture is used to reapproximate the skin edges.

Immediate Postoperative Care

Elbow stability and a stable arc of motion are reassessed once again following soft tissue closure. Congruity of the articular surfaces is evaluated using fluoroscopy with the forearm in the pronated, supinated, and neutral positions. Based on this assessment, the elbow is splinted in a position of stability for 2 weeks.

Patients are prescribed 25 mg of indomethacin 3 times daily for 3 weeks as prophylaxis against heterotopic bone formation, unless otherwise contraindicated.

Rehabilitation and Recovery

Motion is typically initiated at 2 weeks postoperatively. Early range of motion is delayed when stability of the fracture is inadequate. Limiting elbow extension helps to maintain fracture reduction by enabling the radial head to capture the articular fragment. An extension-block splint may be used to facilitate motion within the stable arc.

The integrity of the collateral ligaments is incorporated into a ligament-specific rehabilitation protocol. In the LCL-deficient elbow, joint kinematics are improved with the forearm in pronation,[33] whereas placing the forearm in supination stabilizes the MCL-deficient elbow.[34] If the LCL was repaired and the MCL remains insufficient, an MCL unloading protocol is used (flexion-extension with the forearm supinated). An LCL unloading protocol is used if the LCL is deficient but the MCL remains intact. If both collaterals are deficient or require protection, elbow flexion-extension is initiated with the forearm in neutral rotation. The protected arc of motion is progressively increased on a weekly basis. Forearm rotation is encouraged but performed only with the elbow is flexed beyond 90°. Radiographs are recommended for the first 3 weeks to ensure that the joint remains congruently reduced.

Unrestricted range of motion begins at 6 weeks. Progressive strengthening is initiated at 8 to 10 weeks postoperatively provided there is evidence of clinical and radiographic healing of the fracture. A general approach to rehabilitation is outlined in **Fig. 8**.

CLINICAL RESULTS IN THE LITERATURE

Several treatment options have been proposed for the management of capitellum and trochlea fractures. Selecting the single best option to manage these fractures is challenging for several reasons: (1) The injury pattern is uncommon, and large clinical trials comparing different interventions would be difficult to conduct. (2) The clinical studies available are exclusively case series and have inherent limitations and bias. (3) The utility of available

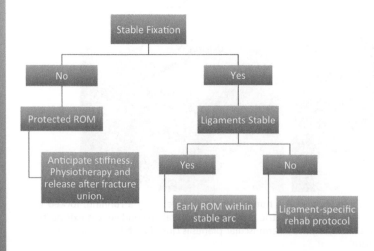

Fig. 8. General approach to rehabilitation following operatively treated capitellum or trochlear fractures. (*Modified from* Faber KJ. Coronal shear fractures of the distal humerus: the capitellum and trochlea. Hand Clin 2004;20(4):462; with permission.)

outcome data is limited by use of various functional scores that cannot be directly compared.

Without high-quality evidence to support treatment decisions, the fracture characteristics and presence of associated periarticular injury generally dictate management. ORIF has been studied most frequently; the results of ORIF as well as fragment excision, closed reduction, and AAIF are summarized in **Table 1**.

Open Reduction and Internal Fixation

ORIF, based on the volume of published literature, is the predominant method for treating displaced capitellum fractures. Most of the reports are noncomparative case series. Definitive treatment recommendations are difficult to establish because existing reports use a variety of fixation methods, fracture classification systems, and varying outcome measures.

In 2006, Dubberley and colleagues[9] reviewed 28 patients with an average follow-up of 56 months. Depending on the fracture characteristics, ORIF was performed using standard cancellous or Herbert screws and supplemented by threaded k-wires or pelvic reconstruction plates. The outcomes were excellent based on the Mayo Elbow Performance Index ([MEPI], average of 91), American Shoulder and Elbow Scores (average of 290), and postoperative range of motion (extension-flexion arc of 19°–138°). According to the proposed classification system, the investigators concluded that type 1 fractures have fewer complications, require less reoperations, and have better outcomes than type 3 patterns.

Subsequent reports have supported the work of Dubberley and colleagues.[9] In 2010, Mighell and colleagues[11] reported on a case series of noncomminuted capitellum fractures (Dubberley 1A and 2A) whereby all fractures united and 17 of 18 patients had good or excellent results according to the Broberg-Morrey scale.[35] Brouwer and colleagues[4] reported on a series of 30 patients, 18 of which had type 3B patterns according to the description of Dubberley and colleagues.[9] At a minimum of 1-year follow-up, 8 of the 18 patients developed a nonunion. The investigators highlighted the difficulty in obtaining rigid fixation and the potential for disrupting the blood supply in the setting of significant posterior comminution.

Fragment Excision

Available studies of patients treated with fragment excision are dated and limited by variability in fracture type (Bryan and Morrey type 1[20] and 2[8]). The largest of the series reported fair to poor results primarily caused by loss of motion, which

averaged 40°.[8] Both Grantham and colleagues[8] and Dushuttle and colleagues[20] warn of the potential for valgus instability and compromised outcomes if the capitellum is excised in the setting of a medial collateral ligament injury.

Closed Reduction

In 1985, Ochner and colleagues[16] described successful closed reduction of 9 capitellum fractures. The investigators detailed a technique requiring general anesthesia with full muscle relaxation. The elbow is placed in full extension and the forearm in supination, which reduces the displaced capitellum. Gentle distraction, flexion, and valgus of the elbow then captures the fragment to stabilize the reduction. No redisplacement following successful reduction was noted. The effectiveness of the technique could not be determined, however, as the total number of patients who underwent attempted closed reduction was not discussed. In the follow-up of 6 patients, ranging from 5 months to 9 years, the investigators reported a slight loss of terminal extension in 3 patients, whereas the remainder regained full range of motion.

Two recent case series with a minimum of 18 months of follow-up reported similarly favorable results in patients with Bryan and Morrey type 1 fractures.[18,36] Both Puloski and colleagues[36] and Cutbush and colleagues[18] reported excellent motion and outcomes based on the Disabilities of the Arm, Shoulder, and Hand (DASH) score.

Arthroscopic-Assisted Reduction and Internal Fixation

AARIF of capitellum fractures is among the expanding indications in minimally invasive elbow surgery[37]; despite this, however, relatively little has been published on the technique. Existing case reports are encouraging, demonstrating excellent range of motion and few complications.[21–23] Proponents of AARIF cite better visualization of associated lesions, improved accuracy of fracture reduction, less risk of devascularizing fracture fragments, and avoidance of trauma to static and dynamic stabilizers of the elbow.[21–23] Despite the theoretic benefits, larger studies and outcome data are required to better understand the role of AARIF in the management of these uncommon fracture patterns.

Arthroplasty

The literature defining the role of arthroplasty in the management of coronal shear fractures is sparse. Fractures of the capitellum and trochlea are among the evolving indications for distal humeral hemiarthroplasty.[25] In 2012, Adolfsson and Nestorson[38] reported the results of 8 patients undergoing hemiarthroplasty for OTA type B3 and C3 fractures of the distal humerus.[38] Primarily good to excellent MEPI scores were reported at an average of 4.5 years of follow-up. Although Kepler and colleagues[39] published a good outcome following radiocapitellar arthroplasty for a capitellum fracture nonunion, larger studies on primary arthroplasty for coronal shear fractures are not available.

Total elbow arthroplasty (TEA) and distal humeral hemiarthroplasty have been recommended for the treatment of comminuted, intra-articular distal humerus fractures not amendable to stable ORIF.[24,25] McKee and colleagues[24] compared TEA with ORIF in a cohort of OTA 13.C fractures. Functional outcomes of TEA were superior to those treated with ORIF in this randomized study of elderly patients.

COMPLICATIONS

Excision of fracture fragments as the primary treatment was described in early studies reporting capitellum and trochlea fractures. The most commonly reported issue was failure to regain full range of motion postoperatively. Valgus instability was seen in 2 of 5 patients reported on by Dushuttle and colleagues[20]; both patients had an associated medial elbow injury.

The complications reported in studies of patients being treated with ORIF are summarized in **Box 1**. The most commonly cited complication was failure to regain full range of motion, particularly the flexion-extension arc. In some of the larger studies, functionally limiting stiffness requiring operative intervention was seen in 21%[9] to 29%[7] of patients. Most patients achieved a functional arc of motion through nonoperative modalities. Although no uniform criteria to determine fracture union exist, the reported rates of fracture union were 73% to 100%. Comminuted fractures extending into the trochlea account for a large portion of the nonunions. Brouwer and colleagues[4] pointed out that 8 of 18 (44%) of Dubberley 3B fractures developed a nonunion. The investigators theorized that the posterior comminution compromised the blood supply and resulted in nonrigid fixation.[4] Several studies identified the formation of heterotopic bone following ORIF.[6,9–11] Although the amount of bone formation was not quantified, most studies reported that the heterotopic ossification was functionally insignificant and did not require treatment (**Fig. 9**). The use of prophylaxis was either not discussed or was administered to selected patients at the surgeon's discretion.

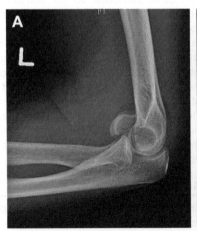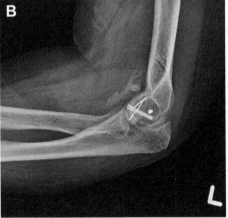

Fig. 9. Heterotopic ossification. (*A*) Preoperative lateral radiograph of a large capitellum-trochlea fracture. (*B*) Six-week postoperative lateral radiograph demonstrating heterotopic bone formation.

SUMMARY

Coronal shear fractures of the distal humerus are uncommon, and the current body of literature is limited to case series whereby it is difficult to draw firm conclusions on treatment and outcomes. Several classification systems exist to describe capitellum and trochlea fractures. They emphasize the continuum of injury severity and complexity. Several treatment options exist and include closed reduction, fragment excision, ORIF, AARIF, and arthroplasty.

An evidence-based management strategy does not exist. For displaced fractures without significant posterior comminution, an attempted closed reduction may be considered. Arthroscopic-assisted management may emerge as an increasingly accepted strategy as arthroscopic techniques continue to evolve. In active, high-demand patients with increasingly complex and displaced fracture patterns, open reduction and stable internal fixation is the preferred strategy. Arthroplasty may be considered in lower-demand and/or elderly patients as well as in situations whereby stable internal fixation cannot be achieved.

REFERENCES

1. Foulk DA, Robertson PA, Timmerman LA. Fracture of the trochlea. J Orthop Trauma 1995;9(6):530–2.
2. Bryan RS, Morrey BF. Fractures of the distal humerus. In: Morrey BF, editor. The elbow and its disorders. Philadelphia: WB Saunders; 1985. p. 302–99.
3. Heck S, Zilleken C, Pennig D, et al. Reconstruction of radial capitellar fractures using fine-threaded implants (FFS). Injury 2012;43(2):163–7.
4. Brouwer KM, Jupiter JB, Ring D. Nonunion of operatively treated capitellum and trochlear fractures. J Hand Surg Am 2011;36(5):804–7.
5. Giannicola G, Sacchetti FM, Greco A, et al. Open reduction and internal fixation combined with hinged elbow fixator in capitellum and trochlea fractures. Acta Orthop 2010;81(2):228–33.
6. Ruchelsman DE. Open reduction and internal fixation of capitellar fractures with headless screws. J Bone Joint Surg Am 2008;90(6):1321.
7. Ring D, Jupiter JB, Gulotta L. Articular fractures of the distal part of the humerus. J Bone Joint Surg Am 2003;85-A(2):232–8.
8. Grantham SA, Norris TR, Bush DC. Isolated fracture of the humeral capitellum. Clin Orthop Relat Res 1981;(161):262–9.
9. Dubberley JH, Faber KJ, Macdermid JC, et al. Outcome after open reduction and internal fixation of capitellar and trochlear fractures. J Bone Joint Surg Am 2006;88(1):46–54.
10. Bilsel K, Atalar AC, Erdil M, et al. Coronal plane fractures of the distal humerus involving the capitellum and trochlea treated with open reduction internal fixation. Arch Orthop Trauma Surg 2013;133(6):797–804.
11. Mighell M, Virani NA, Shannon R, et al. Large coronal shear fractures of the capitellumand trochlea treated with headless compression screws. J Shoulder Elbow Surg 2010;19(1):38–45.
12. Singh AP, Singh AP, Vaishya R, et al. Fractures of capitellum: a review of 14 cases treated by open reduction and internal fixation with Herbert screws. Int Orthop 2010;34(6):897–901.
13. Mahirogullari M, Kiral A, Solakoglu C, et al. Treatment of fractures of the humeral capitellum using Herbert screws. J Hand Surg Br 2006;31(3):320–5.
14. Sano S, Rokkaku T, Saito S, et al. Herbert screw fixation of capitellar fractures. J Shoulder Elbow Surg 2005;14(3):307–11.
15. McKee MD, Jupiter JB, Bamberger HB. Coronal shear fractures of the distal end of the humerus. J Bone Joint Surg Am 1996;78(1):49–54.
16. Ochner RS, Bloom H, Palumbo RC, et al. Closed reduction of coronal fractures of the capitellum. J Trauma 1996;40(2):199–203.
17. Ma YZ, Zheng CB, Zhou TL, et al. Percutaneous probe reduction of frontal fractures of the humeral capitellum. Clin Orthop Relat Res 1984;(183):17–21.
18. Cutbush K, Andrews S, Siddiqui N, et al. Capitellar fractures – is ORIF necessary? J Orthop Trauma 2014. http://dx.doi.org/10.1097/BOT.0000000000000148.
19. Feldman MD. Arthroscopic excision of type II capitellar fractures. Arthroscopy 1997;13(6):743–8.
20. Dushuttle RP, Coyle MP, Zawadsky JP, et al. Fractures of the capitellum. J Trauma 1985;25(4):317–21.
21. Kuriyama K, Kawanishi Y, Yamamoto K. Arthroscopic-assisted reduction and percutaneous fixation for coronal shear fractures of the distal humerus: report of two cases. J Hand Surg Am 2010;35(9):1506–9.
22. Mitani M, Nabeshima Y, Ozaki A, et al. Arthroscopic reduction and percutaneous cannulated screw fixation of a capitellar fracture of the humerus: a case report. J Shoulder Elbow Surg 2009;18(2):e6–9.
23. Hardy P, Menguy F, Guillot S. Arthroscopic treatment of capitellum fracture of the humerus. Arthroscopy 2002;18(4):422–6.
24. McKee MD, Veillette CJ, Hall JA, et al. A multicenter, prospective, randomized, controlled trial of open reduction-internal fixation versus total elbow arthroplasty for displaced intra-articular distal humeral fractures in elderly patients. J Shoulder Elbow Surg 2009;18:3–12.
25. Lapner M, King GJW. Elbow arthroplasty for distal humeral fractures. Instr Course Lect 2014;63:15–26.
26. Doornberg J, Lindenhovius A, Kloen P, et al. Two and three-dimensional computed tomography for

the classification and management of distal humeral fractures. Evaluation of reliability and diagnostic accuracy. J Bone Joint Surg Am 2006;88(8):1795–801.

27. Marsh JL, Slongo TF, Agel J, et al. Fracture and dislocation classification compendium - 2007: Orthopaedic Trauma Association classification, database and outcomes committee. J Orthop Trauma 2007;21(10 Suppl):S1–133.

28. O'Driscoll SW, Bell DF, Morrey BF. Posterolateral rotatory instability of the elbow. J Bone Joint Surg Am 1991;73(3):440–6.

29. Kocher ET. Textbook of operative surgery. 3rd edition. London: Adam & Charles Black; 1911.

30. Boyd HB. Surgical exposure of the ulna and proximal third of the radius through one incision. Surg Gynecol Obstet 1940;7:137–88.

31. Hotchkiss R. Displaced fractures of the radial head: internal fixation or excision? J Am Acad Orthop Surg 1997;5(1):1–10.

32. Elkowitz SJ, Polatsch DB, Egol KA, et al. Capitellum fractures: a biomechanical evaluation of three fixation methods. J Orthop Trauma 2002;16(7):503–6.

33. Dunning CE, Zarzour ZD, Patterson SD, et al. Muscle forces and pronation stabilize the lateral ligament deficient elbow. Clin Orthop Relat Res 2001;(388):118–24.

34. Armstrong AD, Dunning CE, Faber KJ, et al. Rehabilitation of the medial collateral ligament-deficient elbow: an in vitro biomechanical study. J Hand Surg Am 2000;25(6):1051–7.

35. Broberg MA, Morrey BF. Results of delayed excision of the radial head after fracture. J Bone Joint Surg Am 1986;68(5):669–74.

36. Puloski S, Kemp K, Sheps D, et al. Closed reduction and early mobilization in fractures of the humeral capitellum. J Orthop Trauma 2012;26(1):62–5.

37. Yeoh KM, King GJW, Faber KJ, et al. Evidence-based indications for elbow arthroscopy. Arthroscopy 2012;28(2):272–82.

38. Adolfsson L, Nestorson J. The Kudo humeral component as primary hemiarthroplasty in distal humeral fractures. J Shoulder Elbow Surg 2012;21(4):451–5.

39. Kepler CK, Kummer JL, Lorich DG, et al. Radiocapitellar prosthetic arthroplasty for capitellar nonunion. J Shoulder Elbow Surg 2010;19(2):e13–7.

Distal Biceps Injuries

John Haverstock, MD, FRCSC*, George S. Athwal, MD, FRCSC,
Ruby Grewal, MD, MSc, FRCSC

KEYWORDS

- Distal biceps injuries • Distal biceps repair • One-incision repair • Two-incision repair

KEY POINTS

- The diagnosis of partial ruptures of the distal biceps tendon is difficult and should be considered in the differential diagnosis for anterior elbow pain.
- Physical examination is key to the diagnosis, and routine imaging studies are not needed if physical examination is clear.
- Both 1- and 2-incision techniques have excellent results in the literature.
- Two-incision techniques may better re-create supination strength by restoring the windlass effect.

INTRODUCTION

The incidence of distal biceps tendon ruptures (DBTRs) has been estimated to be 1.2 ruptures per 100,000 people per year.[1] These injuries typically occur in the dominant arm, with men aged 30 to 60 years being most commonly affected. Women are very rarely affected. Those women who are, typically present at an older age, with a longer history of prodromal symptoms; may have profound bicipital bursitis; and have a greater chance of incomplete ruptures, in contrast to the complete and acute injuries commonly experienced by men.[2,3]

The preponderance of male DBTR may be related to the increased muscular cross-sectional area creating greater forces across tendons. Patients sustaining an initial DBTR are at increased risk of sustaining a second DBTR; Green and colleagues[4] found an 8% cumulative incidence of bilateral DBTR at an interval of 4.1 years, while Iwamoto and colleagues[5] found an incidence of 13%, both implying a systemic cause.

Theories as to the cause of DBTRs include inflammation, impingement, and hypovascularity. Seiler and colleagues[6] found a hypovascular zone in the middle of the distal biceps tendon (DBT) that may increase the risk of rupture, although this does not explain why most ruptures occur at the tendon insertion on the radial tuberosity. The investigators also found that the space between the proximal ulna and radius decreased by 50% in full pronation and that 85% of the space available was occupied by the DBT. Safran and Graham[1] found a higher rate of DBTR in smokers. The investigators attributed a 7.5 times higher risk of DBTR to a proposed mechanism of repetitive anoxia, combined with hypovascularity and repetitive impingement.

HISTORY

The mechanism of injury is most commonly a sudden eccentric force against a flexed elbow, often during heavy lifting, a fall, or sporting activities with reports of a pop being heard or felt in 35% of cases.[7,8] Within days, there is often edema and ecchymosis, which may vary depending on the severity of bicipital aponeurosis (BA) disruption.[8] In the subacute period, patients may complain of weakness and fatigue in elbow flexion and supination.[7]

Disclosure Statement: The authors have no conflicts of interest that relate to this work on distal biceps tendon injuries.
Roth McFarlane Hand and Upper Limb Centre, London, Ontario, Canada
* Corresponding author. The Hand and Upper Limb Centre, St Joseph's Health Centre, Suite D0-205, 268 Grosvenor Street, London, Ontario N6A 4L6, Canada.
E-mail address: john.haverstock@gmail.com

Hand Clin 31 (2015) 631–640
http://dx.doi.org/10.1016/j.hcl.2015.06.009
0749-0712/15/$ – see front matter © 2015 Elsevier Inc. All rights reserved.

hand.theclinics.com

A partial rupture may lack a clear mechanism of injury suggesting a chronic degenerative cause, or it may have an acute onset as in complete tears.[9–11] A partial biceps tendon rupture and cubital bursitis should be on the differential diagnosis for patients presenting with chronic pain in the antecubital fossa.[11,12]

PHYSICAL EXAMINATION

Inspection of the affected arm reveals an elevated biceps brachii muscle belly in complete injuries with a variable amount of ecchymosis and edema. Range of motion (ROM) and elbow flexion strength are generally preserved, although they may be limited by pain. Weakness of resisted supination is common and may be accompanied by pain.

Pain with resisted supination and tenderness to palpation over the biceps tendon were the most reliable findings for partial biceps tear in a series by Dellaero and Mallon.[11] Those with partial ruptures exhibit tenderness when the bicipital tuberosity is palpated with the forearm in full pronation.[10,13]

The biceps hook test is a simple and effective means to judge whether the DBT is intact. As described by O'Driscoll and colleagues,[14] the examiner attempts to hook the DBT from lateral to medial, while the patient holds the arm in 90° of elbow flexion and supination; an intact tendon allows the examiner to hook the tendon and pull it forward, whereas partially ruptured tendons may show an intact hook test, with pain during the anterior pull.

Harding[15] describes a test by which the examiner observes the contour changes of the distal biceps muscle as the arm is passively supinated and pronated with the elbow in 90° of flexion. An intact DBT causes the biceps muscle belly to rise and fall with supination and pronation, respectively, while a qualitative difference, or complete absence of the rise and fall occurs with varying completeness of DBTR.[15] The authors have found this test to be useful and simple to perform.

An excellent article by ElMaraghy and Devereaux[8] describes the bicipital aponeurosis flex test to detect whether the BA (also known as the lacertus fibrosus) is intact or ruptured with DBT.[8] The patient is asked to make a fist and flex and supinate the wrist. With the elbow in 75° of flexion, the examiner then lightly palpates the antecubital fossa to detect the sharp edge of the tensioned BA, medial and distal to the biceps tendon. An intact BA acts as a secondary restraint, preventing DBT retraction, and may ease repair and minimize the complications associated with a retracted DBT.

ElMaraghy and colleagues[16] also describe the biceps crease interval (BCI) test, in which the distance from the antecubital flexion crease to the cusp of distal descent of the biceps muscle is measured (N = 4.8+/−0.6 cm) and divided by the BCI of the noninjured arm to determine the biceps crease ratio (BCR). A BCI greater than 6.0 cm had a sensitivity of 96% and diagnostic accuracy of 93% in the detection of DBTR, while a BCR of 1.2 was diagnostic for a complete DBTR in 24 of 29 patients.[16]

IMAGING

The physical examination findings for DBTR are often diagnostic, and imaging is not required to confirm the diagnosis. Imaging is indicated if the physical examination findings are unclear or for the characterization of partial injuries. Devereaux and ElMaraghy[7] established a protocol by which the hook test, passive forearm pronation test, and BCI were evaluated. The sensitivity and specificity of unequivocal results in all 3 tests combined was 100% for DBTR, whereas individual tests alone misled the examiner occasionally. If all 3 tests gave positive results for complete rupture, the patient was offered surgical repair; if the results were equivocal, the diagnosis was confirmed with MRI; and if all 3 tests gave negative result, nonoperative management was considered appropriate.

The imaging modalities most commonly used are MRI and ultrasonography (US). Plain radiograph is of little value in the diagnosis of DBTR and is not routinely obtained, although it may be useful if there is a history of previous elbow pathology. MRI for the diagnosis of complete DBTR has been found to have a sensitivity and specificity of 100% and 82.8%, respectively, whereas in cases of partial DBTR, the sensitivity is substantially decreased to 59.1% with a specificity of 100%.[17] When an MRI is needed, it should be obtained with the arm in the flexed, abducted supinated position, referred to as the FABS view.[18] This position puts the tendon in an alignment that facilitates the interpretation for both complete and incomplete tears, which can be difficult in a traditional position.

US can be a cost-effective alternative to MRI; however, the accuracy and diagnostic value is operator dependent, and it is more effective for the detection of complete tears, rather than incomplete tears. US examination has been shown to differentiate complete DBTR from intact partial DBTR with a 95% sensitivity and 71% specificity, but no data comparing intact distal biceps tendons with DBTR are available.[19]

NONOPERATIVE TREATMENT

The literature detailing outcomes of nonoperative treatment is limited. A commonly cited study is that by Morrey and colleagues,[20] which compared operative treatment with nonoperative treatment and found an average loss of 40% supination strength and 30% flexion strength in the nonoperative group compared with the contralateral arm. More recently, Geaney and colleagues[21] found that after 4 years, a small cohort of patients treated nonoperatively had only a 15% loss of supination strength and attributed this relative improvement to immediate physical therapy and a longer follow-up of 4.5 years.

Freeman and colleagues[22] published an excellent article comparing the strength and functional results of nonoperative versus historical operative cases and found that there was a significant difference in terms of mean supination strength (74% vs 101%, $P = .002$) in those treated operatively, but not in terms of mean flexion strength (88% vs 97%, $P = .164$). While examining those treated nonoperatively, those with injuries to the dominant arm experienced significantly weaker supination but not flexion, whereas those with injuries to the nondominant arm experienced significantly weaker flexion but not supination strength.

Patients should be advised of the expected outcomes of both operative and nonoperative therapy. Those requiring supination strength of the dominant arm may be the best candidates for surgical treatment, whereas those who are able to tolerate flexion and supination strength deficits may be considered for nonoperative treatment. Nonoperative treatment can be considered for all patients because the deficits associated with a DBTR have been tolerated in observational and retrospective studies and may represent a minimal disability for some.[21,22]

RESULTS OF OPERATIVE TREATMENT

Surgical treatment of DBTR may be performed through either a 1- or 2-incision technique, with various fixation methods.

The only prospective randomized control trial in DBTR repair was conducted by Grewal and colleagues[23] to compare the outcomes and complications of the 1- versus the 2-incision technique. After following up patients for 2 years, no difference in patient-reported pain or disability between groups was found. Strength and ROM was similar between the 2 groups aside from improved pronation (76.7° vs 72.4°, $P = .08$) in the 1-incision group and greater mean flexion strength (compared with the contralateral arm) in the 2-incision group (104% vs 94%, $P = .01$). Although these 2 measures were found to be statistically significant, the clinical importance of these small differences are not known. The 1-incision group had a greater

incidence of early transient neuropraxia of the lateral antebrachial cutaneous nerve of the forearm (LABCN) (19 vs 3). A single case of very mild heterotopic ossification (HO) that did not limit ROM occurred in each group. It was concluded that both techniques are effective and that the choice should be based on surgeon expertise and patient preference.

The remaining literature consists mostly of case series and retrospective reviews of various fixation techniques, and these generally report similarly favorable reviews. McKee and colleagues[24] retrospectively reviewed the results of a 1-incision repair using 2 suture anchors and found good results in 53 patients, with no reruptures and no patient losing more than 5° of flexion-extension or pronation-supination. Bain and colleagues[25] described the first use of a cortical button to repair DBTR through a 1-incision technique in 12 patients. Early active mobilization was allowed, and all patients were satisfied and regained grade 5 strength without any neurovascular complications or synostosis. Heinzelmann and colleagues[26] reviewed their results using a combination of interference screw with cortical button. A total of 31 patients were reviewed, and 1 patient was found to have HO with decreased pronation-supination, 2 were found to have self-resolving superficial radial nerve palsies, and the average time to return to work was 6.5 weeks.

Biomechanically, the strength of each repair method has been shown to permit early active ROM, although results detailing superiority have been variable and clinical differences seem minimal. A 2-incision repair using No. 5 Ethibond Excel (Ethicon Inc, Somerville, NJ, USA) outlasted a similar repair using FiberWire (Arthrex Corp, Sunnyvale, CA, USA).[27] Pereira and colleagues[28] found that the bone tunnel repair used in 2-incision technique was stronger and stiffer than suture anchor repair in cadavers with good bone quality. Mazzocca and colleagues[29] compared the 4 described fixation methods and found no statistically significant difference in displacement but a significantly greater load to failure with the cortical button compared with the bone tunnel, suture anchor, and interference screw.

Perhaps most importantly, there is concern that the 1-incision techniques may not reestablish full supination strength because it is unable to recreate the windlass mechanism that results from re-creating the anatomic DBT footprint on the rim of the bicipital tuberosity.[30–32] Schmidt and colleagues[33] conducted a follow-up study of 1-incision, cortical button DBTR repairs using both MRI and strength testing and found that the tendon insertion was placed 73° more anteriorly than that of uninjured controls and this likely caused weakness in isometric supination strength (**Figs. 1–3**).

SURGICAL PLANNING

A key consideration when planning surgery and determining the approach is the time from injury to surgery—a longer delay to surgery may result in a retracted tendon adhering to surrounding tissues and obliteration of the track to the tuberosity. A longer delay may also require a larger anterior incision and increase the complications associated with repair.[34] Other patient factors to consider include the size and ROM of the forearm and shoulder.

Advantages of each approach are summarized in **Table 1**.

The authors favor operative treatment for symptomatic individuals with a complete biceps tear and a desire to maximize supination strength and endurance or for those with a high-grade tear that does not improve with a trial of physical therapy (>50%).[9] When preoperative planning does not result in a favored technique, the authors prefer the 2-incision technique.

Several anatomic dissection studies give insight and information to assist with repair. Athwal and colleagues[38] found that the musculotendinous unit externally rotates 90° from origin to insertion so that the long head of the biceps inserts on the proximal portion of the radial tuberosity while the short head inserts on the distal aspect of the tuberosity. Noting that the lacertus fibrosus originates on the proximal aspect of the short head of the distal biceps tendon can help in orientation during a repair.

Both the long and short head have discrete bundles, and within each tendon sheath, there are a series of distinct bands that are connected together by small oblique bands. Purchase with running sutures into the tendon can be maximized by crossing the entire width of the tendon, avoiding a loss of fixation in sutures that grasp only the margins of the tendon.[39]

Author's Preferred Technique—Modified 2-Incision Technique

1. Position patient supine with a standard arm table and sterile tourniquet.
2. Make a 2 cm transverse incision along the elbow flexion crease, identifying and protecting the basilic vein, the LABCN, and the recurrent radial artery. Working in the interval between pronator teres and brachioradialis, use blunt finger dissection to locate the track of the biceps tendon and the bare bicipital tuberosity distally.
3. Proximally, use a milking maneuver in the distal arm to deliver the end of the ruptured biceps tendon, secure it with an Allis clamp, and free it from scar tissue, ensuring adequate excursion (**Fig. 4**).
4. Debride the distal degenerated tendon without overshortening, and then orient the stump to ensure that the short head is distal. Run 2 robust nonabsorbable braided sutures (eg, No. 2 or 3 Ethibond Excel, Cincinnati, OH or Fiberwire, Arthrex, Naples, FL, USA) in 2 rows of running locking Krackow, leaving 4 strands distal to enable suture passage; cutting the sutures from the short head shorter

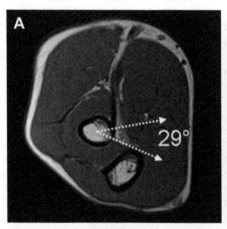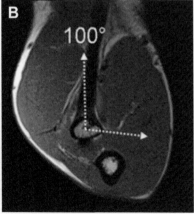

Fig. 1. Axial MRI showing (*A*) the DBT insertion in a healthy volunteer and (*B*) the more anteriorly placed insertion following DBTR; note the windlass effect in the intact tendon of the healthy volunteer. (*From* Schmidt CC, Diaz VA, Weir DM, et al. Repaired distal biceps magnetic resonance imaging anatomy compared with outcome. J Shoulder Elbow Surg 2012;21(12):1629; with permission.)

Anterior

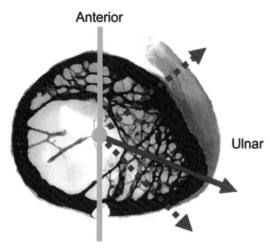

Ulnar

Fig. 2. Cross-sectional image of a bicipital tuberosity that is angulated more posteriorly and will not be repaired anatomically using the 1-incision technique. (*From* Forthman CL, Zimmerman RM, Sullivan MJ, et al. Cross-sectional anatomy of the bicipital tuberosity and biceps brachii tendon insertion: relevance to anatomic tendon repair. J Shoulder Elbow Surg 2008;17(3):524; with permission.)

facilitates orientation after suture passage (**Fig. 5**).

5. Palpate the biceps tuberosity through the anterior incision and pass a curved Kelly retractor (carrying the 4 suture arms) ulnar to it, directing it through the interosseous space toward the dorsal aspect of the forearm. Ensure an assistant is fully pronating the forearm to protect the posterior interosseous nerve (PIN). Pass the curved tip onto the radial

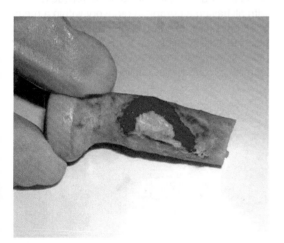

Fig. 3. The long semilunar insertion of the DBT on the ulnar and dorsal aspect of the bicipital tuberosity. (*From* Kulshreshtha R, Singh R, Sinha J, et al. Anatomy of the distal biceps brachii tendon and its clinical relevance. Clin Orthop Relat Res 2007;456:119; with permission.)

tuberosity and run it dorsally between the radius and ulna, taking great care to avoid the ulna. Advance the clamp through the common extensor musculature until it is seen tenting the skin over the dorsal aspect of the proximal forearm (**Fig. 6**).

6. Maintaining the forearm in pronation and flexion, make a longitudinal incision directly over the clamp, exposing the biceps tuberosity through a muscle-splitting technique.

7. Using a burr, prepare a docking site to fit the distal biceps tendon on the ulnar side of the edge of the tuberosity (**Fig. 7**), and ulnar to this, make three 2-mm drill holes, each separated by a minimum of 5 mm to avoid fracture between the holes.[40]

8. Clear away any bone debris with irrigation, and pass the 2 central limbs (one from each running suture) through the trough, exiting through the central drill hole above. Pass the remaining limbs through the remaining 2 holes.

9. With the elbow in 90° flexion and full pronation, pull the sutures, docking the tendon in the radius, and then tie both sutures at full tension (**Fig. 8**).

10. Determine the elbow flexion angle at which the tendon becomes tight to determine whether an extension limit is required to aid in planning postoperative therapy. Repairs requiring up to 90° of flexion are reliably repaired without augmentation.[41]

POSTOPERATIVE CARE

1. There should be a routine prophylaxis for HO with administration of Indocid, 25 mg orally three times a day, and a proton pump inhibitor for 3 weeks unless contraindicated.

2. Splint in 90° and full supination for 1 to 2 days should be provided.

3. A sling or posterior elbow splint at 90° is provided, and the patient begins physiotherapy for active ROM.

4. Patients should not extend the elbow beyond the angle that tightened the tendon intraoperatively.

5. The elbow extension should be increased by 10° each week until full extension is achieved.

6. Unlimited active ROM should be allowed at 6 weeks and strengthening should be started 3 months postoperatively.

COMPLICATIONS

Complications of DBTR repair relate primarily to the approach used (1- vs 2-incision technique)

Table 1
Advantages of the 2- and 1-incision techniques for DBTR

The 2-Incision Technique	The 1-Incision Technique
Smaller anterior incision	No posterior incision
Decreased need for deep retraction and surgical assistance, may be important in patients with larger forearm	—
Lower incidence of LABCN neuropraxia[23,35]	—
Lower implant costs (drill tunnel method)[36]	Familiar implants used
A more anatomic reinsertion point improving the moment arm and restoring the windlass effect to power supination[30,37]	—
Bone-dependent strength and stiffness[28]	Hardware-dependent strength and stiffness
In patients with a limited ability to supinate, the 2-incision technique should be favored to repair the tendon to an anatomically correct position because the bicipital tuberosity will be more difficult to bring anteriorly with the 1-incision technique[30]	In patients with an inability to pronate fully, protecting the PIN during the 2-incision technique is difficult, and the 1-incision technique should be considered
Decreased implant-related complications	Potential for shorter surgical time

Abbreviation: PIN, posterior interosseous nerve.
Data from Refs.[23,28,30,35–37]

and secondarily to the mode of fixation. The original 1-incision approach resulted in neuropraxias secondary to the extensile anterior exposure that was necessary; this prompted Boyd and Anderson[42] to develop a 2-incision repair technique, which minimized nerve injuries. Unfortunately, their approach resulted in a higher rate of HO (44%–62%).[43,44] This result lead Morrey and colleagues[20] to modify the 2-incision technique, using a muscle-splitting approach dorsally and avoiding exposure of the ulna. The 1-incision repair has experienced renewed popularity with the advent of alternative modes of fixation that facilitate the deep reattachment of the biceps tendon without vigorous retraction or a large anterior incision.

Most commonly, the LABCN is injured with the retraction during an anterior approach. The PIN is at risk during the 1-incision technique, with retraction and pressure on the nerve as it winds around the radial neck and through the supinator, and during posterior muscle-splitting approach with the 2-incision technique if the forearm is not pronated. In a large series (n = 280), Nigro and colleagues[45] found a postoperative PIN palsy in 9 patients treated with the 1-incision technique (3.2%), with all having a complete recovery within a mean of 86 days. Use of a cortical button as fixation has also led to PIN injury as it runs in the supinator muscle, opposite the radial tuberosity. Lo and colleagues[46] found that drilling across the radius

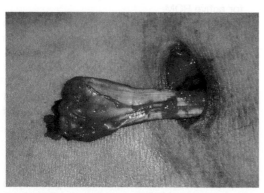

Fig. 4. DBT stump ready before debridement.

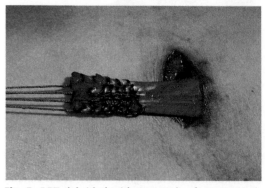

Fig. 5. DBT debrided with 4 strands of suture ready for passage to the posterior incision; note the proximal separation of the tendon into 2 heads.

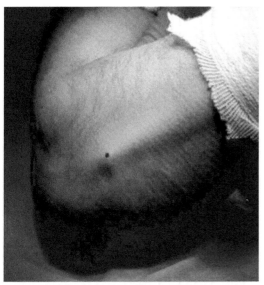

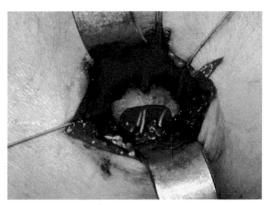

Fig. 8. Posterior muscle-splitting approach to the bicipital tuberosity with sutures ready for docking.

REHABILITATION

Rehabilitation protocols have typically been designed to protect tendon repairs by limiting initial ROM. The period of immobilization in a long-arm splint postoperatively varies from 1 to 6 weeks; this is followed by ROM exercises to gradually extend the elbow and minimize tension across the repair. As reruptures following repair are uncommon, recent studies have questioned the need for immobilization with various early ROM protocols. Cheung and colleagues[49] describe and report the results of an early ROM protocol (postoperative day 1) using a hinged elbow brace. Elbow extension was limited to 60° of flexion initially and decreased by 20° every 2 weeks, achieving full extension at 6 weeks. This protocol resulted in a mean loss of 5.8° of full extension, 3.5° of pronation, and 8.1° of supination. Cil and colleagues[50] report a series of 21 patients treated with a modified mini 2-incision DBTR and allowed early ROM after 1 to 2 days in a sling. By emphasizing early and full ROM, and lifting restricted to 0.45 kg for the first 6 weeks, with full activity after 3 months, no reruptures and good recovery of strength and full ROM were reported (compared with the noninjured extremity).

FUTURE STUDY

Landa and colleagues[51] found that repairing the BA resulted in a significantly greater mean maximum strength on biomechanical testing (256.8 vs 164.5 N, $P = .0058$) and recommend the consideration for the repair of the BA during DBTR. Owing to the proximity of the median nerve and brachial artery, the safety of this will need to be established.

Future work should be aimed at critical examination of specific deficits in supination strength and endurance after both operative and nonoperative

Fig. 6. Prominence of the Kelly clamp in the posterior skin, where the muscle-splitting approach will be made to retrieve sutures and create bone tunnels.

perpendicular to its long axis and aiming 0 to 30° ulnarly reduces this risk by maximizing the distance to the nerve at 16 mm.

Several retrospective studies have assessed the complications rates as a primary outcome.[34,35,47,48] Grewal and colleagues[23] recorded complications in the only prospective study comparing 1- with 2 incisions. Further details regarding the complications reported in these series can be found in **Table 2**.

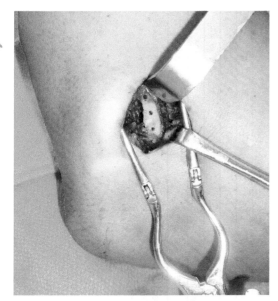

Fig. 7. Posterior muscle-splitting approach showing the prepared docking site in the radius.

Table 2
Complications of 1- and 2-incision DBTRs

		Bisson et al[47]	Kelly et al[34]	Banerjee et al[48]	Cain et al[35]		Grewal et al[23]	
		45[b]	74[b]	27[a]	188[a]	10[b]	47[a]	43[b]
Sample Size								
Nerve Injury	Total	7 (16%)	6 (8%)	6 (15%)	69 (37%)	1 (10%)	19 (40%)	3 (7%)
	LABCN	5 (2 resolved)	3 (2 resolved)	—	51	1	19 (17 resolved)	3 (3 resolved)
	PIN	—	1 (1 resolved)	4 (4 resolved)	7 (6 resolved)	—	—	—
	SRN	—	2 (1 resolved)	2	1	—	—	—
	AIN	1 (1 resolved)	—	—	—	—	—	—
	Ulnar	1	—	—	—	—	—	—
Heterotopic Ossification		3 (6.6%)	4 (5.4%)	3 (11%)	6 (3.1%)	0	1 (2%)	1 (2%)
Stiffness		2 (4.4%)	3 (4%)	NR	3 (2%)	0	NR	NR
Synostosis		3 (6.6%)	0	NR	0	0	0	0
Rerupture		1 (2%)	1 (1.4%)	1 (4%)	4 (2%)	0	3 (6%)	1 (2%)
CRPS		1 (2%)	1 (1.4%)	NR	NR	NR	NR	NR
Hardware Failure		1 (2%)	0	1 (4%)	NR	NR	NR	NR
Persistent pain		1 (2%)	6 (8.1%)	NR	NR	NR	NR	NR

Abbreviations: AIN, anterior interosseous nerve; CRPS, complex regional pain syndrome; NR, not reported; SRN, superficial radial nerve.
[a] One-incision technique.
[b] Two-incision technique.
Data from Refs.[23,34,35,47,48]

treatment because studies have identified persistent deficits that may be due to the inability to restore the windlass effect in current repair techniques.[30,52] The optimization of nonoperative treatment protocols and the full restoration of supination strength and endurance are important goals that will improve patient outcomes.

REFERENCE

1. Safran MR, Graham SM. Distal biceps tendon ruptures: incidence, demographics, and the effect of smoking. Clin Orthop Relat Res 2002;(404):275–83.
2. Jockel CR, Mulieri PJ, Belsky MR, et al. Distal biceps tendon tears in women. J Shoulder Elbow Surg 2010;19(5):645–50.
3. Hinchey JW, Aronowitz JG, Sanchez-Sotelo J, et al. Re-rupture rate of primarily repaired distal biceps tendon injuries. J Shoulder Elbow Surg 2014;23(6): 850–4.
4. Green JB, Skaife TL, Leslie BM. Bilateral distal biceps tendon ruptures. J Hand Surg Am 2012; 37(1):120–3.
5. Iwamoto A, Kearney JP, Goyal G, et al. The incidence of subsequent contralateral distal biceps tendon rupture following unilateral rupture. Orthopedics 2008;31(4):356–8.
6. Seiler JG 3rd, Parker LM, Chamberland PD, et al. The distal biceps tendon. Two potential mechanisms involved in its rupture: arterial supply and mechanical impingement. J Shoulder Elbow Surg 1995;4(3): 149–56.
7. Devereaux MW, ElMaraghy AW. Improving the rapid and reliable diagnosis of complete distal biceps tendon rupture: a nuanced approach to the clinical examination. Am J Sports Med 2013;41(9):1998–2004.
8. ElMaraghy A, Devereaux M. The "bicipital aponeurosis flex test": evaluating the integrity of the bicipital aponeurosis and its implications for treatment of distal biceps tendon ruptures. J Shoulder Elbow Surg 2013;22(7):908–14.
9. Bain GI, Johnson LJ, Turner PC. Treatment of partial distal biceps tendon tears. Sports Med Arthrosc 2008;16(3):154–61.
10. Kelly EW, Steinmann S, O'Driscoll SW. Surgical treatment of partial distal biceps tendon ruptures through a single posterior incision. J Shoulder Elbow Surg 2003;12(5):456–61.
11. Dellaero DT, Mallon WJ. Surgical treatment of partial biceps tendon ruptures at the elbow. J Shoulder Elbow Surg 2006;15(2):215–7.
12. Drosdowech DS, Faber KJ, King GJ. Distal biceps tendon repair: one- and two-incision techniques. Tech Shoulder Elbow Surg 2002;3(2):90–5.
13. Abboud JA, Ricchetti ET, Tjoumakaris FP, et al. The direct radial tuberosity compression test: a sensitive method for diagnosing partial distal biceps tendon ruptures. Curr Orthop Pract 2011;22(1):76–80.
14. O'Driscoll SW, Goncalves LB, Dietz P. The hook test for distal biceps tendon avulsion. Am J Sports Med 2007;35(11):1865–9.
15. Harding WG 3rd. A new clinical test for avulsion of the insertion of the biceps tendon. Orthopedics 2005;28(1):27–9.
16. ElMaraghy A, Devereaux M, Tsoi K. The biceps crease interval for diagnosing complete distal biceps tendon ruptures. Clin Orthop Relat Res 2008; 466(9):2255–62.
17. Festa A, Mulieri PJ, Newman JS, et al. Effectiveness of magnetic resonance imaging in detecting partial and complete distal biceps tendon rupture. J Hand Surg Am 2010;35(1):77–83.
18. Giuffre BM, Moss MJ. Optimal positioning for MRI of the distal biceps brachii tendon: flexed abducted supinated view. AJR Am J Roentgenol 2004; 182(4):944–6.
19. Lobo Lda G, Fessell DP, Miller BS, et al. The role of sonography in differentiating full versus partial distal biceps tendon tears: correlation with surgical findings. AJR Am J Roentgenol 2013;200(1):158–62.
20. Morrey BF, Askew LJ, An KN, et al. Rupture of the distal tendon of the biceps brachii. A biomechanical study. J Bone Joint Surg Am 1985;67(3):418–21.
21. Geaney LE, Brenneman DJ, Cote MP, et al. Outcomes and practical information for patients choosing nonoperative treatment for distal biceps ruptures. Orthopedics 2010;33(6):391.
22. Freeman CR, McCormick KR, Mahoney D, et al. Nonoperative treatment of distal biceps tendon ruptures compared with a historical control group. J Bone Joint Surg Am 2009;91(10):2329–34.
23. Grewal R, Athwal GS, MacDermid JC, et al. Single versus double-incision technique for the repair of acute distal biceps tendon ruptures: a randomized clinical trial. J Bone Joint Surg Am 2012;94(13): 1166–74.
24. McKee MD, Hirji R, Schemitsch EH, et al. Patient-oriented functional outcome after repair of distal biceps tendon ruptures using a single-incision technique. J Shoulder Elbow Surg 2005;14(3):302–6.
25. Bain GI, Prem H, Heptinstall RJ, et al. Repair of distal biceps tendon rupture: a new technique using the Endobutton. J Shoulder Elbow Surg 2000;9(2): 120–6.
26. Heinzelmann AD, Savoie FH 3rd, Ramsey JR, et al. A combined technique for distal biceps repair using a soft tissue button and biotenodesis interference screw. Am J Sports Med 2009;37(5):989–94.
27. Bisson LJ, de Perio JG, Weber AE, et al. Is it safe to perform aggressive rehabilitation after distal biceps tendon repair using the modified 2-incision approach? A biomechanical study. Am J Sports Med 2007;35(12):2045–50.

28. Pereira DS, Kvitne RS, Liang M, et al. Surgical repair of distal biceps tendon ruptures: a biomechanical comparison of two techniques. Am J Sports Med 2002;30(3):432–6.

29. Mazzocca AD, Burton KJ, Romeo AA, et al. Biomechanical evaluation of 4 techniques of distal biceps brachii tendon repair. Am J Sports Med 2007;35(2):252–8.

30. Hansen G, Smith A, Pollock JW, et al. Anatomic repair of the distal biceps tendon cannot be consistently performed through a classic single-incision suture anchor technique. J Shoulder Elbow Surg 2014;23:1898–904.

31. Forthman CL, Zimmerman RM, Sullivan MJ, et al. Cross-sectional anatomy of the bicipital tuberosity and biceps brachii tendon insertion: relevance to anatomic tendon repair. J Shoulder Elbow Surg 2008;17(3):522–6.

32. Kulshreshtha R, Singh R, Sinha J, et al. Anatomy of the distal biceps brachii tendon and its clinical relevance. Clin Orthop Relat Res 2007;456:117–20.

33. Schmidt CC, Diaz VA, Weir DM, et al. Repaired distal biceps magnetic resonance imaging anatomy compared with outcome. J Shoulder Elbow Surg 2012;21(12):1623–31.

34. Kelly EK, Morrey BF, O'Driscoll SW. Complications of repair of the distal biceps tendon with the modified two-incision technique. J Bone Joint Surg Am 2000;82-A(11):1575–81.

35. Cain RA, Nydick JA, Stein MI, et al. Complications following distal biceps repair. J Hand Surg Am 2012;37(10):2112–7.

36. Grant JA, Bissell B, Hake ME, et al. Relationship between implant use, operative time, and costs associated with distal biceps tendon reattachment. Orthopedics 2012;35(11):e1618–24.

37. Jobin CM, Kippe MA, Gardner TR, et al. Distal biceps tendon repair: a cadaveric analysis of suture anchor and interference screw restoration of the anatomic footprint. Am J Sports Med 2009;37(11):2214–21.

38. Athwal GS, Steinmann SP, Rispoli DM. The distal biceps tendon: footprint and relevant clinical anatomy. J Hand Surg Am 2007;32(8):1225–9.

39. Fogg QA, Hess BR, Rodgers KG, et al. Distal biceps brachii tendon anatomy revisited from a surgical perspective. Clin Anat 2009;22(3):346–51.

40. Grewal R, Athwal GS, MacDermid JC, et al. Surgical technique for single and double-incision method of acute distal biceps tendon repair. J BONE JOINT SURG AM Essential Surgical Techniques 2012;2(4):e22.

41. Morrey ME, Abdel MP, Sanchez-Sotelo J, et al. Primary repair of retracted distal biceps tendon ruptures in extreme flexion. J Shoulder Elbow Surg 2014;23(5):679–85.

42. Boyd HB, Anderson LD. A method for reinsertion of the distal biceps brachii tendon. J Bone Joint Surg 1961;43-A:1041–3.

43. Bell RH, Wiley WB, Noble JS, et al. Repair of distal biceps brachii tendon ruptures. J Shoulder Elbow Surg 2000;9(3):223–6.

44. Leighton MM, Bush-Joseph CA, Bach BR Jr. Distal biceps brachii repair. Results in dominant and nondominant extremities. Clin Orthop Relat Res 1995;(317):114–21.

45. Nigro PT, Cain R, Mighell MA. Prognosis for recovery of posterior interosseous nerve palsy after distal biceps repair. J Shoulder Elbow Surg 2013;22(1):70–3.

46. Lo EY, Li CS, Van den Bogaerde JM. The effect of drill trajectory on proximity to the posterior interosseous nerve during cortical button distal biceps repair. Arthroscopy 2011;27(8):1048–54.

47. Bisson L, Moyer M, Lanighan K, et al. Complications associated with repair of a distal biceps rupture using the modified two-incision technique. J Shoulder Elbow Surg 2008;17(1 Suppl):67S–71S.

48. Banerjee M, Shafizadeh S, Bouillon B, et al. High complication rate following distal biceps refixation with cortical button. Arch Orthop Trauma Surg 2013;133(10):1361–6.

49. Cheung EV, Lazarus M, Taranta M. Immediate range of motion after distal biceps tendon repair. J Shoulder Elbow Surg 2005;14(5):516–8.

50. Cil A, Merten S, Steinmann SP. Immediate active range of motion after modified 2-incision repair in acute distal biceps tendon rupture. Am J Sports Med 2009;37(1):130–5.

51. Landa J, Bhandari S, Strauss EJ, et al. The effect of repair of the lacertus fibrosus on distal biceps tendon repairs: a biomechanical, functional, and anatomic study. Am J Sports Med 2009;37(1):120–3.

52. Schmidt CC, Weir DM, Wong AS, et al. The effect of biceps reattachment site. J Shoulder Elbow Surg 2010;19(8):1157–65.

Distal Triceps Tendon Injuries

Jay D. Keener, MD[a],*, Paul M. Sethi, MD[b]

KEYWORDS

- Triceps tendon injury • Triceps rupture • Elbow • Distal triceps • Treatment

KEY POINTS

- Distal triceps ruptures are uncommon injuries.
- Advanced imaging is required for an accurate diagnosis.
- Complete tendon injuries are best managed surgically, whereas some partial tears can be treated conservatively.
- Surgery is successful in restoring function.

INTRODUCTION

Distal triceps tendon injuries are rare and, often, initially unrecognized. In the largest published series of tendon injuries, Anzel and colleagues[1] noted triceps tendon injuries to be the least common, accounting for 1% of tendon injuries. The triceps brachii is the chief extensor of the elbow and is critical for normal upper extremity function. The anatomy of the triceps muscle and tendon architecture has been well described and in recent years renewed interest has occurred in developing surgical repair techniques with better recreation of anatomy and improved biomechanical strength.

Triceps tendon injuries may occur in a variety of clinical scenarios and are most often associated with a distinct event recognized by the patient. There are several well-recognized risk factors that predispose to triceps injuries, both systemic and localized. Like other tendon injuries, triceps tendon ruptures may be partial or complete. The unique anatomy of the elbow extensor mechanism allows some preservation of strength even in the presence of a complete tendon rupture, which can lead to a missed diagnosis and delay in proper treatment. Treatment can be successful both conservatively and surgically in properly selected patients. This article reviews the anatomy of the triceps, the evaluation and treatment of triceps tendon injuries, and the clinical outcomes of treatment.

ANATOMY

The triceps muscle is pennate and composed of 3 distinct muscle bellies: the long, lateral, and medial heads. The triceps is innervated by the radial nerve, which is the terminal branch of the posterior cord of the brachial plexus. The radial nerve is composed of branches of the sixth, seventh, and eighth cervical nerve roots. The long head of the triceps has a broad origin at the infraglenoid tubercle of the scapula and inferior glenohumeral joint capsule.[2] The lateral head has a proximal origin from the humerus just lateral to the teres minor insertion extending distally from the lateral aspect of the spiral groove and lateral intermuscular septum. The medial head originates from the humerus distal to the spiral groove and the medial aspect of the intramuscular septum.

The insertion of the triceps tendon can be divided into the central tendon insertion into the olecranon process and the lateral triceps expansion. The central tendon is thicker medially where a distinct rolled edge is formed by a confluence of the medial and long head tendons (**Fig. 1**).[3]

[a] Department of Orthopaedic Surgery, Washington University, CB# 8233, 660 South Euclid Avenue, St Louis, MO 63110, USA; [b] The ONS Sports and Shoulder Service, 6 Greenwich Office Park, Greenwich, CT 06831, USA
* Corresponding author.
E-mail address: keenerj@wustl.edu

Hand Clin 31 (2015) 641–650
http://dx.doi.org/10.1016/j.hcl.2015.06.010
0749-0712/15/$ – see front matter © 2015 Elsevier Inc. All rights reserved.

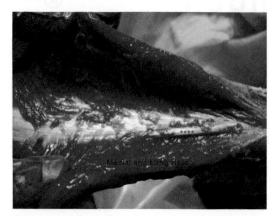

Fig. 1. Deep view of triceps muscle and tendon. The deep muscle has been elevated revealing the central triceps tendon. Note the well-developed rolled edge on the medial side of the deep tendon (*4 asterisks*).

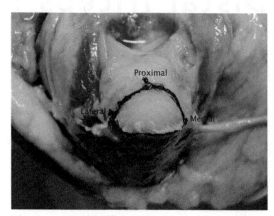

Fig. 3. Insertional footprint of the central triceps tendon. The insertion of the central tendon into the olecranon is broad and dome shaped.

The deep surface of the tendon is covered by muscle fibers from the medial head (**Fig. 2**). Although some investigators think that the medial head tendon has a distinct insertion,[4–6] others have shown that the medial tendon blends with the remaining tendon, forming a single tendon confluence.[3] The total width of the triceps tendon insertion is 4.0 to 4.2 cm.[3,7] The thickness of the central tendon just proximal to the olecranon tip is 6.8 mm.[3] The olecranon footprint tendon insertion is wide and dome shaped (**Fig. 3**). The triceps insertion begins 12 to 14 mm distal to the tip of the olecranon and has a mean width of 20.9 mm and length of 13.4 mm, with dimensions correlating with the size of the boney olecranon.[3] One study showed that the mean area of the footprint insertion was 466 mm^2,[7] whereas another study using

a three-dimensional modeling system suggested that the mean insertion was 646 mm^2.[8]

The lateral triceps expansion serves as an important reinforcement of central tendon and can maintain active elbow extension in the presence of a central tendon rupture. The lateral triceps expansion is thinner than the central tendon covering the anconeus muscle and blends with the extensor carpi ulnaris and dorsal antebrachial fascia, eventually inserting into the dorsolateral ulna (**Fig. 4**). The mean width of the lateral expansion is between 14.4 and 16.8 mm, which is approximately 70% of the width of the central triceps tendon.[3,7]

RISK FACTORS AND INJURY MECHANISM

Triceps tendon injuries are most common in weight lifters and athletes; football players may be at particular risk.[9] Triceps injuries are most common in men.[10] Chronic anabolic steroid[11] and corticosteroid use are considered risk factors given their deleterious effect on tendon strength. Likewise, triceps injuries have been linked to local corticosteroid injections for triceps tendonitis or olecranon bursitis.[11,12] A variety of systemic disorders, including renal osteodystrophy, hyperparathyroidism, and diabetes mellitus, can predispose to triceps injuries.

Triceps tendon ruptures usually occur as a result of a forceful eccentric contraction of the triceps, such as a fall on the outstretched hand or during weight lifting. Usually the injury occurs at the level of the tendon insertion into bone; however, musculotendinous ruptures can occur. Direct blunt trauma to the posterior arm is a less common mechanism and generally requires high energy. Even less commonly, lacerations can lead to direct transection of the tendon.

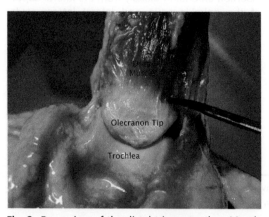

Fig. 2. Deep view of the distal triceps tendon. Muscle fibers covering the deep layer of the tendon originate primarily from the medial head of the triceps.

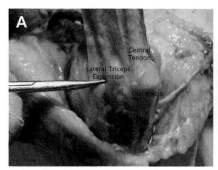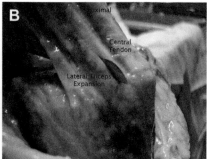

Fig. 4. Superficial appearance of the triceps tendon insertion. (*A*) The lateral triceps expansion is continuous with the anconeus muscle and lateral antebrachial fascia inserting distally into the dorsolateral ulna. (*B*) The lateral triceps expansion is broad and thinner than the central tendon, and is approximately 70% of the width of the central tendon.

CLINICAL EVALUATION

Most injuries result from a recognizable event by the patient, often accompanied by a painful pop or tearing sensation. A subjective loss of elbow extension strength is common. Acute injuries are accompanied by variable amounts of swelling of the olecranon bursa and localized bruising. Physical examination usually reveals localized tenderness and swelling and often a palpable defect in the tendon confirming the diagnosis. Usually full elbow range of motion is present, and posterior pain may be present with terminal flexion motion. Inability to extend the elbow against gravity is a sign of a complete rupture; however, the converse is not always true. Because of the integrity of the lateral triceps expansion complete central tendon rupture often preserves antigravity elbow extension. Therefore, accurate diagnosis can be misleading by clinical examination alone. One study showed that approximately half of acute triceps tendon ruptures were initially misdiagnosed.[13] Both partial and full-thickness rupture has loss of elbow extension power compared with the opposite extremity.

A modification of the Thompson calf squeeze test has been proposed to rule out complete triceps tendon ruptures.[14] During this test the upper arm is placed on a table surface with the patient prone and the forearm allowed to hang freely over table edge. The triceps muscle is manually squeezed with the arm relaxed. Similar to the ankle during the Thompson test, when the muscle is squeezed the elbow should extend slightly.

DIAGNOSTIC IMAGING

Plain radiographs should be obtained on presentation and include anteroposterior, lateral, and oblique views of the elbow. The presence of a small avulsion fracture from the olecranon process (flake sign) is pathognomonic of a triceps rupture (**Fig. 5**).

Advanced studies such as MRI, computed tomography scan, or ultrasonography (US) are usually necessary to confirm the diagnosis and can give some idea of the chronicity of injury. Both MRI and US can distinguish partial from complete tendon injuries.[9,15–19] MRI can be particularly helpful to identify associated soft tissue injuries. The triceps tendon is best visualized on the sagittal images (**Fig. 6**). Complete discontinuity of the central tendon from the olecranon indicates a full-thickness tear, often associated with a fluid gap on T2 imaging. Partial tears appear as an area of increased T1 and proton density signal within the tendon and, when acute, have increased T2 signal intensity.[17] Partial tears may include either the deep or superficial layers. Partial tears may be

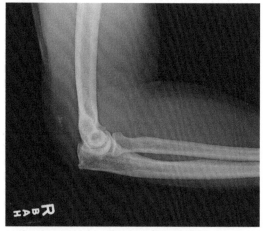

Fig. 5. Flake sign. Lateral radiograph of an elbow with a triceps tendon tear. Note the displaced avulsion of an osteophyte from the olecranon tip indicating a triceps tendon injury.

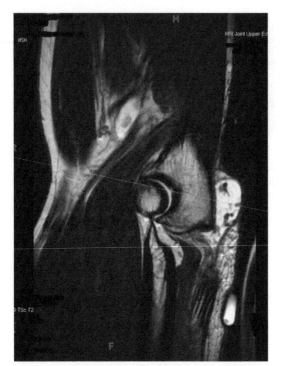

Fig. 6. Sagittal T2-weighted MRI of a displaced acute triceps tendon injury; a complete rupture with only a few fibers of the deep central triceps tendon intact.

more common at the medial aspect of the tendon.[6,9]

TREATMENT RECOMMENDATIONS

Because there exists no classification system for triceps tendon ruptures, injuries are generally described by severity and location: partial versus complete ruptures and tendon versus musculotendinous injuries. Most triceps tendon injuries occur at the tendon insertion. Advanced imaging is usually necessary to confirm the severity of injury and the recommended treatment is dictated by the injury severity and the age and physical demands of the patient. In general, partial tears with minimal strength loss can be managed nonsurgically and complete ruptures are treated with surgical repair.

Conservative Treatment

Tears of the triceps occurring within the muscle or musculotendinous junction are thought to have good healing potential and are generally treated conservatively. Partial tears of the tendon are more controversial. In sedentary individuals, all partial tears can be managed conservatively. When partial tears are not associated with tendon retraction, strength is usually preserved and conservative treatment is preferred. Treatment includes a brief period (3–4 weeks) of immobilization at 30° flexion followed

by progressive elbow flexion mobilization.[15,20,21] Progression of elbow motion is allowed as tolerated beyond 4 weeks.

There is little literature regarding outcomes of conservative treatment of partial triceps tendon injuries. Mair and colleagues[9] reported the results of 10 partial triceps injuries in football players treated conservatively. The tears involved between 30% and 75% of the tendon. Four elbows eventually required surgery, 3 because of residual weakness and 1 because of early full tendon rupture. The remaining 6 elbows recovered with no residual symptoms.

Surgical Treatment

Most complete triceps tendon injuries should be managed with surgical repair.[15,22] The exceptions include very low demand patients or those not medically fit for surgery. Partial tendon injuries that are high grade (involving >50% of the tendon), associated with tendon retraction and extension weakness, or that have failed conservative treatment are also recommended for surgical repair (**Fig. 7**). These indications are particularly applicable in active individuals and athletes. Ideally, surgery should be performed within 2 to 3 weeks for acute complete tears with tendon retraction. Primary repair can be performed in a delayed

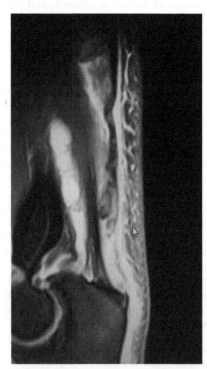

Fig. 7. Sagittal MRI of high-grade partial tear of the distal triceps tendon. The superficial tendon is torn, whereas the deep tendon remains intact. *Arrow* point to retracted superficial tendon and surrounding fluid.

fashion and may be more feasible with injuries associated with less tendon retraction.

SURGICAL TECHNIQUE

A variety of techniques have been described for triceps tendon repair. There is no clear superior technique in terms of clinical outcomes but each has theoretic advantages. All techniques focus on reattachment of the torn central tendon to the olecranon. In addition, any disruption of the lateral triceps expansion should be performed and helps to augment the primary repair. In cases in which there is a significant amount of olecranon bone attached to the displaced triceps tendon, it may be favorable to reattach the bone fragment with either heavy sutures or anchors rather than to excise the bone.

Perhaps the most historically popular triceps repair technique involves the creation of bone tunnels in the olecranon. Purchase of the central tendon is achieved with high-tensile, braided sutures in a running, locked (Krackow) fashion or with use of a Bunnell-type suture configuration. The strands of suture are threaded through bone tunnels; both crossing tunnels[13] (**Fig. 8**) and

3 parallel tunnels[23] (**Fig. 9**) have been described. The sutures are then tied over the olecranon as a bone bridge with the elbow held in near full extension. Alternatively, the triceps may be reattached with the use of suture anchors placed within the olecranon tip.[21,24–26] With these techniques, side-to-side sutures are recommended to reinforce the edges of the repair.

Modified repair techniques have recently become more popular in attempts to restore a larger, native anatomic footprint and improve the mechanical strength of the repair. The strength of the native triceps tendon has been shown to rival that of the patellar tendon at roughly 1700 N in cadavers.[27,28] Yeh and colleagues[7] showed significantly greater repair strength (under cyclical loading) with a transosseous-equivalent repair compared with both traditional bone tunnel and suture anchor repairs. In addition, the transosseous-equivalent repair gave a better recreation of the native triceps footprint qualitatively compared with the other techniques, although this was not quantified. With the transosseous-equivalent repair, 2 anchors are positioned in the proximal olecranon approximately 12 mm from

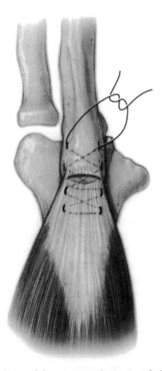

Fig. 8. Traditional bone tunnel repair of the triceps tendon. Bunnell-type suture configuration securing the central triceps tendon through crossing tunnels in the olecranon. (*Reproduced* with permission from the Mayo Foundation of Medical Education and Research, Rochester, MN.)

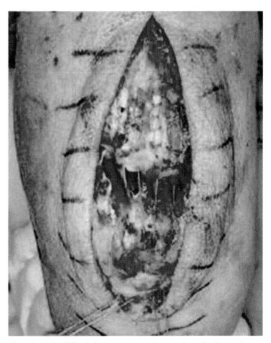

Fig. 9. Modified bone tunnel repair of the triceps tendon. Krackow-type suture configuration in the triceps tendon. The tendon is secured through 3 parallel tunnels passed through the olecranon tip. (*From* Sierra RJ, Weiss NG, Shrader MW, et al. Acute triceps ruptures: case report and retrospective chart review. J Shld Elbow Surg 2006;15(1):131; with permission.)

the olecranon tip. Sutures from these anchors are then passed through the tendon creating horizontal mattress stitches. These sutures, along with the tails of a Krackow-type suture weaved through the triceps tendon, are then secured to 2 anchors placed more distally on the dorsal aspect of the ulna (**Fig. 10**).[7] This arrangement effectively compresses the distal tendon footprint against the bone, creating a larger area of boney apposition and better recreating the large area of the native triceps footprint. Alternatively, medial mattress stitches from anchors can be combined with a central tendon Bunnell-type suture secured through crossing bone tunnels.[29]

Knotless repair constructs have recently been studied and show favorable biomechanical strength.[30,31] In addition, this type of repair can be performed with 1 anchor, thereby creating less expense than transosseous repair techniques. Clark and colleagues[31] studied an anatomic knotless repair compared with a traditional cruciate bone tunnel repair in cadaveric elbows. The knotless repair showed significantly less displacement under cyclic loading and better peak load to failure and yield strength than the traditional repair. With the anatomic knotless

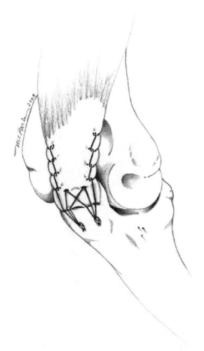

Fig. 10. Double-row triceps tendon repair. Repair of the triceps tendon with a double-row technique. (*From* Yeh PC, Dodds SD, Smart LR, et al. Distal triceps rupture. J Am Acad Orthop Surg 2010;18(1):31–40; with permission.)

repair, 2 core high-tensile, braided sutures are woven through the central triceps tendon, creating 4 repair strands (2 medial and lateral suture ends) (**Fig. 11**). A shuttle suture is passed through the distal tendon on both the medial and lateral aspects of the tendon as well. Two parallel bone tunnels are created at the medial and lateral aspects of the olecranon, exiting the dorsal aspect of the ulna. The 3 strands of suture are passed through the olecranon bone tunnel on both the medial and lateral sides. Next, each shuttle suture is used to repass the free ends of the Krackow suture back through each of the bone tunnels, creating a cruciate repair (1 limb from the medial and lateral sides are crossed into the opposite tunnel). All slack is taken out of the 4 Krackow strands and the elbow is extended. All 4 strands are then secured to an interference fit–type anchor placed after predrilling into the dorsal apex of the olecranon, angled away from the articular surface.

POSTOPERATIVE CARE

Most protocols recommend immobilization of the elbow at 30° to 45° for a short period (1–2 weeks) to allow skin healing and protect the repair.[15,22] Gentle active elbow flexion and passive or gravity-assisted extension starts at 2 weeks and continues until full range of motion has returned. Active elbow extension is initiated at 4 weeks. Light strengthening begins at 6 weeks with slow progression until 3 months. Heavy lifting and weight training should be delayed until 4 to 6 months following surgery.[13] With the advent of stronger repair constructs, some investigators have recommended a more accelerated rehabilitation protocol. We prefer to place the arm in a sling rather than a splint and begin immediate active and passive range of motion of the elbow and forearm unrestricted. Patients should avoid lifting more than 2.3 kg (5 pounds) during this phase. Light triceps strengthening is initiated 6 weeks after surgery and advanced as tolerated. Direct comparisons between rehabilitation timelines have not been performed, therefore the advantages and safety of accelerated rehabilitation protocols have not been established.

REVISION, CHRONIC, OR DIFFICULT ACUTE REPAIRS

In some instances, primary repair of the tendon can be difficult either because of a fixed retracted position of the tendon, which may be seen in cases of chronic rupture (>6 weeks), or in cases of deficient or poor-quality tissue, such as a revision repair. In cases in which direct primary repair is

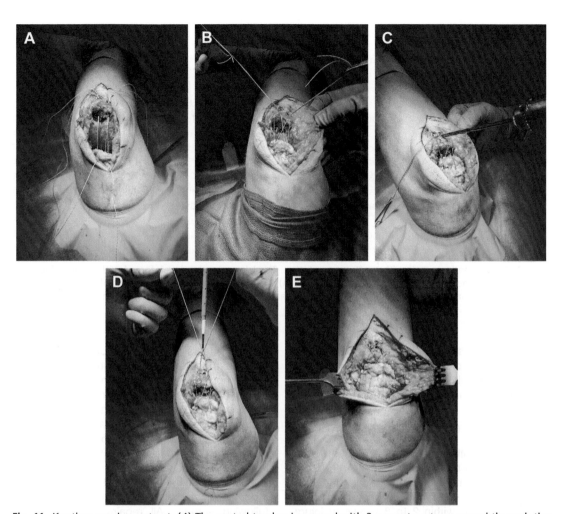

Fig. 11. Knotless repair construct. (*A*) The central tendon is secured with 2 separate sutures passed through the tendon in a Krackow configuration creating 4 separate strands (2 medial and 2 lateral sutures). In addition, a shuttle suture is passed through the medial and lateral aspects of the distal tendon. Three strands of suture are passed through a medial and lateral longitudinal bone tunnel in the olecranon. (*B*) Each shuttle suture is used to repass the free ends of both the medial and lateral Krackow sutures back through each of the bone tunnels, creating a cruciate repair. (*C*) A bone tunnel is created distal to the olecranon tip on the dorsal surface of the bone, away from the articular surface. (*D*) The 4 limbs of suture are passed through an interference fit–type anchor to be secured into the bone tunnel. Note the extended position of the elbow to facilitate reduction of the tendon. (*E*) Secured knotless cruciate repair of the triceps tendon.

suspected to be difficult, potential tendon augmentation should be discussed with the patient before surgery. A variety of tendon augmentation procedures have been described and include allograft or autograft hamstring tendon augmentation, rotational anconeus flap, Achilles tendon augmentation, and ligament augmentation devices.[15,32–34] The method of reconstruction in these cases depends on several factors, including surgeon preference, tendon mobility and tissue quality, and a variety of host factors.

Repair augmentation with tendon can substantially improve the repair strength compared with primary repair. Petre and colleagues[27] compared the biomechanical strength of the intact triceps tendon with direct tendon repair and repairs augmented with flexor carpi radialis tendon. Although neither repair construct was a strong as the native tendon, the augmented repairs were nearly twice as strong as the repairs without augmentation. In scenarios with deficient or poor-quality tissue, hamstring augmentation can be used to reinforce the repair or gain tendon length. The tendon is woven in a Bunnell fashion through the residual tendon (**Fig. 12**). A transverse bicortical tunnel is drilled 1 cm from the olecranon

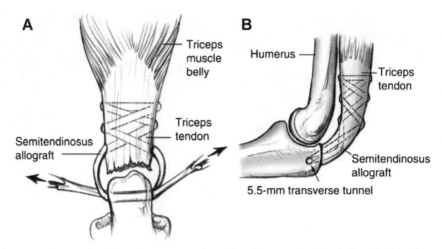

Fig. 12. Triceps tendon repair with graft augmentation. The triceps tendon is reinforced with a hamstring graft woven through the tendon in a Bunnell-type manner (*A*). The tendon is fixated through the olecranon through a transverse bone tunnel (*B*). (*From* Yeh PC, Dodds SD, Smart LR, et al. Distal triceps rupture. J Am Acad Orthop Surg 2010;18(1):31–40; with permission.)

tip. The free ends of the graft are passed through the tunnel from opposite directions. An interference screw is placed, securing the graft within the tunnel with the elbow in extension.

CLINICAL OUTCOMES AND COMPLICATIONS

The clinical results of acute distal triceps tendon repairs are generally good; however, reruptures have been described to occur in up to 20% of cases.[13] Successful repair is more predictable when performed within 2 to 3 weeks of injury. One series noted that a primary repair was feasible in only 6 of 15 cases when surgery was performed more than 25 days after the injury.[13] Most studies reporting the outcomes of triceps tendon repair are retrospective and consist of small case series without control groups or direct comparisons of various repair constructs. In addition, outcomes are not reported in a consistent fashion and often lack validated scales of upper extremity function.

Van Riet and colleagues[13] showed peak strength of 92% (range of 75%–106%) and loss of extension of 8° compared with the uninjured side at 1 year postoperatively in 14 acute tears (average of 63 days before surgery) that were primarily repaired using the transosseous cruciate technique. Mair and colleagues[9] treated 11 acute complete triceps tears in professional football players with immediate repair. All but 1 missed an entire season. There was 1 tendon rerupture. The remaining patients were doing well at 3 years postoperatively with no pain or subjective weakness. Bava and colleagues[24] noted good results

in 5 acute tears repaired with suture anchors at a mean 32 months following surgery. Function was nearly normal in these patients with a mean DASH (Disabilities of the Arm, Shoulder, and Hand) score of 1.4, American Shoulder and Elbow Surgeons elbow score of 99.2, and a mean Mayo Elbow Performance Index of 95.8. The results of more anatomic repair constructs are largely unknown. Kokkalis and colleagues[29] reported the results of 11 acute triceps tendon tears repaired with a double-row technique at a mean of 21 months following surgery. All repairs were performed within 3 weeks of injury. The mean visual analog scale pain score decreased from 8.5 preoperatively to 2.4 at follow-up. The mean loss of elbow extension was 7° and the mean arc of elbow motion was 136°. Elbow extension strength was significantly improved but not quantified. Nine of the 11 patients were completely satisfied with the surgery and had returned to full activity.

Results of repairs of chronic ruptures often lack quantitative data and objective outcome measures. However, Van Riet and colleagues[13] measured the outcomes of 9 chronic ruptures (average of 163 days before surgery) that underwent reconstructions. These patients showed, on average, 66% peak elbow extension strength (range of 35%–100%) and loss of elbow extension of 13°. Despite the wide range of peak strength, this report shows that reconstructions of chronic tears are inferior to primary repairs of acute tears. The results of repairs and reconstructions from 3 recurrent rupture cases by van Riet and colleagues[13] were functionally equivalent to results of first-time primary repairs.

Common complications of triceps tendon repairs include olecranon bursitis, localized soft tissue irritation from sutures or wires, residual mild elbow flexion contracture, and elbow extension weakness. In addition, rerupture remains a concern, especially with poor-quality tissue or delayed repairs performed under tension.

SUMMARY

Acute triceps ruptures are an uncommon entity, occurring mainly in athletes, weight lifters (especially those taking anabolic steroids), and following elbow trauma. Accurate diagnosis is made clinically, although MRI may aid in confirmation and surgical planning. Acute ruptures are classified on an anatomic basis based on tear location and the degree of tendon involvement. Most complete tears are treated surgically in medically fit patients. Partial-thickness tears are managed according to the tear severity, functional demands, and response to conservative treatment. Surgical repair offers predictable return of function with a small risk of loss of elbow motion. Even surgical treatment of chronic tears has shown improved elbow extension strength and patient satisfaction. We favor an anatomic footprint repair of the triceps to provide optimal tendon-to-bone healing and, ultimately, functional outcome.

REFERENCES

1. Anzel SH, Covey KW, Weiner AD, et al. Disruption of muscles and tendons; an analysis of 1, 014 cases. Surgery 1959;45(3):406–14.
2. Handling MA, Curtis AS, Miller SL. The origin of the long head of the triceps: a cadaveric study. J Shoulder Elbow Surg 2010;19(1):69–72.
3. Keener JD, Chafik D, Kim HM, et al. Insertional anatomy of the triceps brachii tendon. J Shld Elbow Surg 2010;19(3):399–405.
4. Madsen M, Marx RG, Millett PJ, et al. Surgical anatomy of the triceps brachii tendon: anatomical study and clinical correlation. Am J Sports Med 2006; 34(11):1839–43.
5. Belentani C, Pastore D, Wangwinyuvirat M, et al. Triceps brachii tendon: anatomic-MR imaging study in cadavers with histologic correlation. Skeletal Radiol 2009;38(2):171–5.
6. Athwal GS, McGill RJ, Rispoli DM. Isolated avulsion of the medial head of the triceps tendon: an anatomic study and arthroscopic repair in 2 cases. Arthroscopy 2009;25(9):983–8.
7. Yeh PC, Stephens KT, Solovyova O, et al. The distal triceps tendon footprint and a biomechanical analysis of 3 repair techniques. Am J Sports Med 2010;38(5):1025–33.
8. Capo JT, Collins C, Beutel BG, et al. Three-dimensional analysis of elbow soft tissue footprints and anatomy. J Shld Elbow Surg 2014;23(11):1618–23.
9. Mair SD, Isbell WM, Gill TJ, et al. Triceps tendon ruptures in professional football players. Am J Sports Med 2004;32(2):431–4.
10. Stucken C, Ciccotti MG. Distal biceps and triceps injuries in athletes. Sports Med Arthrosc 2014;22(3): 153–63.
11. Sollender JL, Rayan GM, Barden GA. Triceps tendon rupture in weight lifters. J Shld Elbow Surg 1998;7(2):151–3.
12. Stannard JP, Bucknell AL. Rupture of the triceps tendon associated with steroid injections. Am J Sports Med 1993;21(3):482–5.
13. van Riet RP, Morrey BF, Ho E, et al. Surgical treatment of distal triceps ruptures. J Bone Joint Surg Am 2003;85-A(10):1961–7.
14. Viegas SF. Avulsion of the triceps tendon. Orthop Rev 1990;19(6):533–6.
15. Yeh PC, Dodds SD, Smart LR, et al. Distal triceps rupture. J Am Acad Orthop Surg 2010;18(1):31–40.
16. Downey R, Jacobson JA, Fessell DP, et al. Sonography of partial-thickness tears of the distal triceps brachii tendon. J Ultrasound Med 2011;30(10): 1351–6.
17. Wenzke DR. MR imaging of the elbow in the injured athlete. Radiol Clin North Am 2013;51(2):195–213.
18. Thornton R, Riley GM, Steinbach LS. Magnetic resonance imaging of sports injuries of the elbow. Top Magn Reson Imaging 2003;14(1):69–86.
19. Kaempffe FA, Lerner RM. Ultrasound diagnosis of triceps tendon rupture. A report of 2 cases. Clin Orthop Relat Res 1996;(332):138–42.
20. Bos CF, Nelissen RG, Bloem JL. Incomplete rupture of the tendon of triceps brachii. A case report. Int Orthop 1994;18(5):273–5.
21. Farrar EL 3rd, Lippert FG 3rd. Avulsion of the triceps tendon. Clin Orthop Rel Res 1981;(161):242–6.
22. Tom JA, Kumar NS, Cerynik DL, et al. Diagnosis and treatment of triceps tendon injuries: a review of the literature. Clin J Sport Med 2014;24(3):197–204.
23. Sierra RJ, Weiss NG, Shrader MW, et al. Acute triceps ruptures: case report and retrospective chart review. J Shld Elbow Surg 2006;15(1):130–4.
24. Bava ED, Barber FA, Lund ER. Clinical outcome after suture anchor repair for complete traumatic rupture of the distal triceps tendon. Arthroscopy 2012;28(8):1058–63.
25. Bach BR Jr, Warren RF, Wickiewicz TL. Triceps rupture. A case report and literature review. Am J Sports Med 1987;15(3):285–9.
26. Pina A, Garcia I, Sabater M. Traumatic avulsion of the triceps brachii. J Orthop Trauma 2002;16(4): 273–6.
27. Petre BM, Grutter PW, Rose DM, et al. Triceps tendons: a biomechanical comparison of intact and

repaired strength. J Shld Elbow Surg 2011;20(2): 213–8.

28. Adams DJ, Mazzocca AD, Fulkerson JP. Residual strength of the quadriceps versus patellar tendon after harvesting a central free tendon graft. Arthroscopy 2006;22(1):76–9.

29. Kokkalis ZT, Mavrogenis AF, Spyridonos S, et al. Triceps brachii distal tendon reattachment with a double-row technique. Orthopedics 2013;36(2):110–6.

30. Paci JM, Clark J, Rizzi A. Distal triceps knotless anatomic footprint repair: a new technique. Arthrosc Tech 2014;3(5):e621–6.

31. Clark J, Obopilwe E, Rizzi A, et al. Distal triceps knotless anatomic footprint repair is superior to transosseous cruciate repair: a biomechanical comparison. Arthroscopy 2014;30(10):1254–60.

32. Wagner JR, Cooney WP. Rupture of the triceps muscle at the musculotendinous junction: a case report. J Hand Surg Am 1997;22(2):341–3.

33. Sanchez-Sotelo J, Morrey BF. Surgical techniques for reconstruction of chronic insufficiency of the triceps. Rotation flap using anconeus and tendo achillis allograft. J Bone Joint Surg Br 2002;84(8):1116–20.

34. Weistroffer JK, Mills WJ, Shin AY. Recurrent rupture of the triceps tendon repaired with hamstring tendon autograft augmentation: a case report and repair technique. J Shld Elbow Surg 2003;12(2):193–6.

Arthroscopic Management of Elbow Fractures

Leslie A. Fink Barnes, MD, Bradford O. Parsons, MD*,
Michael Hausman, MD

KEYWORDS

- Elbow trauma • Elbow arthroscopy • Arthroscopic-assisted fracture treatment • Coronoid
- Lateral condyle • Medial condyle

KEY POINTS

- Keep pump pressure low (25–30 mm Hg) to avoid postfracture compartment syndrome.
- Joint distension, proximally placed portals, and gentle elbow flexion increase working space from nerves.
- Assess fracture alignment after reduction, then introduce fixation percutaneously with Kirschner wires (K-wires), cannulated screws, or suture lasso configuration.
- Elbow stability should be evaluated after fracture fixation to determine whether ligament repair is required.
- Fracture healing should be prioritized rather than motion in cases of severe comminution or questionable fixation.

INTRODUCTION: NATURE OF THE PROBLEM

Fractures and trauma about the elbow are challenging to treat, in that exposure to certain parts of the elbow may destabilize the elbow or put neurovascular structures at risk. Further, stiffness is a frequent complication, ranging from capsular fibrosis to heterotopic ossification with a bony block to motion. Therefore, arthroscopic-assisted fracture management about the elbow has several advantages, including improved visualization, better wound healing, preservation of collateral ligaments and critical soft tissue structures, and the opportunity for early motion to minimize complications from stiffness. In affording a view of the entire articular surface through small portals, arthroscopy facilitates visualization of intra-articular fractures, and assessment of all joint surfaces for concurrent chondral injury and of cartilaginous pediatric fractures not readily seen on radiographs. Arthroscopic assistance for percutaneous fixation of lateral condyle fractures is especially useful in pediatric patients in whom much of the condyle is radiolucent cartilage.[1,2] Arthroscopic treatment of elbow trauma has shown good results in the pediatric population, and may minimize insult to the epiphyseal blood supply because of less soft tissue stripping than in open surgery.[3]

Elbow arthroscopy has attendant risks and the potential for complications. The overall complication rate has been reported to be as low as 2%

Disclosures: Dr B.O. Parsons is a paid consultant for Arthrex and Zimmer. Dr M. Hausman is an unpaid consultant for Checkpoint Surgical NDI, a paid consultant for Stryker, and receives royalties from Smith & Nephew. Dr L.A. Fink Barnes reports no conflicts of interest.
Leni and Peter W. May Department of Orthopaedics, Icahn School of Medicine at Mount Sinai Medical Center, 5 East 98th Street, Box 1188, New York, NY 10029, USA
* Corresponding author.
E-mail address: bradford.parsons@mountsinai.org

Hand Clin 31 (2015) 651–661
http://dx.doi.org/10.1016/j.hcl.2015.06.011
0749-0712/15/$ – see front matter © 2015 Elsevier Inc. All rights reserved.

among experienced surgeons, but included in the complication rate is the potential for major nerve transection.[4] Other series have reported major and minor complications at a rate of 12%, which included joint space infection, and transient nerve palsies of the ulnar nerve, posterior interosseous nerve, and sensory cutaneous nerves but no permanent neurologic deficits.[5] Therefore, knowledge of elbow anatomy and arthroscopic techniques is essential for successful management of these injuries. As with all new techniques, a learning curve entailing additional time is a disadvantage of this technique.[6]

Several types of elbow fractures are amenable to arthroscopic or arthroscopic-assisted fracture fixation, including coronoid fractures, lateral condyle fractures, capitellum fractures, and coronal shear fractures of the distal humerus. Arthroscopic radial head fracture treatment has been described but, in our experience, is technically challenging and treatment is not facilitated or improved with arthroscopy. In addition, arthroscopy can be used for assessment of valgus instability before open repair or reconstruction.

SURGICAL TECHNIQUE
Preoperative Planning

Preoperative planning includes radiographs of bilateral elbows, including stress radiographs where appropriate to detect terrible triad injuries or collateral ligament instability. Advanced imaging, such as a computed tomography (CT) scan, is usually indicated for articular fractures; in skeletally immature patients, MRI may be preferred. Three-dimensional reconstructions are helpful. In the operating room before surgery, a stress examination under anesthesia is a helpful adjunct to assess instability using the minifluoroscope.[7,8] Regional anesthesia may be used for postoperative pain management, but some surgeons prefer to avoid this in order to obtain an immediate postoperative neurologic assessment.

PREPARATION AND PATIENT POSITIONING

Elbow arthroscopy can be performed in the lateral decubitus or supine positions, and a tourniquet is used. For lateral decubitus positioning, patients are positioned using an inflatable beanbag with a padded axillary roll. The upper arm is supported by an arm holder attached to the side of the operating table (Western elbow holder, Smith & Nephew, Nashville, TN) with the triceps and olecranon facing upwards. For supine positioning, a sterile arm holder is used to secure the elbow, such as a McConnell arm holder (McConnell Orthopedic Manufacturing Co, Greenville, TX) or a pneumatic arm holder (Spider, Smith & Nephew, Nashville, TN), so that the forearm is raised superiorly and the olecranon is facing the surgeon (**Fig. 1**).[9] Some surgeons prefer lateral patient positioning because it affords easier access to the posterior elbow joint. However, most of the work for fracture procedures

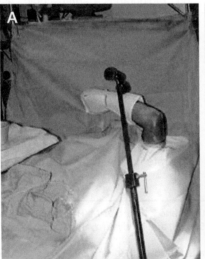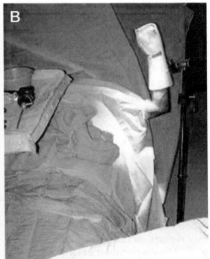

Fig. 1. The preferred patient positioning for elbow arthroscopy: supine with a McConnell arm positioner. (*A*) Positioned for access to the posterior compartment. (*B*) Positioned for anterior elbow access. (*From* Hsu JW, Gould JL, Fonseca-Sabune H, et al. The emerging role of elbow arthroscopy in chronic use injuries and fracture care. Hand Clin 2009;25(3):306; with permission.)

is done anteriorly. Supine positioning may also allow for easier conversion to open surgery if necessary. Further, supine positioning enables ease of adjustment in the degree of elbow flexion at different portions of the procedure, which is useful in fracture procedures. However, surgeons should choose the position that is most comfortable and familiar to them.

SURGICAL APPROACH

The major surface topology is marked and the position of the ulnar nerve is carefully palpated. If the nerve's position cannot be confirmed, a medial portal may be contraindicated. Entry into the joint is usually straightforward, because the capsule is pliant and normal and the joint is predistended by fracture hematoma. Standard precautions for elbow arthroscopy apply.[10] The safest portals are the midlateral (soft spot portal), proximal lateral, transtriceps, distal posterolateral, and anteromedial portals.[11]

A standard 4-mm 30° arthroscope is routinely used, but a 70° scope can be useful for coronoid and capitellar fractures. Occasionally a smaller 3.5-mm arthroscope is helpful for radial head fractures and in the assessment of the proximal radioulnar joint (PRUJ).

If an adequate reduction and fixation cannot be obtained arthroscopically, a limited open incision can be made for open fixation with a plate or screws. After fixation, reduction and stability are evaluated arthroscopically and fluoroscopically. Any additional ligamentous repair can be performed in a traditional open technique or with an arthroscopic imbrication.[12,13]

SURGICAL PROCEDURE: CORONOID FRACTURES

For fixation of coronoid fractures, a standard elbow arthroscopy setup is used according to the surgeon's preference (**Figs. 2** and **3**).

Step 1. An anteromedial viewing portal is established first, followed by a proximal anterolateral working portal, with the potential for the addition of another anterolateral portal for use of retractors. A 70° scope may also be useful.

Step 2. After lavage and debridement, the coronoid fracture is assessed. Especially in type II and III coronoid fractures, assessment of concurrent injuries is important.

Step 3. Guidewires for cannulated screws or suture passage are inserted from the posterior, subcutaneous border of the proximal ulna. An anterior cruciate ligament

(ACL)-type drilling guide and the minifluoroscopy are helpful. Correct positioning of the wires is confirmed by direct arthroscopic viewing.

Step 4. The fracture is then reduced and a method of fixation is chosen.[14,15] Common fixation techniques include suture lasso, and lag screws placed indirectly from posterior to anterior or under direct visualization from anterior to posterior.[16] Reduction techniques include using arthroscopic graspers or ring curettes placed through the anterolateral portal, or an over-the-top ACL guide placed in the medial portal while viewing is switched to the lateral portal.

Step 5. After confirmation of reduction, a calibrated posterior-to-anterior guidewire is inserted percutaneously. A second guidewire may be helpful for derotational purposes when necessary. A 3.5-mm cannulated screw of appropriate length is then inserted over the guidewire.

Step 6. Screw fixation can be reinforced with arthroscopic suture fixation, or suture fixation can be used in the presence of fragment comminution. Using the anteromedial working portal, a mattress suture is passed through the anterior capsule, near its insertion on to the coronoid, using an arthroscopic suture passing system (ie, Spectrum System, Linvatec Corp, Largo, FL).

Step 7. Through a small incision on the dorsal ulna, a Freer elevator is then used to dissect the soft tissue off the medial ulna, with care taken to stay deep to the ulnar nerve. A Hewson suture passer is used to retrieve one end of the suture medially.

Step 8. Laterally, an 18-G needle is introduced through the soft spot portal into the PRUJ. Following arthroscopic confirmation of placement, a Hewson suture passer, or equivalent, is used to retrieve the lateral limb of the suture, which is then passed subcutaneously into the dorsal incision.

SURGICAL PROCEDURE: RADIAL HEAD FRACTURES

Step 1. For radial head fractures, a posterolateral viewing portal is first established for diagnostic and joint visualization purposes, and a lateral soft spot portal is created for the working portal. If the fracture fragment is anterior, an anteromedial portal may need for viewing. Fracture reduction with an elevator and fixation can then be undertaken from the lateral side. Flexion of the

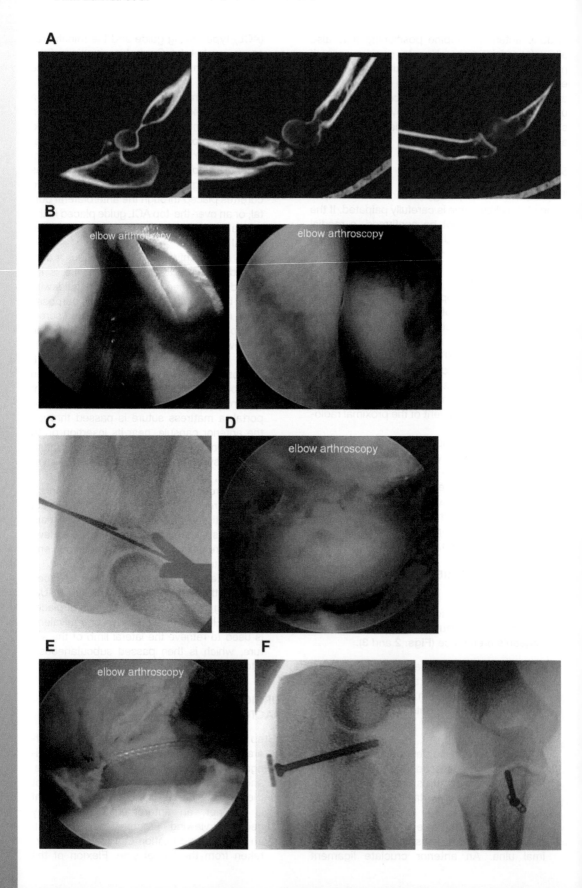

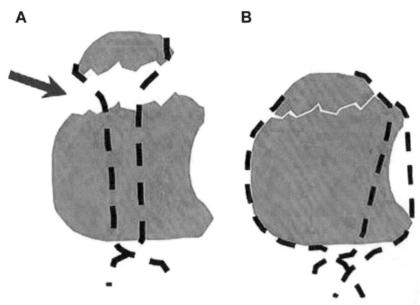

Fig. 3. The preferred suture placement to avoid the suture anchor effect, which prevents firm, precise coaptation of the fragments. Sutures passed through the fracture bed (*A*) result in the anchor effect (*B*). (*From* Hausman MR, Klug RA, Qureshi S, et al. Arthroscopically assisted coronoid fracture fixation: a preliminary report. Clin Orthop Relat Res 2008;466(12):3150; with permission.)

elbow and supination of the forearm optimize the working field.

Step 2. The radiocapitellar joint should be carefully inspected for osteochondral lesions and loose bodies through the anteromedial portal, the posterior radiocapitellar portal, or looking from a posterior portal with a 70° arthroscope. A partial anterolateral debridement is likely to be necessary to see the radial head. In addition, the arthroscope should be transferred to the midlateral (soft spot portal) or posterolateral portal to enable visualization of the olecranon fossa. Loose bodies are frequently encountered in the fossa after fracture of the radial head.[17]

Step 3. Fracture fixation is achieved with headless cannulated screws placed over a guidewire from the anterolateral portal.

For excision of radial head fractures, the portals used are the proximal medial, anterolateral, and the midlateral (soft spot) portal. The anterior three-quarters of the radial head and 2 to 3 mm of the radial neck are resected with a stonecutting abrader in the anterolateral portal and the arthroscope in the proximal medial portal. For resection of the posterior portion of the radial head, the burr may be transferred to the midlateral portal, which permits resection of the remnants of the radial head posteriorly and also at the PRUJ.[17]

SURGICAL PROCEDURE: CAPITELLAR FRACTURES

Step 1. Capitellar fractures characteristically displace proximally, and the procedure begins with reduction of the proximally displaced fragment (**Fig. 4**). Using standard anteromedial, anterolateral, and posterolateral portals, full visualization and easy access to all involved joints can be established. A proximal anterolateral portal is established under fluoroscopic control to allow insertion of a trocar proximal to the fragment.

Step 2. The capitellar fracture is then reduced by extending the elbow and, if necessary,

Fig. 2. (*A*) CT image of a terrible triad injury, showing a displaced coronoid fracture and radial head fracture. (*B*) Arthroscopic views from the proximal anterolateral portal, looking medially, showing debridement and reduction of the coronoid fracture. (*C*) Lateral fluoroscopic view of percutaneous Kirschner wire (K-wire) fixation through the coronoid fracture, placed retrograde. (*D*) Arthroscopic view showing introduction of the FiberWire suture and a curved suture lasso (*arrow*) used to shuttle the suture around a type II coronoid fracture. (*E*) Arthroscopic view showing the FiberWire suture capturing the coronoid fragment. (*F*) Anteroposterior (*right*) and lateral (*left*) fluoroscopic images showing final reduction and fixation of the coronoid fracture with a percutaneous screw, and suture lasso technique tied posteriorly over a cortical button.

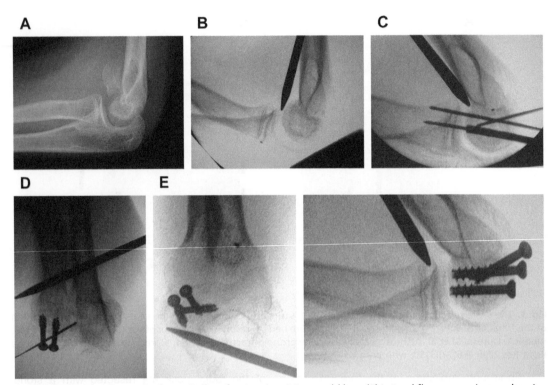

Fig. 4. (*A*) Lateral radiograph of a capitellum fracture in a 14-year-old boy. (*B*) Lateral fluoroscopy image showing arthroscopic-assisted reduction of a capitellum fracture. (*C*) Lateral fluoroscopy image showing arthroscopic-assisted reduction and percutaneous fixation of the capitellum fracture. (*D*) Posteroanterior fluoroscopy image showing arthroscopic-assisted reduction and percutaneous fixation of the fracture. (*E*) Posteroanterior (*left*) and lateral fluoroscopy images (*right*) showing final fixation of a capitellum fracture.

pushing the fragment distally with the trocar. The elbow is flexed more than 90° so that the radial head locks the capitellum into position. If flexing the elbow displaces the fragment, then the trocar, or a Freer elevator, is inserted like a shoehorn into the radiocapitellar joint to keep the fragment in place and to glide the radial head over the capitellum as the elbow is fully flexed. Displaced type 2 fractures are more challenging. The reduction maneuver may be similar, or may require retrieval and distal traction on the fragment with a small skin hook through the posterior radiocapitellar portal. A 70° scope may be useful.

Step 3. Proximal anteromedial and posterior portals are used to visualize and debride the fracture. An accessory posterior radiocapitellar portal may be necessary. There is frequently some comminution or plastic deformation of the distal humerus that prevents anatomic reduction and these bone fragments must be debrided from the posterior radiocapitellar portal.

Step 4. For type 1 capitellar fractures, guidewires for cannulated 3.5-mm screws are then placed percutaneously under fluoroscopic guidance perpendicular to the fracture, from posterior to anterior. The position and length of the screws can be confirmed by direct arthroscopic inspection of the guidewire.

Step 5. After measuring the requisite length of the screws, the wires are advanced, to prevent inadvertent pullout, the holes are drilled, and the screws inserted.

For reducible type 2 fractures, the osseous fragment is usually too thin for screw fixation and must be fixed with transosseous sutures as follows: a distal posterolateral portal is used for visualization. The fracture is stabilized with a Freer elevator anteriorly while a guidewire for a cannulated drill is introduced percutaneously from the posterior humerus into the center of the fragment. A tunnel is then created over the guidewire with the cannulated drill through the humerus. The soft tissue guide is left in place while the drill and guidewire are removed, and 2 free ends of suture are passed through the guide and tunnel into the joint then retrieved with a grasper. Through the posterolateral portal, a 2.5-mm drill is used to create a bone tunnel proximomedial to the fracture for passage of mattress sutures. An 18-G spinal needle is then introduced into the joint via the anteromedial working portal, along with 1 end of a shuttling suture such as 0 or 2-0 polydioxanone suture (PDS). A loop is tied into the steel wire or shuttling suture and the suture is placed into the loop. The wire loop is then cinched down onto the PDS, and used to guide the PDS back into the joint and out through the proximal drill hole to sit outside the arm. These steps are repeated for a PDS passed through a proximolateral bone tunnel. Two more PDS ends are passed through the lesion into the joint. An 18-G needle is introduced through the soft spot into the PRUJ. Steel wire, or a suture shuttle, as described earlier, is used to retrieve the PDS out through the soft spot. This step is repeated for a suture brought out via the posterolateral capsule. The Freer elevator is used to tunnel under the soft tissue and retrieve all the sutures via the posterior wound. The suture pairs are then tied posteriorly to firmly fix the osteochondral fragment with multiple mattress sutures.

For unreducible type 2 and type 3 capitellar fractures, fragment excision is preferred. This procedure can be approached through a lateral open incision or arthroscopically, which offers the dual advantages of minimized risk of nerve and ligamentous damage and allowing full examination of all elbow compartments. Standard anteromedial (viewing) and anterolateral (working) portals can be used. After hematoma evacuation and lavage, the fracture fragments are identified. If the fragments are too small for fixation, they can be debrided as loose bodies. Other joint surfaces, in particular the radial head, should be inspected for traumatic defects. Early range of motion exercises are advocated postoperatively to prevent arthrofibrosis.

SURGICAL PROCEDURE: PEDIATRIC LATERAL CONDYLE

Step 1. A standard anteromedial viewing portal is established, and an anterolateral working portal is used (**Fig. 5**). A standard 4.5-mm arthroscope is used for patients older than 3 years.

Step 2. Manual pressure over the lateral condyle is used to reduce the fracture under arthroscopic visualization, and percutaneous 1.6-mm (0.062-inch) Kirschner wires (K-wires) are inserted in a retrograde manner for use as joysticks laterally.

Step 3. After adequate fracture reduction, 2 K-wires are advanced proximally and medially from the distal lateral portion of the fragment, engaging the medial cortex proximal to the fracture.

Step 4. A third K-wire is placed percutaneously at the level of the center of the capitellum in a posterior-to-anterior direction for rotational control.

Step 5. The position and trajectory of the K-wires are confirmed fluoroscopically, whereas the maintenance of an anatomic articular reduction is confirmed through arthroscopic visualization.

Immediate Postoperative Care

Postoperative care depends on the procedure performed, the fracture type, and the fixation stability. The elbow may be splinted as necessary and active motion is initiated according to the fracture and circumstances, similar to open surgery.

REHABILITATION AND RECOVERY

The goals of rehabilitation after arthroscopic fracture fixation in the elbow are preservation of motion while protecting the fracture until healing occurs. Forearm supination may be considered during rehabilitation following coronoid fixation for added stability.[15] For radial head fractures, elbow range of motion should begin 3 days after surgery because stiffness is an especially important concern in these scenarios.[18] For capitellar fractures, postoperative management should consist of early range of motion to prevent stiffness.

At the start of physical therapy, gentle passive range-of-motion exercises are begun at 25° to 100° of flexion, gradually increasing by 5° of flexion and 10° of extension per week within a stable range. Patients should be aware that shoulder elevation, abduction or internal rotation can produce varus or valgus forces across the elbow as well.[19] By week 3 of therapy, the goal for elbow range of motion is 20° to 110° and active range of motion is initiated without resistance. Active shoulder range of motion and periscapular exercises may also be performed at this time.

At 4 weeks after surgery, the goal of elbow range of motion should be 0° to 125° and light resistive exercises can begin. By 6 weeks, full elbow range of motion should be obtained and formal strengthening of the elbow can begin, gradually increasing weights by 2.3 kg (5 lb) per week as tolerated. Contact sports should not be initiated until full strength is achieved, which is defined as strength

658

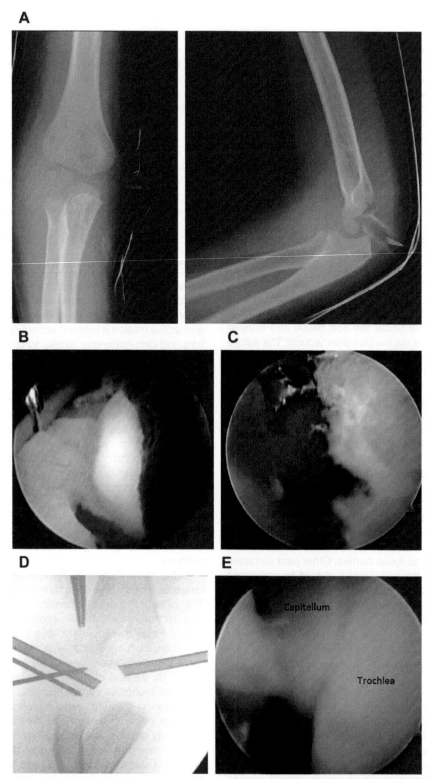

Fig. 5. (*A*) Lateral radiograph showing a pediatric lateral condyle fracture. (*B*) Arthroscopic view of the lateral condyle fragment from the medial portal, preparing to advance the medial cannula to the fracture site for pin placement in the lateral condyle. (*C*) Arthroscopic view from the medial portal to confirm the position of the K-wire in the fragment, then reduce and advance the K-wire. (*D*) Anteroposterior radiograph showing provisional fixation with prepositioned K-wires. (*E*) Arthroscopic view from the lateral portal, showing reduced capitellar fragment.

F

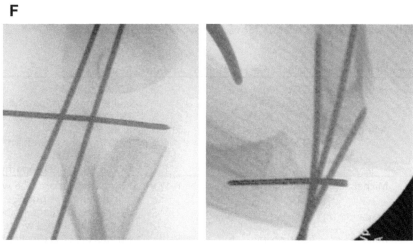

Fig. 5. (*continued*). (*F*) Corresponding anteroposterior (*left*) and lateral (*right*) radiographs showing reduction and fixation with K-wires. The transcondylar K-wire significantly increases stability and resistance to rotation.

comparable with the contralateral side if normal. This strength is generally achieved after 8 weeks from surgery.

CLINICAL RESULTS IN THE LITERATURE

Most current clinical results in the literature on these techniques come in the form of small case series, and more research is needed to evaluate the efficacy of arthroscopic fracture fixation techniques compared with other treatment.[20] However, the available evidence supports the use of elbow arthroscopy in the management of intra-articular elbow fractures.[21]

Visualization of the coronoid for fixation is especially challenging, and arthroscopic-assisted fixation offers the advantage of improved visibility.[14,15,22,23] Other techniques for fixation include the direct anterior approach, lateral approaches after radial head excision, indirect posterior-to-anterior fixation, or nonoperative management if the elbow is stable.[16,24] There are special considerations in overhead athletes with coronoid fractures, in whom type I coronoid fractures have been reported to result in loose body formation and hypertrophic fibrous nonunion requiring arthroscopic excision.[25] **Table 1** provides a summary of the clinical results for arthroscopic-assisted fracture fixation in the elbow.

Radial head fractures have been treated nonoperatively, with open reduction with internal fixation (ORIF), with arthroscopic-assisted fixation, with open or arthroscopic excision, or with radial head replacement.[17,26–30] In select, nondisplaced Mason type 2 fractures with no block to motion,

nonoperative treatment has yielded results comparable with open surgery.[29] For displaced type 2 fractures, Rolla and colleagues[26] fixed these arthroscopically with a single cannulated screw, placed from an anterolateral portal perpendicular to the fracture line. Their short-term results yielded no complications, and all patients returned to premorbid activity within 6 months. Excision is indicated for comminuted fractures or for small fragments less than 25% of the articular surface, in low-demand patients with no concomitant elbow or forearm disorder.[27]

Capitellar fractures have been treated arthroscopically as well.[31,32] Coronal shear fractures of the distal humerus are particularly challenging to assess adequately with radiography, and arthroscopy has been shown to improve outcomes in these fractures to avoid fishtail deformity.[33,34] Open treatment puts the posterior interosseous nerve and lateral collateral ligament at risk in this approach. An arthroscopic approach to these fractures minimizes risk to the lateral ligaments, allows better visualization of all joint spaces of the elbow, and facilitates earlier rehabilitation.

Arthrofibrosis following fracture can also be treated arthroscopically with chondral debridement and capsular release. This technique has been shown to increase the arc of motion by approximately 20° to 30° on average.[35,36] This technique may be favored to minimize stiffness following contracture release in case early rehabilitation is possible. Other posttraumatic conditions of the elbow can be treated with arthroscopic debridement, such as debridement of fishtail deformity of the distal humerus with or without

Table 1
Results of arthroscopic-assisted fixation for various types of elbow fracture

Fracture Type	First Author	Journal (Year)	No. of Patients	Follow-up (mo)	Results
Coronoid	Hausman[22]	CORR (2008)	4	12–23	ROM 2.5°–140° Full pronation/supination No recurrent instability
	Adams[23]	Arthroscopy (2007)	6	31.8	ROM 9°–133° 87°/79° pronosupination Mayo score 100 HO and ulnar neuropathy
Radial head	Michels[30]	Knee Surg (2007)	14	1–11 y	Mayo elbow score 97.6 with 79% excellent/21% good Associated cartilage lesions in capitellum fared worse
	Rolla[26]	Arthroscopy (2006)	6	6–18	Mayo score 50% excellent/50% good
Radial head (excision)	Wijeratna[27]	Int Orthop (2012)	15	5–47	Average Quick-DASH 24.7 AROM 9°–138°/63°/62°
Lateral condyle	Hausman[1]	J Pediatr Orthop (2007)	6	5–11	Full AROM No deformity AVN in 1 case
	Perez Carro[2]	Arthroscopy (2007)	4	2–3	Full AROM No complications
Capitellum (excision)	Feldman[32]	Arthroscopy (1997)	2	15–17	Full AROM in 1 patient AROM 0°–125°, 90°/90° in the other with grade IV chondral damage to radius No complications
Capitellum	Hardy[31]	Arthroscopy (2002)	1	3	AROM 15°–140°, 90°/90°
	Kuriyama[33]	J Hand Surg (2010)	2	17–20	AROM 0°–5°/125°–160°/85°–90°/90° AVN in 1 case, no pain

Abbreviations: AROM, active range of motion; AVN, avascular necrosis; CORR, Clinical Orthopaedics and Related Research; DASH, disabilities of the arm, shoulder and hand; HO, heterotopic ossification.
   Data from Refs.[1,2,22,23,26,27,30–33]

hemiepiphysiodesis after posttraumatic osteonecrosis.[34] In general, removal of loose bodies and mechanical blocks to motion produces better results than chondroplasty.[37]

SUMMARY

Many fractures about the elbow can be treated with arthroscopic assistance, including fractures of the coronoid, radial head, capitellum, and lateral condyle. Advantages to arthroscopic-assisted internal fixation for these fractures include improved visualization and less soft tissue trauma. However, the techniques are challenging and have potential complications. Furthermore, most current clinical research on these techniques has been from small case series, and more research is needed to evaluate the efficacy compared with other treatment.

REFERENCES

1. Hausman MR, Qureshi S, Goldstein R, et al. Arthroscopically-assisted treatment of pediatric lateral humeral condyle fractures. J Pediatr Orthop 2007; 27(7):739–42.
2. Perez Carro L, Golano P, Vega J. Arthroscopic-assisted reduction and percutaneous external fixation of lateral condyle fractures of the humerus. Arthroscopy 2007;23(10):1131.e1–4.
3. Micheli LJ, Luke AC, Mintzer CM, et al. Elbow arthroscopy in the pediatric and adolescent population. Arthroscopy 2001;17(7):694–9.
4. Reddy AS, Kvitne RS, Yocum LA, et al. Arthroscopy of the elbow: a long-term clinical review. Arthroscopy 2000;16(6):588–94.
5. Kelly EW, Morrey BF, O'Driscoll SW. Complications of elbow arthroscopy. J Bone Joint Surg Am 2001; 83(1):25–34.

6. Atesok K, Doral MN, Whipple T, et al. Arthroscopy-assisted fracture fixation [review]. Knee Surg Sports Traumatol Arthrosc 2011;19(2):320–9.

7. Field LD, Altchek DW. Evaluation of the arthroscopic valgus instability test of the elbow. Am J Sports Med 1996;24(2):177–81.

8. O'Driscoll SW, Morrey BF, Korinek S, et al. Elbow subluxation and dislocation. A spectrum of instability. Clin Orthop Relat Res 1992;280:186–97.

9. Hsu JW, Gould JL, Fonseca-Sabune H, et al. The emerging role of elbow arthroscopy in chronic use injuries and fracture care [review]. Hand Clin 2009; 25(3):305–21.

10. Lynch GJ, Meyers JF, Whipple TL, et al. Neurovascular anatomy and elbow arthroscopy: inherent risks. Arthroscopy 1986;2:190–7.

11. Dodson CC, Nho SJ, Williams RJ 3rd, et al. Elbow arthroscopy. J Am Acad Orthop Surg 2008;16(10): 574–85.

12. Regan W, Morrey B. Fractures of the coronoid process of the ulna. J Bone Joint Surg Am 1989;71(9): 1348–54.

13. Beingessner DM, Dunning CE, Stacpoole RA, et al. The effect of coronoid fractures on elbow kinematics and stability. Clin Biomech (Bristol, Avon) 2007; 22(2):183–90.

14. O'Brien MJ, Savoie FH 3rd. Arthroscopic and open management of posterolateral rotatory instability of the elbow. Sports Med Arthrosc 2014; 22(3):194–200.

15. Reichel LM, Milam GS, Reitman CA. Anterior approach for operative fixation of coronoid fractures in complex elbow instability. Tech Hand Up Extrem Surg 2012;16(2):98–104.

16. Savoie FH 3rd, Field LD, Gurley DJ. Arthroscopic and open radial ulnohumeral ligament reconstruction for posterolateral rotatory instability of the elbow. Hand Clin 2009;25(3):323–9.

17. Menth-Chiari WA, Poehling GG, Ruch DS. Arthroscopic resection of the radial head. Arthroscopy 1999;15(2):226–30.

18. Paschos NK, Mitsionis GI, Vasiliadis HS, et al. Comparison of early mobilization protocols in radial head fractures. J Orthop Trauma 2013;27(3):134–9.

19. Pipicelli JG, Chinchalkar SJ, Grewal R, et al. Rehabilitation considerations in the management of terrible triad injury to the elbow [review]. Tech Hand Up Extrem Surg 2011;15(4):198–208.

20. Van Tongel A, Macdonald P, Van Riet R, et al. Elbow arthroscopy in acute injuries [review]. Knee Surg Sports Traumatol Arthrosc 2012;20(12):2542–8.

21. Yeoh KM, King GJ, Faber KJ, et al. Evidence-based indications for elbow arthroscopy [review]. Arthroscopy 2012;28(2):272–82.

22. Hausman MR, Klug RA, Qureshi S, et al. Arthroscopically assisted coronoid fracture fixation: a preliminary report. Clin Orthop Relat Res 2008;466(12): 3147–52.

23. Adams JE, Merten SM, Steinmann SP. Arthroscopic assisted treatment of coronoid fractures. Arthroscopy 2007;23(10):1060–5.

24. Papatheodorou LK, Rubright JH, Heim KA, et al. Terrible triad injuries of the elbow: does the coronoid always need to be fixed? Clin Orthop Relat Res 2014;472(7):2084–91.

25. Liu SH, Henry M, Bowen R. Complications of type I coronoid fractures in competitive athletes: report of two cases and review of the literature. J Shoulder Elbow Surg 1996;5(3):223–7.

26. Rolla PR, Surace MF, Bini A, et al. Arthroscopic treatment of fractures of the radial head. Arthroscopy 2006;22(2):233.e1–6.

27. Wijeratna M, Bailey KA, Pace A, et al. Arthroscopic radial head excision in managing elbow trauma. Int Orthop 2012;36(12):2507–12.

28. Lapner M, King GJ. Radial head fractures [review]. J Bone Joint Surg Am 2013;95(12):1136–43.

29. Lindenhovius AL, Felsch Q, Ring D, et al. The long-term outcome of open reduction and internal fixation of stable displaced isolated partial articular fractures of the radial head. J Trauma 2009;67(1): 143–6.

30. Michels F, Pouliart N, Handelberg F. Arthroscopic management of Mason type 2 radial head fractures. Knee Surg Sports Traumatol Arthrosc 2007;15(10): 1244–50.

31. Hardy P, Menguy F, Guillot S. Arthroscopic treatment of capitellum fracture of the humerus. Arthroscopy 2002;18(4):422–6.

32. Feldman MD. Arthroscopic excision of type II capitellar fractures. Arthroscopy 1997;13(6):743–8.

33. Kuriyama K, Kawanishi Y, Yamamoto K. Arthroscopic-assisted reduction and percutaneous fixation for coronal shear fractures of the distal humerus: report of two cases. J Hand Surg Am 2010;35(9): 1506–9.

34. Glotzbecker MP, Bae DS, Links AC, et al. Fishtail deformity of the distal humerus: a report of 15 cases. J Pediatr Orthop 2013;33(6):592–7.

35. Timmerman LA, Andrews JR. Arthroscopic treatment of posttraumatic elbow pain and stiffness. Am J Sports Med 1994;22(2):230–5.

36. Lapner PC, Leith JM, Regan WD. Arthroscopic debridement of the elbow for arthrofibrosis resulting from nondisplaced fracture of the radial head. Arthroscopy 2005;21(12):1492.

37. Andrews JR, St Pierre RK, Carson WG Jr. Arthroscopy of the elbow. Clin Sports Med 1986;5(4): 653–62.

Elbow Trauma in the Athlete

Lauren H. Redler, MD*, Joshua S. Dines, MD

KEYWORDS

- Medial epicondyle avulsion fracture • Medial ulnar collateral ligament injury (MCL)
- Distal biceps rupture • Triceps rupture • Olecranon stress fracture

KEY POINTS

- Less displacement in medial epicondyle fractures is tolerated in valgus stress athletes, including pitchers and gymnasts.
- Surgical reconstruction of the medial ulnar collateral ligament gets athletes back to their previous level of play more than 80% of the time and has more favorable outcomes compared with primary repair.
- The choice of surgical approach and method of tendon fixation for repair of distal biceps tendon ruptures should be dictated by surgeon experience and comfort.
- Potential complications of triceps tendon repairs include olecranon bursitis and irritation from underlying internal fixation, which often requires removal of hardware.
- Aggressive early fixation of olecranon stress fractures is necessary in the competitive athlete because they often fail to respond to nonoperative treatment.

MEDIAL EPICONDYLE AVULSION FRACTURE IN THE ADOLESCENT ATHLETE

Introduction

An important anatomic characteristic unique to the elbows of young athletes is the timeline of skeletal maturity. Fusion of the capitellum (1–2 years), radial head (2–5 years), elbow trochlea (8–10 years), olecranon process (10–11 years), lateral epicondyle (11–13 years), and the medial epicondyle (15–16 years) occurs in a somewhat predictable but variable manner. These 6 ossification centers correspond to potential elbow injury sites, because the epiphyseal plates are weaker than the surrounding bone.[1]

Medial epicondyle fractures make up approximately 10% to 20% of all elbow fractures in children and adults.[2] Males patients represent nearly three-fourths of those injured, with a peak age of 11 to 12 years.[3] Before skeletal maturity, valgus overload stress more predictably leads to medial epicondyle avulsion fractures.[4] With closure of the medial epicondyle physis, there is a shift from growth plate injuries to ligamentous and flexor-pronator muscle injury.[1] With repeated microtrauma or acute elbow dislocation, athletes generally report feeling sudden pain and hearing a pop.[5,6] On physical examination, patients will present with loss of motion, local soft tissue swelling, and point tenderness over the medial epicondyle. Standard anteroposterior, lateral, and oblique radiographs demonstrate the avulsed fragment with varying displacement.[7,8]

Fractures through the physeal plate can have 2 distinct patterns[9] (**Table 1**). The fracture fragment is usually displaced distally due to the traction

Hospital for Special Surgery, Sports Medicine and Shoulder Service, 535 East 70th Street, New York, NY 10021, USA
* Corresponding author.
E-mail address: Lauren.redler@gmail.com

Hand Clin 31 (2015) 663–681
http://dx.doi.org/10.1016/j.hcl.2015.07.002
0749-0712/15/$ – see front matter © 2015 Elsevier Inc. All rights reserved.

Table 1
Classification of pediatric medial epicondyle avulsion fractures

Type	Age	Characteristics	Treatment
1	Younger	• Large fragment (often entire epicondyle) • Often displaced anteriorly and distally • Can become entrapped in joint	Usually requires operative fixation
2	Adolescent	• Small fracture fragment • Medial epicondylar fragmentation	Depends on elbow stability

From Safran MR. Elbow injuries in athletes. A review. Clin Orthop Relat Res 1995;(310):264; with permission.

forces of the common origin of the wrist flexors and medial collateral ligament attachments on the medial epicondyle (**Fig. 1**). Intra-articular incarceration of the fragment happens in 15% to 18%, usually with type 1 fractures.[10]

Mechanisms for acute fracture include

- Direct force applied to the medial epicondyle
- Avulsion force from valgus or extension loading

- Elbow dislocation

Indications for nonoperative treatment include

- Less than 2-mm displacement on radiographs

Indications for surgical treatment include[2,7,8,10–15]

- Greater than 5- to 15-mm displacement (lower threshold in valgus stress athletes: pitcher, gymnast)
- Fragment incarceration in the joint
- Open fracture
- Gross instability
- Ulnar nerve involvement/entrapment (relative)

These indications are slightly altered for the high-performance athlete who requires a stable elbow for participation in their sport. The dependence on the medial epicondyle to withstand valgus stress in these athletes has led many authors to advocate for surgical treatment, even in the setting of minimal displacement.[16,17]

Surgical Technique

Goals of operative fixation are to maximize the possibility of early return to full function and high-level activity and to minimize late deformity and the likelihood of stiffness (as with prolonged cast immobilization).

Surgical techniques include

- Kirschner (K) wire fixation
- Screw fixation (**Fig. 2**)
- Suture
- Excision of fragment with soft tissue repair

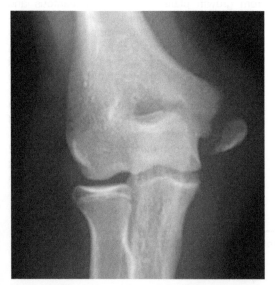

Fig. 1. Medial epicondyle avulsion fracture. Type 1 fracture with a large fragment displaced distally.

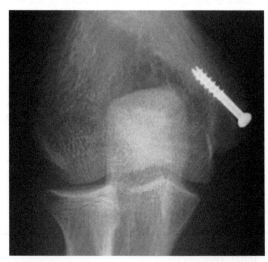

Fig. 2. Open reduction internal fixation of a medial epicondyle avulsion fracture. Screw is oriented perpendicular to the fracture and proximally to avoid penetrating the coronoid fossa.

- Tension band wiring
- Palmer nails
- Closed reduction and percutaneous pinning (caution due to proximity of ulnar nerve)

Fragment excision and reattachment of the soft tissue of the medial elbow have been described for cases with comminution and instability.[18]

Preoperative planning

The size of the fracture fragment helps guide the appropriate strategy for internal fixation. It is important to note the presence or absence of preoperative ulnar nerve symptoms and any concomitant injuries.

Preparation and patient positioning

- Supine position with the entire operative extremity extended onto a hand table
- A lateral position used based on surgeon preference
- Nonsterile tourniquet placed as far proximal as possible
- General anesthesia

Surgical approach/procedure

- Exsanguinate limb and elevate tourniquet to 250 mm Hg
- A 4-cm incision just posterior to the medial epicondyle (this gives access to visualize and protect the ulnar nerve as well as prevents later discomfort if the scar is centered over the prominence)
- Free the ulnar nerve, protect with a vessel loop
- Ensure removal of any soft tissue obstructions to anatomic fracture reduction
- Reduce fragment; towel clip, Alice clamp, or Esmarch bandage applied distally to proximally to gently milk the fracture fragment to its donor site
- Guidewire for 4.0-mm cannulated partially threaded screw placed in the center of the fragment in a superomedial and posterior to anterior trajectory
- Fluoroscopy to confirm position of guidewire

Pearls

- To aid in reduction, ensure the wrist is fully flexed with the fingers flexed and relaxed
- Use a peripheral K-wire or 18-gauge needle for provisional fixation and to prevent spinning
- Retro drill the fracture fragment to ensure you are in the center with the guidewire

- Medial epicondyle is a posterior structure (the trajectory of guidewire and screw will be from posterior to anterior)
- Do not overcompress

Pitfalls

- Do not place screw in the olecranon fossa
- If screw is overcompressed, the fragment can be split: use sutures or small K-wires to keep together and keep patient in a cast longer
- Do not penetrate the lateral column with the guidewire: risk wrapping up the radial nerve

Immediate postoperative care

Patients are immobilized at 70 to 90° of flexion and neutral forearm rotation for 7 to 10 days to allow for soft tissue healing.

Rehabilitation and Recovery

Subsequently, the arm is placed in a posterior splint, which patients remove under controlled conditions to perform gentle passive range of motion 3 to 5 times per day. Alternatively, a hinged elbow brace with free range can be used for the first 4 to 6 weeks. Active range of motion is initiated when palpation of the medial epicondyle is pain-free. Physical therapy is initiated at 6 to 8 weeks only if full range of motion has not been achieved and is usually required in about half of the patients.[19] Return to full sports and throwing may occur at 3 months.

Clinical Results in the Literature

Long-term data from Farsetti and colleagues[13] have shown that operative and nonoperative treatment of medial epicondyle fractures with displacement ranging from 5 to 15 mm had comparable results at a mean follow-up of greater than 30 years. However, in a systematic review, operative fixation was found to provide a higher union rate, while both pain symptoms and ulnar nerve complications were not significantly different between the nonoperative and operative groups.[10] In a recent series, Lawrence and colleagues[19] noted that regardless of nonoperative or operative treatment, all athletes were able to return to competitive sports at their previous level of play. For a full list of clinical results, see **Table 2**.[11,13,14,19–29]

MEDIAL ULNAR COLLATERAL LIGAMENT INJURY
Introduction

The anterior bundle of the medial ulnar collateral ligament (MCL) is the primary stabilizer to valgus stress during the throwing motion. High tensile

Table 2
Clinical outcomes for pediatric medial epicondyle fractures

Author, Year	No. of Patients (M/F)	Mean Age (Range) (y)	Average F/U, mo	Nonoperative Treatment	Operative Treatment	Union Nonop./Total Nonop.	Union Op./Total Op.
Lawrence et al,[19] 2013	20 (13/7)	Nonop: 11.5 ± 2.4; Op: 12.8 ± 2.6	43.2	6	14	6/6 (100%)	14/14 (100%)
Ip & Tsang,[24] 2007	24 (15/9)	13 (9–17)	27.4	4	20	3/4 (75%)	17/20 (85%)
Haxhija et al,[23] 2006	14 (15/10)	12 (7–15)	36	0	14	All op.	14/14 (100%)
Lee et al,[25] 2005	25 (18/7)	13.7 (7.5–17.4)	27.2	0	25	All op.	25/25 (100%)
Farsetti et al,[13] 2001	42 (27/15)	12 (8–15)	408	19	23	2/19 (10.5%)	17/17 (100%)
Pimpalnerkar et al,[26] 1998	14 (12/2)	9.7 (6–16)	17.2	0	12	All op.	6/14 (43%)
Duun et al,[21] 1994	33 (16/17)	12 (7–15)	96	0	33	All op.	30/33 (91%)
Skak et al,[27] 1994	23 (13/11)	10.3 (4–14)	86.4	3	21	0/3 (0%)	20/21 (95%)
Fowles et al,[22] 1990	28 (27/5)	12 (6–16)	Nonop: 17.9; Op: 20	19	9	13/19 (68.4%)	8/9 (89%)
Wilson et al,[29] 1988	43 (26/17)	Nonop: 11.8 (7–16.2); Op: 12 (7.3–16.1)	55.2	20	23	11/20 (55%)	20/23 (87%)
Hines et al,[11] 1987	31 (no data)	12.7 (7–16)	49.2	0	31	All op.	30/31 (97%)
Dias et al,[20] 1987	20 (6/14)	13 (9–16)	42	20	0	0/20 (0%)	All nonop.
van Niekerk & Severijnen,[28] 1985	20 (10/10)	10	24	9	10	8/9 (89%)	10/11 (91%)
Papavasiliou,[14] 1982	91 (76/15)	11.5 (5–17)	Range 36–216	28	63	23/28 (82%)	63/63 (100%)

Abbreviations: F/U, follow-up; nonop, nonoperative; op, operative.
Data from Refs.[11,13,14,19–29]

stresses particularly during the late cocking phase can exceed the failure strength of the ligament, leading to attenuation or rupture.[16]

Indications for surgery include

- Complete tear of the anterior bundle in athletes wishing to return to throwing sports
- Partial tear in athletes who have failed a comprehensive rehabilitation program
- Occasional nonthrowing athletes who remain symptomatic after nonoperative treatment

Surgical Technique (Docking Technique)

Preoperative planning

It is imperative to check for the presence or absence of the ipsilateral palmaris longus tendon for use as a tendon graft. If not present, use of the contralateral palmaris, gracilis, plantaris, or toe extensor tendon can be considered. In addition, patients should be examined for ulnar neuropathy or ulnar nerve instability.

Preparation and patient positioning

- Supine on the operating table with elbow centered on a hand table
- Nonsterile tourniquet placed as far proximal as possible
- General anesthesia

Surgical approach/procedure

In a landmark article, Jobe and colleagues[30] published the first results of an MCL reconstructive technique with submuscular transposition of the ulnar nerve. Over the years, the technique has been modified from the original flexor-pronator mass detachment,[30,31] to elevation,[32–35] and now

via a muscle-splitting approach.[36–43] A variety of tunnel configurations and fixation techniques are described in the literature, including suture anchors, bone tunnels, docking technique, and tenodesis screw fixation.

The procedure is started by exsanguinating the limb and elevating the tourniquet to 250 mm Hg followed by graft harvest via 3 small incisions on the volar forearm. Care must be taken to assure harvest of the palmaris and not the similar-looking flexor carpi radialis or median nerve.

Surgical steps include[36]

- A medial incision centered over the medial epicondyle
- Identification and protection of the medial antebrachial cutaneous nerve with a vessel loop
- If planning to do an ulnar nerve transposition, the ulnar nerve release must continue proximally to the arcade of Struthers and distally to its branch to the flexor carpi ulnaris, and a portion of the medial intermuscular septum is removed to prevent tenting of the transposed nerve. Carefully dissect and protect the ulnar nerve with a vessel loop or Penrose drain.
- Use a muscle-splitting approach (**Fig. 3**) through the flexor mass to expose the anterior bundle of the MCL.
- Incise the ligament longitudinally (**Fig. 4**) to visualize the deeper portion and the joint.
- Two 3.5-mm bur holes are made anterior and posterior to the sublime tubercle, 5 to 10 mm distal to the articular surface of the coronoid process, separated by 1 cm, and then connected with a curved curette.

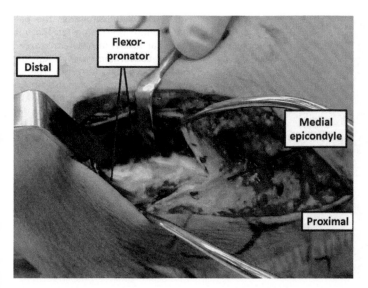

Fig. 3. Flexor-pronator muscle splitting approach. The flexor-pronator muscle mass is split to expose the MCL. This avoids the need to elevate the muscle mass completely off its origin.

Distal

Flexor-pronator

Medial epicondyle

Proximal

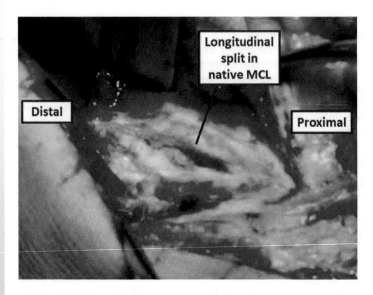

Longitudinal
split in
native MCL

Distal

Proximal

Fig. 4. Longitudinal incision in the native MCL. This provides visualization of the joint and allows access to the deep portion of the medial epicondyle for preparation and tunnel drilling.

- Two antegrade 1.5-mm medial epicondylar connecting tunnels are placed along the proximal portion of the epicondyle separated by 1 cm and converge with a 4.0 mm × 15 mm retrograde tunnel at the origin of the MCL.
- Shuttle the graft with the aid of looped sutures through the ulna.
- Repair the native ligament with nonabsorbable sutures for supplemental stability.
- The posterior limb is then docked in the anterior humeral tunnel.
- Determine the length of graft needed in the second limb after the first limb is docked in the anterior humeral tunnel.

- Excise excess tendon and whipstitch tendon for the estimated length to be positioned in the humeral tunnel. Alternatively, after docking, this excess graft can come back out the humeral tunnel and be sewn to the anterior limb of the graft for augmentation.
- Dock the graft and tie sutures over a bone bridge along the proximal portion of the medial epicondyle with the elbow in 30° of flexion, supination, and application of a varus force on the elbow (Fig. 5).
- Secure the graft with multiple side-to-side nonabsorbable sutures.

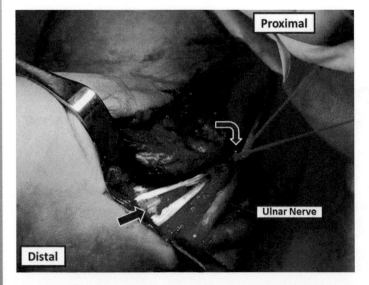

Proximal

Ulnar Nerve

Distal

Fig. 5. Docking technique. The palmaris longus graft is passed through the ulnar tunnel (arrow) and docked in the converging tunnels on the medial epicondyle (asterisk). The sutures are tied over a bone bridge (curved arrow). In this patient, the ulnar nerve was decompressed for planned transposition.

- If an ulnar nerve transposition is indicated: fascial sling from the flexor-pronator muscle fascia, tensioned loosely.

Immediate postoperative care

The elbow is splinted at 90° and neutral forearm rotation for 7 to 10 days to allow for soft tissue healing. Patients are switched to a hinged elbow brace at postoperative week 1.

Rehabilitation and Recovery

A supervised postoperative rehabilitation protocol is imperative. The patient starts with active wrist, elbow, and shoulder range of motion. Strength exercises do not begin until 1 to 2 months postoperatively. A throwing program is initiated at 4 months starting with tossing the ball short distances. The program progresses to throwing from the pitching mound at up to 70% of maximum effort at 8 months. Return to competition is discouraged until 1 year after surgery.

Clinical Results in the Literature

In the series by Jobe and colleagues,[30] 63% of athletes returned to their previous level of participation in sports, but there was a high incidence of complications related to the ulnar nerve requiring reoperation. For this reason, there was a transition from submuscular transposition[30,31] to obligatory subcutaneous transposition.[32–35] Currently, subcutaneous transposition is favored but only done if patients have preoperative motor symptoms or persistent sensory symptoms.[36–42,44,45] A recent systematic review noted that surgical reconstruction gets athletes back to their previous level of play more than 80% of the time.[46] For a full list of clinical results of ulnar collateral ligament reconstruction, see **Table 3**.[30–45]

Primary repair of proximal or distal injuries of the MCL is a viable alternative in the non-high-level athlete and can have favorable outcomes with a rapid return to sports.[47] Overall, however, repair has shown inferior results as compared with reconstruction.[16,31–33]

DISTAL BICEPS RUPTURE
Introduction

The typical presentation is a middle-aged man with sudden onset severe pain and often an audible pop when performing an eccentric contraction of the biceps.[48] Patients will experience a loss of flexion and supination strength, and if the tear is complete, will have proximal displacement of the distal biceps tendon with a bulge (a Popeye deformity). There may be pre-existing degenerative changes within the tendon, because there is usually a history of prodromal symptoms.[9]

The hook test, which assesses for continuity of the tendon in the antecubital fossa, can be used to diagnose complete tears. There is little controversy in the treatment of these injuries, because restoration of full function requires operative repair.[49] Classification of complete tears can be seen in **Fig. 6**. After 4 weeks, the biceps muscle atrophies, and the tendon scars and may lose length.[49]

Surgical Technique
Preoperative planning

- Determine the available length of biceps tendon based on preoperative MRI; if inadequate length is anticipated, ensure that allograft is available for reconstruction if necessary.

Preparation and patient positioning

- Supine with elbow centered on a hand table
- Nonsterile tourniquet as proximal as possible
- If 2-incision technique is planned, ensure the patient has adequate ipsilateral shoulder internal rotation to gain access to the posterior aspect of the ulna with the arm in full pronation.

Surgical approach/procedure

- Procedure ideally done within 2 to 3 weeks to prevent scar formation in the biceps tendon sheath.[49]
- Fixation options include suturing through bone tunnels, suture anchors, cortical buttons, and tenodesis screws.
- Traditionally, single-incision technique is associated with a high incidence of radial nerve palsies secondary to dissection, and the 2-incision technique is associated with radioulnar synostosis and heterotopic ossification.[49]
- Now with similar results,[50,51] the choice of surgical approach and method of tendon should be dictated by surgeon preference and comfort.

Single-incision technique is as follows:

- Three-centimeter transverse incision just distal to the elbow flexion crease
- The lateral antebrachial cutaneous (LABC) nerve identified and protected with a vessel loop

Table 3
Clinical outcomes for ulnar collateral ligament reconstruction

Author, Year	No. of Ulnar Collateral Ligament Reconstructions	No. of Excellent Results (%)	Mean Age (Range) (y)	No. of Patients by Sport	Average F/U (Range) (y)	Mean Time to Return to Play (Range) (mo)
Jones et al,[45] 2014	55	48/55 (87%)	17.6 (15–18)	47 baseball, 3 gymnastics, 5 javelin	2.6 (2–3.1)	11.5 (9–14)
Dines et al,[44] 2012	10	9/10 (90%)	18.5 (18–21)	10 javelin	2.4 (2–3.8)	15 (NR)
Hechtman et al,[39] 2011	34	29/34 (85%)	18.7 (15–23)	34 baseball	6.9 (4.2–8.7)	10 (7–13)
Cain et al,[34] 2010	1281 (743 F/U)	617/743 (83%)	21.5 (14–59)	1213 baseball, 15 javelin, 13 football, 9 softball, 7 tennis, 4 cheerleading, 2 wrestling, 2 soccer, 2 gymnastics, 1 pole-vaulting	3.2 (2–10.8)	11.6 (3–72)
Bowers et al,[36] 2010	21	19/21 (90%)	20 (16–27)	21 baseball	2.3 (2–4.1)	NR
Dines et al,[37] 2007	22	19/22 (86%)	20.1 (16–24)	20 baseball, 1 hockey, 1 football	3 (1.6–4.6)	NR
Koh et al,[40] 2006	20 (19 F/U)	18/19 (95%)	21.7 (17–25)	20 baseball	3.5 (0.5–5.6)	13.1 (NR)
Dodson et al,[38] 2006	100	90/100 (90%)	22 (16–43)	96 baseball, 2 football, 2 tennis	3 (2–5)	NR
Paletta & Wright,[41] 2006	25	23/25 (92%)	24.5 (19–27)	25 baseball	2.5 (2–NR)	11.5 (10–16)
Petty et al,[35] 2004	31 (27 F/U)	20/27 (74%)	17.4 (15–19)	27 baseball	2.92 (1.5–6.25)	11 (NR)
Rohrbough et al,[42] 2002	36	33/36 (92%)	23 (15–57)	33 baseball, 1 lacrosse, 1 tennis, 1 golf	3.3 (2.1–5.3)	NR
Thompson et al,[43] 2001	83 (33 F/U)	27/33 (82%)	24.3 (NR)	78 baseball, 2 javelin, 1 football, 1 platform diving, 1 softball	3.1 (2–4)	13 (6–18)
Azar et al,[33] 2000	78	53/67 (79%)	21.6 (15–39)	85 baseball, 3 football, 1 tennis, 1 wrestling, 1 farm-related	2.95 (1–6)	9.8 (NR)
Andrews & Timmerman,[32] 1995	12 (9 F/U)	7/9 (78%)	NR	NR	NR	NR
Conway et al,[31] 1992	56	38/56 (68%)	23.7 (15–24)	52 baseball, 3 javelin, 1 tennis	6.3 (2–15)	12.5 (8–21)
Jobe et al,[30] 1986	16	10/16 (63%)	NR (20–31)	14 baseball, 2 javelin	4.3 (2–9.75)	NR (11–19)

Abbreviations: F/U, follow-up; NR, not reported.
Data from Refs.[30–45]

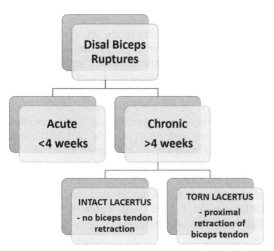

Fig. 6. Classification of distal biceps tendon ruptures.

- The stump of the biceps located subcutaneously with blunt finger dissection
- The tendon stump debrided and whipstitched with a no. 2 braided nonabsorbable suture
- The radial recurrent vessels ligated in the interval between the brachioradialis and pronator teres
- Tuberosity visualized and cleared of any remaining soft tissue
- While placing fixation into the tuberosity (interference screw, suture anchors, or a cortical button), ensure the forearm is in full supination to protect the posterior interosseous nerve (PIN) from injury

Suture anchor technique

- Placed on the ulnar edge of the tuberosity, 1 proximal and the second 5 to 10 mm distal
- Tendon tied down to the suture anchors
- Advantage: no drilling of the far cortex, reducing the risk of PIN injury
- Disadvantage: inferior fixation strength compared with suspensory fixation[52]

Cortical button technique

- Guidewire placed bicortically through the midpoint of the ulnar border of the tuberosity
- Drill in a 30° ulnar trajectory to be farthest from the PIN[53]
- Endobutton reamer passed bicortically over the guidewire
- 7.0-mm or 8.0-mm reamer passed through the near cortex only
- Button added to suture construct connected to the biceps tendon
- With an inserter, the button is then delivered to the far cortex, and the sutures are toggled to lock the button in place

- Confirm appropriate positioning of the button with intraoperative fluoroscopy

Interference screw technique

- Guide pin placed into the tuberosity
- Near cortex reamed with a 5.0-mm reamer
- Sutures sewn into the tendon are passed through a tenodesis screw and screwdriver
- With proper tensioning, the distal end of the tendon is brought to the tip of the screwdriver
- The tendon is then dunked into the bone socket and the tenodesis screw is advanced until it is flush with the tuberosity

The 2-incision technique is as follows[49]:

- A 3-cm transverse incision is made just distal to the elbow flexion crease.
- The LABC nerve is identified and protected with a vessel loop.
- The stump of the biceps is located subcutaneously with blunt finger dissection.
- The tendon stump is debrided and whipstitched with a no. 2 braided nonabsorbable suture.
- The radial recurrent vessels are ligated in the interval between the brachioradialis and pronator teres.
- Blunt finger dissection is used in this interval to identify the bicipital tuberosity.
- A large curved clamp is then passed just ulnar to the bicipital tuberosity, through the interosseous space, and tents the skin on the dorsolateral forearm.
- A longitudinal incision is made over the curved clamp.
- Tuberosity is exposed with the forearm in maximal pronation via a muscle-splitting approach.
- A bur is then used to create a 10- to 15-mm oval-shaped trough in the ulnar aspect of the tuberosity.
- Three 2.0-mm drill holes are placed through the dorsal radial cortex into the base of the trough.
- A long curved clamp is passed from the posterior incision, along the bicipital tendon sheath, and out the anterior incision, and is used to retrieve the sutures previously placed in the biceps.
- Sutures from the biceps are then passed from inside the bony trough out through the drill holes to dock the biceps tendon.
- The anterior wound is then closed.
- These sutures are then tensioned and tied over the bony bridge.
- The wound is thoroughly irrigated to remove any bony debris.

Immediate postoperative care

Patients are placed in a well-padded splint at 90° of flexion and full supination for 7 to 10 days to allow for soft tissue healing.

Rehabilitation and Recovery

After splint removal, patients are placed in a range-of-motion brace for 2 to 4 weeks, followed by the initiation of physical therapy. Full range of motion is expected by 6 to 8 weeks.[49] Resisted range of motion is started at 8 weeks will full strength expected to return between 3 and 6 months.

Clinical Results in the Literature

El-Hawary and coworkers[50] compared single-incision with a modified dual-incision technique and found no difference between the groups with respect to supination motion, supination strength, or flexion strength. Recovery of strength was initially more rapid for the 2-incision group. Grewal and colleagues,[51] in a level 1 randomized, controlled trial comparing 1- and 2-incision techniques, found no difference in outcomes as measured by American Shoulder Elbow Surgeons; Disabilities of the Arm, Shoulder, and Hand; and Patient-Rated Elbow Evaluation scores. These investigators did note a 10% advantage in flexion strength at 1 year for the 2-incision group (104% vs 94%). The single-incision group was associated with a higher complication rate of LABC nerve palsies, but there was no difference found with regards to heterotopic ossification.

For a full table of clinical outcomes and associated nerve injuries of single- and double-incision distal biceps repairs, see **Table 4**[50,54–62] and **Table 5**,[50,63–72] respectively.

TRICEPS RUPTURE
Introduction

The triceps muscles allow for many activities of daily living (ADLs), including getting up from a chair. It is among the least common of reported

Table 4
Clinical outcomes for single-incision distal biceps repair

Author, Year	No. of Patients	Fixation	Results	Nerve Injuries
Silva et al,[62] 2010	29 (30 surgeries)	Bio-Tenodesis screw	Flexion and supination strength 4/5	10 transient radial sensory nerve palsies, 2 permanent radial sensory nerve palsies, 9 transient LABC nerve dysesthesias
Peeters et al,[61] 2009	23	Cortical button	MEPS 94, 91% flexion, 80% supination vs CL	None
Heinzelmann et al,[57] 2009	32	Tenodesis screw with cortical button	Normal flexion strength in 30/32, normal supination strength in 28/32	2 temporary superficial radial nerve palsies
Fenton et al,[55] 2009	14	Tenodesis screw	MEPS 96.8, 96% flexion vs CL	None
Khan et al,[59] 2008	18	Suture anchors	82% flexion, 82% supination vs CL	1 transient superficial radial nerve palsy
John et al,[58] 2007	53	Suture anchors	46 excellent, 7 good results	1 transient PIN palsy
McKee et al,[60] 2005	53	Suture anchors	96% flexion, 93% supination vs CL	2 transient LABC nerve dysesthesias, 1 transient PIN palsy
El-Hawary et al,[50] 2003	9	Cortical button	96% flexion, 91% supination vs CL	3 transient LABC nerve dysesthesias
Greenberg et al,[56] 2003	14	Cortical button	97% flexion, 82% supination vs CL	3 transient LABC nerve dysesthesias
Bain et al,[54] 2000	12	Cortical button	"All 5/5 strength"	None

Abbreviations: CL, contralateral arm; MEPS, Mayo Elbow Performance Score.
Data from Refs.[50,54–62]

Table 5
Clinical outcomes for double-incision distal biceps repair

Author, Year	No. of Patients	Approach	Fixation	Results	Nerve Injuries
Cil et al,[66] 2009	21	Muscle split	TO tunnels	112% flexion, 89% supination vs CL	None
Weinstein et al,[72] 2008	32	Muscle split	Suture anchors	Strength within 5% of CL	2 LABC nerve dysesthesias
Hartman et al,[68] 2007	33	Muscle split	TO tunnels	MEPS 96.5 for acute repairs	None
Cheung et al,[65] 2005	13	Muscle split	TO tunnels	91% flexion, 89% supination vs CL	1 LABC neuritis
El-Hawary et al,[50] 2003	10	Muscle split	TO tunnels	97% flexion, 85% supination vs CL	1 transient superficial radial nerve dysesthesia
Moosmayer et al,[71] 2000	9	Boyd-Anderson	TO tunnels	87% flexion, 81% supination vs CL	2 transient PIN palsies
Bell et al,[64] 2000	21	Boyd-Anderson	TO tunnels, suture anchors and screws	Slight loss of flexion strength in dominant arm repairs, supination strength in nondominant arm repairs vs CL	None
Karunakar et al,[69] 1999	21	Boyd-Anderson	TO tunnels	14% elbows with flexion deficit, 48% elbows with supination deficit vs CL	1 transient LABC nerve dysesthesia
Davison et al,[67] 1996	8	Boyd-Anderson	TO tunnels	Full flexion, range 24%–83% supination weakness vs CL	None
Leighton et al,[70] 1995	9	Boyd-Anderson	TO tunnels	Full strength in dominant arm repairs, 86% flexion and supination vs CL in nondominant arm repairs	None
Baker & Bierwagen,[63] 1985	10	Boyd-Anderson	TO tunnels	109% flexion, 113% supination vs CL	None

Abbreviations: CL, contralateral arm; MEPS, Mayo Elbow Performance Score; TO, transosseous tunnels.
Data from Refs.[50,63–72]

tendon injuries.[73] There is a male predominance of 2:1, and the injury usually occurs after a sudden eccentric load is applied to a contracting triceps muscle.[74] For this reason, this injury is common in professional body builders, particularly those who use anabolic steroids.[75–77] Triceps ruptures usually occur at or near the insertion of the tendon onto the olecranon.[78–81] Over a 10-year span, only 12 cases were recorded in the National Football League.[79]

Surgical repair is generally performed for active individuals with complete ruptures or partial ruptures with impaired strength. The deeper head can pull off independently. With the superficial fibers intact, the patient will have normal extension strength near full extension but will exhibit weakness in deeper flexion. Some patients with complete disruption of the triceps tendon are still able to actively extend the elbow due to an intact lateral expansion.[74] A cadaveric study[73] showed the lateral expanse to be roughly half the average width of the tendon itself and noted that it should be repaired. They hypothesized that it was analogous to repairing the medial retinaculum in quadriceps tendon ruptures.

Several risk factors have been identified[49]

- Chronic renal failure
- Endocrine disorders
- Metabolic bone disease
- Steroid use

Nonoperative management[74,82]
- Any tear less than 50%
- Partial tears at the muscle belly, musculotendinous junction, or tendon insertion with insignificant loss of extension strength
- Tear greater than 50% in sedentary or debilitated/elderly patients

Operative indications include[74,78,79,83]

- Partial tears in an elderly patient still active enough for ADLs
- Partial tears in active individuals
- Partial tears in patients who have failed nonoperative management
- Complete tears

Surgical Technique

Preoperative planning

- Lateral radiographs may show a fleck of avulsed olecranon
- MRI is useful to distinguish between partial and complete tears

Preparation and patient positioning

- Lateral decubitus position, arm rest
- No tourniquet is used due to risk of inhibiting triceps tendon mobilization during repair

Surgical approach/procedure

- Posterolateral approach to the elbow so that wound healing is not an issue (prominent olecranon tip in flexion)
- Expose distal enough to visualize the entire insertion of the tendon onto the olecranon
- Extend incision 2 cm distal down ulnar shaft for planned fixation
- Soft tissue removed from bony insertion site (**Fig. 7**)
- Tendon end minimally debrided

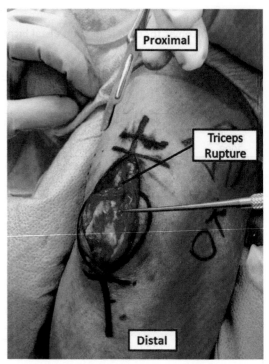

Fig. 7. Triceps tendon rupture. Ensure soft tissue is removed from the insertion point on the olecranon to prepare the bony bed for repair.

- Krackow-type whipstitch with no. 2 nonabsorbable suture, 4 passes on each side
- Cruciate repair[78]
  - Two crossing transosseous drill holes are made on the olecranon parallel to the joint surface.
  - Each strand of suture is shuttle through each drill hole from proximal to distal and tied over a bone bridge.
- Suture anchor repair[73] (**Fig. 8**)
  - Two metal 4.5-mm suture anchors are placed in the middle of the footprint, with the use of the dead man's angle, aimed away from the joint.
  - Each strand from the whipstitch is tied down to each suture anchor with 5 alternating half-hitch knots.
- Anatomic double row repair[73]
  - A similar 4-throw Krackow-type whipstitch is used, but with the free ends proximally rather than distally.
  - Two 3.0-mm bioabsorbable anchors are placed on the proximal end of the footprint, 1 medial and 1 lateral, 13 mm distal to the tip of the olecranon, directed distally to avoid joint penetration (analogous to the medial row of a rotator cuff repair).

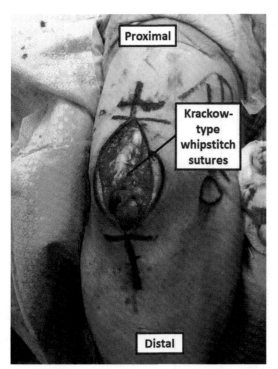

Fig. 8. Triceps rupture repair. Krackow-type whipstitch with no. 2 nonabsorbable suture with 4 passes on each side.

○ A mattress suture from each anchor is placed in the distal tendon 2 cm from the ruptured end.
○ Two pilot holes are created just distal to the anatomic footprint.
○ One tail from each anchor and 1 limb of the free Krackow (total of 3 sutures) are then threaded into an anchor for the distal row (analogous to the lateral row of a rotator cuff repair).
○ With tension held on the sutures to reduce the tendon to its desired position on the footprint, the distal anchors are advanced until flush.

Immediate postoperative care

The elbow is splinted at 30 to 45° for 7 to 10 days to allow for soft tissue healing. During this time, the patient is allowed to perform wrist, hand, and shoulder range of motion exercises.

Rehabilitation and Recovery

- Immediately after splint removal, range-of-motion exercises, including passive extension and guided active flexion, as well as pronation/supination, are initiated.
- Active range of motion is begun at 4 weeks.
- Weight lifting is avoided for 4 to 6 months.

Clinical Results in the Literature

Most published reports do not include detailed quantitative data or subjective outcomes based on standardized measures. Most are case reports,[81,84–87] and many reports are not concerning athletes. For a complete list of clinical results, see **Table 6**.[75,78,79,88] There are no clinical studies comparing outcomes between the various repair techniques. However, in a cadaveric evaluation of 3 techniques (cruciate, suture anchor, anatomic), Yeh and colleagues[73] identified statistically greater cyclic loading performance with the anatomic repair.

OLECRANON STRESS FRACTURE
Introduction

Olecranon stress fractures are a rare injury in baseball pitchers and have been reported in javelin throwers, gymnasts, divers, and weight lifters.[89] These fractures may occur as a result of repetitive microtrauma caused by olecranon impingement or excessive triceps tensile stress.[16] Clinical findings include a long history of posterolateral olecranon pain that recurs when throwing is resumed. Early radiographs may be normal. When throwing, athletes present with unusual posterior elbow pain and no significant findings on radiographs; a computed tomography (CT) scan should be performed. MRI, bone scan, and CT are often diagnostic.[89] Initial treatment includes active rest, throwing cessation, and possible bone growth stimulation. Although there are some reports of successful nonoperative management,[90] early surgical fixation is advocated in the competitive athlete because they often fail to respond to extended nonoperative treatment.[16]

Surgical Technique

Preoperative planning

- Imaging should be reviewed to determine orientation of fracture and appropriate size screw based on the patient's anatomy.
- Proximal fractures are usually transverse in nature.[89]
- Midproximal fractures are usually obliquely oriented: proximal medial to distal lateral (**Fig. 9**).

Preparation and patient positioning

- Prone or sloppy lateral positioning with a bean bag elbow holder (similar to arthroscopy)
- Alternatively, the patient can be positioned supine with the arm on a hand table

Table 6
Clinical outcomes for distal triceps repair

Author, Year	No. of # Patients	Tears	Average Age (Range)	Average F/U (Range) (y)	Operative Technique	Outcome
Mair et al,[79] 2004	19 (21 tears)	11 complete, 10 partial	29 (22–36)	Complete: 3; partial: 2.7	Transosseous drill holes	All players returned to play at least one season; 6/10 partial tears healed nonoperatively
van Riet et al,[78] 2003	13	8 complete, 15 partial	47 (21–69)	7.75 (0.5–22)	Transosseous drill holes	Peak strength avg. 92% of the untreated extremity
Sollender et al,[75] 1998	4	4 complete	NR (middle-aged men)	6.7 (0.92–12)	Transosseous drill holes	Full ROM, 1 rerupture, minimal residual weakness in elbow extension
Levy,[88] 1987	9	9 complete, 8 with avulsion fragment	NR (35–60)	3.5 (0.8–6)	Mersilene tape and bone tunnel	Full function

Abbreviations: NR, not reported; ROM, range of motion.
Data from Refs.[75,78,79,88]

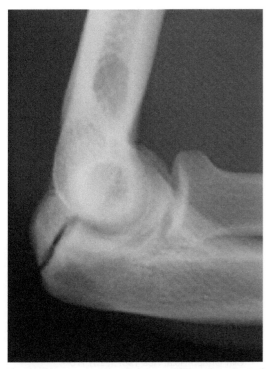

Fig. 9. Olecranon stress fracture. Obliquely oriented midproximal fracture.

- Ensure easy access of intraoperative fluoroscopy
- Nonsterile tourniquet as far proximal as possible

Surgical approach/procedure

- Under c-arm fluoroscopy control
- A small nick is made in the skin just posterior to the olecranon process
- A guidewire for a 6.5-mm or 7.3-mm cannulated screw is placed
  - Perpendicular to the proximal transverse-oriented fracture
  - Down the intramedullary canal for midproximal oblique-oriented fracture
- Screw is placed after appropriate sized reaming
- Tourniquet is deflated before wound closure to prevent hematoma formation

Immediate postoperative care

The elbow is splinted at 90° for 7 to 10 days to allow for soft tissue healing. During this time, the patient is allowed to perform wrist, hand, and shoulder range-of-motion exercises.

Table 7
Clinical outcomes for operative fixation of olecranon stress fractures

Author, Year	No. of Patients	Sport	Mean Age (Range) (y)	Time to Healing (Range) (wk)	Outcomes
Paci et al,[89] 2013	18	Baseball	20 (16.1–23.8)	8.4 (3.9–17.9)	94% (17/18) returned to previous level of play at avg. 29 wk, 33% (6/18) required hardware removal, 11% (2/18) required reoperation for infection
Fujioka et al,[91] 2012	6	5 Baseball, 1 softball	18.2 (16–21)	NR	Headless cannulated double-threaded screw. Return to play at avg. 21 wk.
Rao et al,[93] 2001	1	Weight lifter	20	16	Returned to weight-lifting at 6 mo.
Nuber & Diment,[90] 1992	2	Baseball pitchers	22 (21–23)	8.5 (5–12)	Healed with nonoperative treatment
Hulkko et al,[92] 1986	4	Javelin	NR	Nonop: 72; tension band: 12	1 refracture at 11 mo
Tullos et al,[94] 1972	1	Baseball pitcher	NR	NR	Bone grafting required for nonunion

Abbreviations: avg, average; NR, not reported.
  Data from Refs.[89–94]

Rehabilitation and Recovery

A multiphase rehabilitation protocol is as follows[89]:

- Early postoperative elbow range of motion is initiated after splint removal.
- Unlimited passive range of motion and active pronation/supination are allowed immediately.
- Active flexion beyond 90° is avoided for 6 weeks.
- Strengthening and a throwing program are initiated at 8 weeks.
- Advanced throwing program is started at 12 weeks.
- Throwing from the mound is initiated after the patient completes a long toss program to 120 to 145 feet without any elbow symptoms.

Clinical Results in the Literature

Very few clinical studies have been published on the treatment of olecranon stress fractures.[89–94] For a list of available clinical results, see **Table 7**. Patients should be informed that there is a significant risk of the need for hardware removal after fixation and that there is a slightly greater risk for infection compared with fixation of traumatic olecranon fractures, possibly due to the subcutaneous position of the screw head.[89]

SURGICAL PEARLS

These helpful tips can be used in all operative cases of elbow trauma in the athlete:

- Simulation of surgical movements during setup can minimize competition with the patient's body, contralateral arm, or arm holder for access to the operative field.
- Medial and lateral aspects of the elbow can be labeled to avoid confusion that may be caused by reversed anatomy in lateral or prone positioning, particularly if the hand is covered.
- A nonsterile tourniquet is usually used, except in the case of distal triceps repairs because it may impede tendon mobilization.

REFERENCES

1. Gregory B, Nyland J. Medial elbow injury in young throwing athletes. Muscles Ligaments Tendons J 2013;3(2):91–100.
2. Gottschalk HP, Eisner E, Hosalkar HS. Medial epicondyle fractures in the pediatric population. J Am Acad Orthop Surg 2012;20(4):223–32.
3. Kamath AF, Cody SR, Hosalkar HS. Open reduction of medial epicondyle fractures: operative tips for technical ease. J Child Orthop 2009;3(4):331–6.
4. Hang DW, Chao CM, Hang YS. A clinical and roentgenographic study of Little League elbow. Am J Sports Med 2004;32(1):79–84.
5. Greiwe RM, Saifi C, Ahmad CS. Pediatric sports elbow injuries. Clin Sports Med 2010;29(4):677–703.
6. Klingele KE, Kocher MS. Little league elbow: valgus overload injury in the paediatric athlete. Sports Med 2002;32(15):1005–15.
7. Makhni EC, Jegede KA, Ahmad CS. Pediatric elbow injuries in athletes. Sports Med Arthrosc 2014;22(3):e16–24.
8. Edmonds EW. How displaced are "nondisplaced" fractures of the medial humeral epicondyle in children? Results of a three-dimensional computed tomography analysis. J Bone Joint Surg Am 2010;92(17):2785–91.
9. Safran MR. Elbow injuries in athletes. A review. Clin Orthop Relat Res 1995;(310):257–77.
10. Kamath AF, Baldwin K, Horneff J, et al. Operative versus non-operative management of pediatric medial epicondyle fractures: a systematic review. J Child Orthop 2009;3(5):345–57.
11. Hines RF, Herndon WA, Evans JP. Operative treatment of medial epicondyle fractures in children. Clin Orthop Relat Res 1987;(223):170–4.
12. Louahem DM, Bourelle S, Buscayret F, et al. Displaced medial epicondyle fractures of the humerus: surgical treatment and results. A report of 139 cases. Arch Orthop Trauma Surg 2010;130(5):649–55.
13. Farsetti P, Potenza V, Caterini R, et al. Long-term results of treatment of fractures of the medial humeral epicondyle in children. J Bone Joint Surg Am 2001;83-A(9):1299–305.
14. Papavasiliou VA. Fracture-separation of the medial epicondylar epiphysis of the elbow joint. Clin Orthop Relat Res 1982;(171):172–4.
15. Smith FM. Medial epicondyle injuries. J Am Med Assoc 1950;142(6):396–402. illust.
16. Cain EL Jr, Dugas JR, Wolf RS, et al. Elbow injuries in throwing athletes: a current concepts review. Am J Sports Med 2003;31(4):621–35.
17. Woods GW, Tullos HS. Elbow instability and medial epicondyle fractures. Am J Sports Med 1977;5(1):23–30.
18. Kobayashi Y, Oka Y, Ikeda M, et al. Avulsion fracture of the medial and lateral epicondyles of the humerus. J Shoulder Elbow Surg 2000;9(1):59–64.
19. Lawrence JT, Patel NM, Macknin J, et al. Return to competitive sports after medial epicondyle fractures in adolescent athletes: results of operative and nonoperative treatment. Am J Sports Med 2013;41(5):1152–7.
20. Dias JJ, Johnson GV, Hoskinson J, et al. Management of severely displaced medial epicondyle fractures. J Orthop Trauma 1987;1(1):59–62.
21. Duun PS, Ravn P, Hansen LB, et al. Osteosynthesis of medial humeral epicondyle fractures in children.

8-year follow-up of 33 cases. Acta Orthop Scand 1994;65(4):439–41.

22. Fowles JV, Slimane N, Kassab MT. Elbow dislocation with avulsion of the medial humeral epicondyle. J Bone Joint Surg Br 1990;72(1):102–4.

23. Haxhija EQ, Mayr JM, Grechenig W, et al. Treatment of medial epicondylar apophyseal avulsion injury in children. Oper Orthop Traumatol 2006;18(2):120–34 [in German].

24. Ip D, Tsang WL. Medial humeral epicondylar fracture in children and adolescents. J Orthop Surg (Hong Kong) 2007;15(2):170–3.

25. Lee HH, Shen HC, Chang JH, et al. Operative treatment of displaced medial epicondyle fractures in children and adolescents. J Shoulder Elbow Surg 2005;14(2):178–85.

26. Pimpalnerkar AL, Balasubramaniam G, Young SK, et al. Type four fracture of the medial epicondyle: a true indication for surgical intervention. Injury 1998; 29(10):751–6.

27. Skak SV, Grossmann E, Wagn P. Deformity after internal fixation of fracture separation of the medial epicondyle of the humerus. J Bone Joint Surg Br 1994;76(2):297–302.

28. van Niekerk JL, Severijnen RS. Medial epicondyle fractures of the humerus. Neth J Surg 1985;37(5): 141–4.

29. Wilson NI, Ingram R, Rymaszewski L, et al. Treatment of fractures of the medial epicondyle of the humerus. Injury 1988;19(5):342–4.

30. Jobe FW, Stark H, Lombardo SJ. Reconstruction of the ulnar collateral ligament in athletes. J Bone Joint Surg Am 1986;68(8):1158–63.

31. Conway JE, Jobe FW, Glousman RE, et al. Medial instability of the elbow in throwing athletes. Treatment by repair or reconstruction of the ulnar collateral ligament. J Bone Joint Surg Am 1992;74(1): 67–83.

32. Andrews JR, Timmerman LA. Outcome of elbow surgery in professional baseball players. Am J Sports Med 1995;23(4):407–13.

33. Azar FM, Andrews JR, Wilk KE, et al. Operative treatment of ulnar collateral ligament injuries of the elbow in athletes. Am J Sports Med 2000;28(1):16–23.

34. Cain EL Jr, Andrews JR, Dugas JR, et al. Outcome of ulnar collateral ligament reconstruction of the elbow in 1281 athletes: results in 743 athletes with minimum 2-year follow-up. Am J Sports Med 2010; 38(12):2426–34.

35. Petty DH, Andrews JR, Fleisig GS, et al. Ulnar collateral ligament reconstruction in high school baseball players: clinical results and injury risk factors. Am J Sports Med 2004;32(5):1158–64.

36. Bowers AL, Dines JS, Dines DM, et al. Elbow medial ulnar collateral ligament reconstruction: clinical relevance and the docking technique. J Shoulder Elbow Surg 2010;19(2 Suppl):110–7.

37. Dines JS, ElAttrache NS, Conway JE, et al. Clinical outcomes of the DANE TJ technique to treat ulnar collateral ligament insufficiency of the elbow. Am J Sports Med 2007;35(12):2039–44.

38. Dodson CC, Thomas A, Dines JS, et al. Medial ulnar collateral ligament reconstruction of the elbow in throwing athletes. Am J Sports Med 2006;34(12): 1926–32.

39. Hechtman KS, Zvijac JE, Wells ME, et al. Long-term results of ulnar collateral ligament reconstruction in throwing athletes based on a hybrid technique. Am J Sports Med 2011;39(2):342–7.

40. Koh JL, Schafer MF, Keuter G, et al. Ulnar collateral ligament reconstruction in elite throwing athletes. Arthroscopy 2006;22(11):1187–91.

41. Paletta GA Jr, Wright RW. The modified docking procedure for elbow ulnar collateral ligament reconstruction: 2-year follow-up in elite throwers. Am J Sports Med 2006;34(10):1594–8.

42. Rohrbough JT, Altchek DW, Hyman J, et al. Medial collateral ligament reconstruction of the elbow using the docking technique. Am J Sports Med 2002; 30(4):541–8.

43. Thompson WH, Jobe FW, Yocum LA, et al. Ulnar collateral ligament reconstruction in athletes: muscle-splitting approach without transposition of the ulnar nerve. J Shoulder Elbow Surg 2001;10(2): 152–7.

44. Dines JS, Jones KJ, Kahlenberg C, et al. Elbow ulnar collateral ligament reconstruction in javelin throwers at a minimum 2-year follow-up. Am J Sports Med 2012;40(1):148–51.

45. Jones KJ, Dines JS, Rebolledo BJ, et al. Operative management of ulnar collateral ligament insufficiency in adolescent athletes. Am J Sports Med 2014;42(1):117–21.

46. Vitale MA, Ahmad CS. The outcome of elbow ulnar collateral ligament reconstruction in overhead athletes: a systematic review. Am J Sports Med 2008; 36(6):1193–205.

47. Savoie FH 3rd, Trenhaile SW, Roberts J, et al. Primary repair of ulnar collateral ligament injuries of the elbow in young athletes: a case series of injuries to the proximal and distal ends of the ligament. Am J Sports Med 2008;36(6):1066–72.

48. Keener JD. Controversies in the surgical treatment of distal biceps tendon ruptures: single versus double-incision repairs. J Shoulder Elbow Surg 2011;20(2 Suppl):S113–25.

49. Stucken C, Ciccotti MG. Distal biceps and triceps injuries in athletes. Sports Med Arthrosc 2014;22(3): 153–63.

50. El-Hawary R, Macdermid JC, Faber KJ, et al. Distal biceps tendon repair: comparison of surgical techniques. J Hand Surg Am 2003;28(3):496–502.

51. Grewal R, Athwal GS, MacDermid JC, et al. Single versus double-incision technique for the repair of

acute distal biceps tendon ruptures: a randomized clinical trial. J Bone Joint Surg Am 2012;94(13): 1166–74.

52. Mazzocca AD, Burton KJ, Romeo AA, et al. Biomechanical evaluation of 4 techniques of distal biceps brachii tendon repair. Am J Sports Med 2007;35(2): 252–8.

53. Lo EY, Li CS, Van den Bogaerde JM. The effect of drill trajectory on proximity to the posterior interosseous nerve during cortical button distal biceps repair. Arthroscopy 2011;27(8):1048–54.

54. Bain GI, Prem H, Heptinstall RJ, et al. Repair of distal biceps tendon rupture: a new technique using the Endobutton. J Shoulder Elbow Surg 2000; 9(2):120–6.

55. Fenton P, Qureshi F, Ali A, et al. Distal biceps tendon rupture: a new repair technique in 14 patients using the biotenodesis screw. Am J Sports Med 2009; 37(10):2009–15.

56. Greenberg JA, Fernandez JJ, Wang T, et al. Endo-Button-assisted repair of distal biceps tendon ruptures. J Shoulder Elbow Surg 2003;12(5):484–90.

57. Heinzelmann AD, Savoie FH 3rd, Ramsey JR, et al. A combined technique for distal biceps repair using a soft tissue button and biotenodesis interference screw. Am J Sports Med 2009;37(5):989–94.

58. John CK, Field LD, Weiss KS, et al. Single-incision repair of acute distal biceps ruptures by use of suture anchors. J Shoulder Elbow Surg 2007;16(1):78–83.

59. Khan AD, Penna S, Yin Q, et al. Repair of distal biceps tendon ruptures using suture anchors through a single anterior incision. Arthroscopy 2008;24(1): 39–45.

60. McKee MD, Hirji R, Schemitsch EH, et al. Patient-oriented functional outcome after repair of distal biceps tendon ruptures using a single-incision technique. J Shoulder Elbow Surg 2005;14(3):302–6.

61. Peeters T, Ching-Soon NG, Jansen N, et al. Functional outcome after repair of distal biceps tendon ruptures using the endobutton technique. J Shoulder Elbow Surg 2009;18(2):283–7.

62. Silva J, Eskander MS, Lareau C, et al. Treatment of distal biceps tendon ruptures using a single-incision technique and a Bio-Tenodesis screw. Orthopedics 2010;33(7):477.

63. Baker BE, Bierwagen D. Rupture of the distal tendon of the biceps brachii. Operative versus nonoperative treatment. J Bone Joint Surg Am 1985; 67(3):414–7.

64. Bell RH, Wiley WB, Noble JS, et al. Repair of distal biceps brachii tendon ruptures. J Shoulder Elbow Surg 2000;9(3):223–6.

65. Cheung EV, Lazarus M, Taranta M. Immediate range of motion after distal biceps tendon repair. J Shoulder Elbow Surg 2005;14(5):516–8.

66. Cil A, Merten S, Steinmann SP. Immediate active range of motion after modified 2-incision repair in acute distal biceps tendon rupture. Am J Sports Med 2009;37(1):130–5.

67. Davison BL, Engber WD, Tigert LJ. Long term evaluation of repaired distal biceps brachii tendon ruptures. Clin Orthop Relat Res 1996;(333):186–91.

68. Hartman MW, Merten SM, Steinmann SP. Mini-open 2-incision technique for repair of distal biceps tendon ruptures. J Shoulder Elbow Surg 2007; 16(5):616–20.

69. Karunakar MA, Cha P, Stern PJ. Distal biceps ruptures. A followup of Boyd and Anderson repair. Clin Orthop Relat Res 1999;(363):100–7.

70. Leighton MM, Bush-Joseph CA, Bach BR Jr. Distal biceps brachii repair. Results in dominant and nondominant extremities. Clin Orthop Relat Res 1995;(317):114–21.

71. Moosmayer S, Odinsson A, Holm I. Distal biceps tendon rupture operated on with the Boyd-Anderson technique: follow-up of 9 patients with isokinetic examination after 1 year. Acta Orthop Scand 2000; 71(4):399–402.

72. Weinstein DM, Ciccone WJ 2nd, Buckler MC, et al. Elbow function after repair of the distal biceps brachii tendon with a two-incision approach. J Shoulder Elbow Surg 2008;17(1 Suppl):82S–6S.

73. Yeh PC, Stephens KT, Solovyova O, et al. The distal triceps tendon footprint and a biomechanical analysis of 3 repair techniques. Am J Sports Med 2010;38(5):1025–33.

74. Yeh PC, Dodds SD, Smart LR, et al. Distal triceps rupture. J Am Acad Orthop Surg 2010;18(1):31–40.

75. Sollender JL, Rayan GM, Barden GA. Triceps tendon rupture in weight lifters. J Shoulder Elbow Surg 1998;7(2):151–3.

76. Sherman OH, Snyder SJ, Fox JM. Triceps tendon avulsion in a professional body builder. A case report. Am J Sports Med 1984;12(4):328–9.

77. Herrick RT, Herrick S. Ruptured triceps in a powerlifter presenting as cubital tunnel syndrome. A case report. Am J Sports Med 1987;15(5):514–6.

78. van Riet RP, Morrey BF, Ho E, et al. Surgical treatment of distal triceps ruptures. J Bone Joint Surg Am 2003;85-A(10):1961–7.

79. Mair SD, Isbell WM, Gill TJ, et al. Triceps tendon ruptures in professional football players. Am J Sports Med 2004;32(2):431–4.

80. Madsen M, Marx RG, Millett PJ, et al. Surgical anatomy of the triceps brachii tendon: anatomical study and clinical correlation. Am J Sports Med 2006; 34(11):1839–43.

81. Bach BR Jr, Warren RF, Wickiewicz TL. Triceps rupture. A case report and literature review. Am J Sports Med 1987;15(3):285–9.

82. Vidal AF, Drakos MC, Allen AA. Biceps tendon and triceps tendon injuries. Clin Sports Med 2004; 23(4):707–22, xi.

83. Strauch RJ. Biceps and triceps injuries of the elbow. Orthop Clin North Am 1999;30(1):95–107.

84. Brumback RJ. Compartment syndrome complicating avulsion of the origin of the triceps muscle. A case report. J Bone Joint Surg Am 1987;69(9): 1445–7.

85. Levy M, Goldberg I, Meir I. Fracture of the head of the radius with a tear or avulsion of the triceps tendon. A new syndrome? J Bone Joint Surg Br 1982;64(1):70–2.

86. Sharma SC, Singh R, Goel T, et al. Missed diagnosis of triceps tendon rupture: a case report and review of literature. J Orthop Surg (Hong Kong) 2005; 13(3):307–9.

87. Tsourvakas S, Gouvalas K, Gimtsas C, et al. Bilateral and simultaneous rupture of the triceps tendons in chronic renal failure and secondary hyperparathyroidism. Arch Orthop Trauma Surg 2004;124(4): 278–80.

88. Levy M. Repair of triceps tendon avulsions or ruptures. J Bone Joint Surg Br 1987;69(1):115.

89. Paci JM, Dugas JR, Guy JA, et al. Cannulated screw fixation of refractory olecranon stress fractures with and without associated injuries allows a return to baseball. Am J Sports Med 2013;41(2):306–12.

90. Nuber GW, Diment MT. Olecranon stress fractures in throwers. A report of two cases and a review of the literature. Clin Orthop Relat Res 1992;(278):58–61.

91. Fujioka H, Tsunemi K, Takagi Y, et al. Treatment of stress fracture of the olecranon in throwing athletes with internal fixation through a small incision. Sports Med Arthrosc Rehabil Ther Technol 2012;4(1):49.

92. Hulkko A, Orava S, Nikula P. Stress fractures of the olecranon in javelin throwers. Int J Sports Med 1986;7(4):210–3.

93. Rao PS, Rao SK, Navadgi BC. Olecranon stress fracture in a weight lifter: a case report. Br J Sports Med 2001;35(1):72–3.

94. Tullos HS, Erwin WD, Woods GW, et al. Unusual lesions of the pitching arm. Clin Orthop Relat Res 1972;88:169–82.

Complications of Elbow Trauma

Emilie V. Cheung, MD[a],*, Eric J. Sarkissian, MD[b]

KEYWORDS

- Complications • Heterotopic ossification • Stiffness • Instability • Wound infection

KEY POINTS

- Complications of elbow trauma include stiffness associated with heterotopic ossification (HO), instability or subluxation, and wound infection.
- HO may develop after intra-articular fractures or fracture-dislocations; treatment with capsular release and excision of heterotopic bone is effective in restoring motion.
- Instability patterns following elbow trauma are associated with fracture patterns involving the coronoid process, including posterolateral rotatory instability (PLRI) and varus posteromedial instability.
- Wound complications may arise because of the thin soft-tissue envelope at the olecranon.

STIFFNESS AND HETEROTOPIC OSSIFICATION

The elbow is at risk for stiffness after trauma.[1–3] Reasons for loss of elbow motion may be intrinsic (such as intra-articular incongruity) or extrinsic (extra-articular incongruity). Extrinsic sources of contracture arise from soft-tissue contracture,[1,4] HO, or both. HO is a well-known sequela of injury to the elbow.[5] Direct trauma to the elbow is the most commonly reported cause of HO around the elbow, with an incidence of 3% being reported for simple elbow dislocations and up to 89% for those with periarticular fractures with traumatic brain injury.[6,7] Some have hypothesized that complex fracture patterns involving the coronoid and terrible triad injuries, which therefore necessitated ligament repair, combined medial and lateral approaches, or both, would show a higher rate of ectopic bone formation even after controlling for fracture type. Theoretically, complex fracture patterns, such as those requiring concomitant ligament repair, may subject the elbow to the additional trauma of the added surgical dissection.

The largest historical series that studied the incidence of posttraumatic elbow HO and stiffness was by Thompson and Garcia,[8] which reported a 3% incidence of posttraumatic HO about the elbow in 1314 patients. This study reviewed a heterogeneous group of elbow injuries, including distal humeral fractures, Monteggia fractures, olecranon fractures, isolated radial head fractures, simple dislocations of the elbow, and fracture-dislocations. The researchers reported a 17.6% incidence of HO in 136 patients who had fracture-dislocations of the elbow. Multiple attempts at closed reduction were suggested to be a risk factor.

More recently, in an analysis of patients undergoing surgical treatment of intra-articular elbow fractures, distal humeral fractures were significantly correlated with both the presence and size of HO, as well as return to the operating room for capsule resection, ectopic bone excision, or both.[6] Postoperative radiographs at 2 weeks showed the presence of ectopic bone in 86% of cases. Furthermore, all patients who underwent

Sources of Funding, Support, or Other Conflicts of Interest: None.
[a] Orthopedic Surgery, Stanford University, 450 North Broadway Street, MC 6342, Redwood City, CA 94304, USA; [b] Department of Orthopaedic Surgery, Stanford University Hospital and Clinics, 300 Pasteur Drive, Room R144, Stanford, CA 94305-5341, USA
* Corresponding author.
E-mail address: evcheung@stanford.edu

further surgical management for HO resection, capsular release, or both had ectopic bone noted on the 2-week postoperative radiographs. Based on these findings, patients with major elbow trauma may be counseled at the 2-week postoperative mark regarding their risk for ectopic bone and return to surgery for HO resection, capsular release, or both. If no ectopic bone was present at that time, patients had a negligible chance of an additional operation (**Fig. 1**).

One factor that might play a role in the development of HO after distal humerus fractures is the surgical approach. Chen and colleagues[9] found a 12% incidence of ectopic bone formation in distal humerus fractures treated with an olecranon osteotomy compared with no significant HO in those patients treated with a triceps-sparing approach. This finding seems to make logical sense because olecranon osteotomy by definition is disruptive to the intra-articular aspect of the elbow joint. However, in distal humeral fractures, the approach affords the best visualization and maneuverability about the fracture, and the risks of using this approach (ie, nonunion, malunion, stiffness) must be weighed against its primary benefit. One must remember that the primacy of the operation is to achieve near-anatomic alignment of the fracture fragments. Subsequent operations can be performed to treat stiffness, but secondary operations cannot rescue a joint that is not anatomically fixed from the beginning.

A recent study reported an incidence of 37% of elbows developing HO after surgical treatment of fractures involving the proximal ulna and radius.[10]

Ectopic bone was preferentially located at the origin of torn soft-tissue structures or around fracture sites, and it was particularly common around the posterior aspect of the ulna and the neck of the radius. HO interfered with motion in 20% of elbows, and 10% of elbows underwent additional surgery to remove heterotopic bone to improve motion. Elbow subluxation or dislocation at the time of presentation, an open fracture, a severe chest injury, and a delay in definitive surgical treatment were risk factors for development of HO. Another study found that HO continues to be a substantial complication after internal fixation for distal humerus fractures (**Fig. 2**).[11] HO was identified in 42% of elbows, mostly around the humerus and along the course of the medial collateral ligament (MCL) in this series. The development of HO was significantly associated with sustaining a head injury, delayed surgery, the method of fracture fixation, and the use of bone graft or substitute. One study examined surgically treated elbow fracture-dislocations and found an incidence of HO in 43%.[3] The only factor found to be significantly associated with HO formation was the performance of multiple reductions.

Treatment of elbow stiffness involves open capsular release and circumferential excision of heterotopic bone.[12,13] The studies reported in the literature have supported this as an effective means of restoring motion.[14,15] Complications of this procedure include recurrence of HO, hematoma formation, infection, and ulnar neuropathy.[12,13] One large series reported on 77 patients treated with circumferential elbow capsulectomy, HO excision, hardware removal, and ulnar nerve

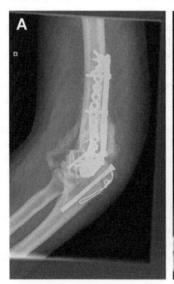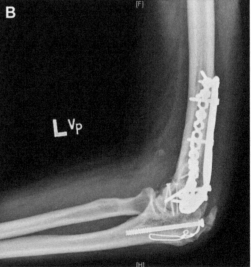

Fig. 1. A 40-year-old man who underwent surgical fixation of distal humeral fracture at an outside hospital, presenting with stiffness (*A*). Range of motion was 60° to 100°. Patient then underwent HO excision and capsular release with improvement in range of motion to 30° to 130° (*B*).

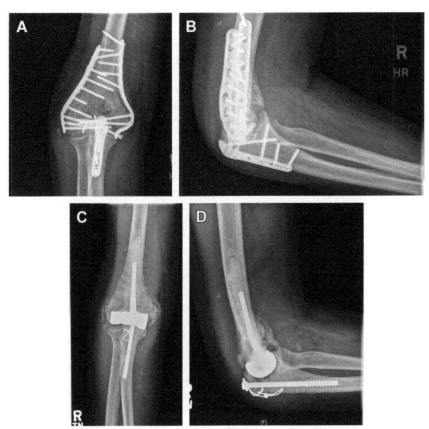

Fig. 2. A 65-year-old man who had failure of fracture fixation of the distal humerus 4 months prior (*A, B*). Distal humeral hemiarthroplasty was performed as a salvage operation with good improvement in range of motion and pain relief (*C, D*).

neurolysis.[12] At a mean follow-up of 12 months, 69% of patients achieved a minimum 100° functional elbow arc of motion. Recurrent HO occurred in 6% of patients. Salazar and colleagues[13] found that hypertension, obesity, and absence of intraoperative anterior ulnar nerve transposition were associated with an adverse effect on change from preoperative to final arc of motion. Patients with partially and completely restricted range of motion (ROM) showed substantial improvement in postoperative ROM. Surgery combined with postoperative prophylaxis and a regimented rehabilitation program are feasible modalities to treat patients with HO of the elbow.

INSTABILITY

Instability describes a spectrum of joint incongruity, from subtle dynamic instability to frank dislocation. PLRI is the most common pattern after elbow trauma[16] and can arise from soft-tissue or bony injury. Varus posteromedial instability is associated with disruption of the lateral soft tissues and

the anteromedial coronoid facet (AMCF). Varus posteromedial instability often results from untreated or malunited fractures of the anteromedial face of the coronoid.

The keystone of stability of the ulnohumeral joint is the coronoid. The coronoid process, which consists of a tip, body, anterolateral facet, and anteromedial facet (AMF), acts as an anterior buttress of the ulnohumeral articulation. The tip is often involved in posterolateral instability patterns such as in terrible triad injuries. Large basilar fractures of the coronoid process are associated with posterior olecranon fracture dislocations. The anteromedial portion of the coronoid process extends from the proximal ulnar metaphysis as a unsupported process and is vulnerable to injury, particularly with a varus injury force and can result in posteromedial instability.[2]

Posterolateral Rotatory Instability

Posterolateral elbow instability occurs over a spectrum, from disruption of the lateral collateral ligament (LCL) alone to the terrible triad and complex elbow dislocations. Clinical evidence suggests that at least 50% of the coronoid must be present for the ulnohumeral joint to be stable.[17] Biomechanical studies have been conflicting. One study suggested that in the setting of an intact radial head and collateral ligaments, a transverse fracture through 50% of the coronoid does not increase instability.[18] In another study, after prosthetic head replacement, with intact ligaments, the elbow remained unstable with 50% of the coronoid removed, and fixation of the coronoid resolved instability.[19]

Papatheodorou and colleagues[20] reported on 26 patients without fixation of type I and II coronoid process fractures in terrible triad injuries. After fixation of the LCL and radial head or radial head replacement, the elbows demonstrated intraoperative stability, and the coronoid fractures were treated without fixation. Mean Broberg-Morrey and DASH (Disability of Arm Shoulder, Arm, Hand) scores were 90 and 14, respectively, with a minimum follow-up of 2 years.

Varus Posteromedial Instability

In O'Driscoll type 2 fractures, the elbow may remain unstable after fixation of the AMCF fragment indicating a coexisting MCL tear.[21] In their series of 19 patients, Park and colleagues[21] noted 3 patients with a humeral avulsion of the MCL with persistent instability after fragment fixation. The MCL injuries were repaired.

Doornberg and Ring[17] described 18 patients with AMF fractures with an average follow-up of 26 months. Six of these patients had limited stability of the AMF, resulting in joint instability and early-onset arthritis with a fair or poor functional result. The remaining 12 patients had secure fixation of the AMF fracture, resulting in good or excellent function and full ROM of the elbow.

Sanchez-Sotelo and colleagues[22] reported an excellent result in a patient with a malunited AMCF fracture and rotatory instability treated with buttress plating and LCL reconstruction. Lee and colleagues[23] reported good to excellent results in 15 patients with type II or type III coronoid process fractures who were treated with plate fixation and ligament repair. Previous clinical studies have emphasized the necessity of internal fixation and collateral ligament repair, without regard to the size or classification. Pollock and colleagues[24] performed a biomechanical study of AMCF fractures and suggested fixation of larger (5-mm) coronoid fractures. They suggested that smaller (2.5-mm) AMCF fractures with deficient LCL but intact MCL may be amenable to nonoperative interventions if strict rehabilitation protocols were followed.

Complex fracture-dislocation

Appropriately termed the terrible triad, the combination of ligamentous injury with coronoid and radial head fractures has been found to have a high complication rate.[25] The most effective method to stabilize these injuries requires surgical intervention to allow for return to early motion. Closed reduction often results in redislocation, which may risk further damage. This type of injury can be appropriately assessed with 3-dimensional computed tomographic (CT) reconstructions to help address each component of the injury. Goals of surgery include restoration of the anterior bony buttress, which consists of the coronoid process and radial head, and repair of the MCL and the lateral unlar collateral ligament (LUCL). Even small coronoid fractures should be repaired, if possible, because the repair adds an additional reinforcement against dislocation and restoration of function of the anterior capsule.[26] The coronoid can be secured with suture fixation and/or screw fixation. After repair or replacement of the radial head, the radial extensor mass and LUCL can be reattached to the lateral condyle of the humerus; this is immediately followed by an assessment of stability through a full ROM. If there is redislocation during elbow extension before reaching 30° to 40° from full extension, it may be necessary to repair the MCL and apply a hinged external fixator.[27]

Chronic posterolateral rotatory instability

Although many structures are disrupted in an elbow dislocation, chronic instability is primarily owing to a deficiency in the LCL resulting in PLRI. Some studies have reported that nearly one-third of patients with a simple dislocation of the elbow treated by closed reduction had long-term symptoms of instability.[28,29] Often, these patients present with a history of persistent, recurring pain and clicking, catching, or subluxation within the ROM. Patients generally recall one episode of trauma that may or may not have resulted in a dislocation. Posterolateral instability may also ensue iatrogenically, if the lateral ligament complex is disrupted.[30]

ROM in these patients is usually pain free, with negative valgus and varus stress testing. The lateral pivot shift test is the most sensitive test for clinical diagnosis of PLRI and is often performed under general anesthesia.[31] To recreate the mechanism of instability, the patient lays supine on the examination table and has the involved arm overhead with the shoulder in external rotation. Next, the elbow is placed in extension with the forearm in supination while a valgus load is simultaneously applied. The elbow is then slowly brought from extension into flexion, and the radial head is felt to slip back in place. The test result is positive if a visible or palpable clunk is elicited. Even simpler, the patient can be asked to push up from a chair with their forearms in supination. If pain or instability is felt as the elbow proceeds to extension, the test result is positive. Another test known as the posterolateral rotatory drawer test has the elbow placed in 40° to 90° of flexion while applying an anteroposterior force on the radius and ulna[31]; this is done to subluxate the forearm away from the humerus on the lateral side. The test result is considered positive if subluxation or apprehension is elicited.

Stress radiographs or fluoroscopy may also be useful to confirm the diagnosis of elbow instability.[31] When the lateral pivot shift test is performed, the elbow is placed in maximal rotatory subluxation and the ulnohumeral joint space is seen to be widened on lateral and anteroposterior views. In addition, the lateral view can show posterior subluxation of the radial head. If necessary, magnetic resonance arthrography and diagnostic elbow arthroscopy can be used to visualize damage to the LCL complex and radial head subluxation, respectively.[32,33]

Generally, patients with less severe symptoms can be managed with extensor strengthening exercises or athletic neoprene sleeves, whereas patients with more severe symptoms and signs of chronic instability require surgery.[34] Patients requiring an operation often need reconstruction of the LUCL, usually with an autograft or allograft tendon. Various operative techniques successfully using different tendon graft sites have been investigated in the literature, including the palmaris longus, plantaris, gracilis, and semitendinosus.[35]

Chronic elbow dislocation

Neglected elbow dislocations or inadequate assessment after an attempted reduction can lead to a chronic dislocation of the elbow. Arthritic changes occur rapidly if the elbow is not reduced. Radiographs can be readily used to make the diagnosis; however, CT evaluation should be considered to help with surgical planning. The goal of treatment can be conflicting, because it involves restoring both a stable concentric joint while also facilitating early motion within a satisfactory arc of motion. In the younger population, treatment options vary depending on the degree of posttraumatic arthritis present. If there is mild to moderate arthritis, then open reduction, reconstruction of MCL and LCL, and placement of a hinged external fixator is an option. There is a risk of redislocation, even with hinged external fixation, and a temporary internal plate may be needed to keep the

joint concentrically reduced albeit at the expense of total joint motion. If there is more severe arthritis, distraction interpositional arthroplasty or joint fusion may be considered. In the older age group, total elbow arthroplasty is also a good potential option.

Nerve and vessel injury

Approximately 25% of dislocations are complicated by a nerve injury, the most common being that of the ulnar nerve.[36] This injury is generally owing to a valgus stretching of the nerve. Median nerve involvement occurs secondary to stretch injuries or as a result of compression from swelling. Children and adolescents may be more susceptible to intra-articular entrapment of the median nerve because approximately 30% of elbow dislocations in skeletally immature patients are associated with avulsion injury to the medial epicondyle epiphyses.[37] The most common symptom is a transient paresthesia. However, a permanent deficit may result if the nerve is entrapped within the joint. Heightened awareness is necessary to avoid permanent neurologic deficits. A thorough physical examination includes evaluation of individual nerve distributions before and after reduction, as well as during passive ROM.[38] Radiographs may reveal medial joint space widening or fracture of the medial condyle.[39] MRI may also be used to detect nerve entrapment. Surgical indications for open exploration and decompression include electromyographic evidence of denervation, progression of symptoms, or persistence of symptoms for more than 3 months.[38]

Injury to the brachial artery is rare with elbow dislocation. One study found the incidence of brachial artery injury associated with elbow dislocation to be 13%.[40] Posterior dislocations in particular may compromise the brachial artery because the vessel may become entrapped between the bicipital aponeurosis and the humerus.[41] Injuries to the brachial artery can include spasm, thrombosis, intimal damage, or rupture. Immediate closed reduction may restore distal pulses. If pulses remain absent or decreased in comparison with the contralateral side, Doppler ultrasonography is a quick, inexpensive, and effective noninvasive screening study, whereas angiography remains the diagnostic gold standard.[38] In the presence of clear signs of ischemia, surgical exploration of suspected vascular injuries should not be delayed and may include arterial reconstruction, stabilization of the joint, and even fasciotomy for compartment syndrome. Primary repair of brachial artery injuries are preferred but not possible at times. Platz and colleagues[42] reported good long-term results in patients after primary repair after closed elbow dislocation with reversed saphenous vein graft and immediate reconstruction of ligamentous injuries.

WOUND COMPLICATIONS AND INFECTION

Wound dehiscence with exposed hardware or exposed bone at the tip of the olecranon is not an uncommon complication associated with surgical approaches to the elbow that involve a posterior skin incision. The thin soft-tissue envelope at the posterior elbow predisposes this area to wound complications. Soft-tissue irritation from hardware prominence after open reduction internal fixation of olecranon fractures has been reported in up to 80% of cases.[43,44] In one study on the operative fixation of complex distal humerus fractures, 12% of patients had postoperative wound complications.[45] Other studies demonstrated a 4% to 6% wound complication rate after open reduction internal fixation of a distal humerus fracture.[46–49] In a recent study, wound-healing problems accounted for 10% of non–implant-related complications and 5% of cases required a return to the operating room after total elbow arthroplasty.[50]

Significant morbidity can result from wound dehiscence. At the least, this complication delays the rehabilitation that is necessary for optimal elbow motion. At the worst, it may lead to deep periprosthetic infection and multiple surgical procedures. In a report of 89 distal humerus fractures treated with internal fixation, 15.7% developed major wound complications requiring a range of 1 to 6 additional surgical procedures.[51] Six patients required plastic surgical soft-tissue coverage. Significant risk factors for poor wound healing were grade III open fractures and the use of an olecranon osteotomy stabilized with a plate. Fracture healing rates and functional elbow ROM were not significantly affected by major wound complications after implementation of proper soft-tissue coverage techniques.

Treatment of such wound complications depends on the extent of the wound. At times, local wound care managed in an outpatient setting may be sufficient. However, mobilization of subcutaneous tissues to allow for adequate excursion to achieve primary closure or more complicated and morbid procedures such as a flap requiring microvascular technique may be necessary.

Normal wound healing is divided into 3 overlapping phases: (1) the inflammation phase, which occurs immediately and involves chemotaxis and phagocytosis; (2) the tissue formation phase, which begins in 2 to 3 days and is characterized by angiogenesis, collagen deposition, granulation tissue formation, and wound contraction; and (3) the tissue remodeling phase, which begins at 3 weeks and can last up to 2 years.[52] A well-vascularized bed of tissue, such as a muscular wound bed, provides the ideal environment for wound healing during the early phases of healing.[53] Patients with a devascularized bony bed or hardware at the tip of the olecranon do not have

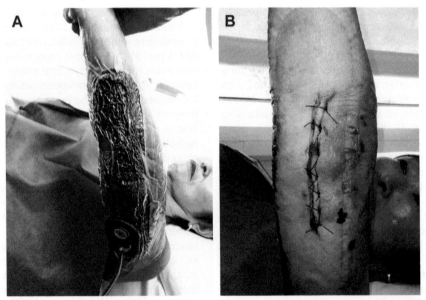

Fig. 3. A 70-year-old woman who underwent total elbow arthroplasty for complex distal humeral fracture. An incisional wound vacuum device was placed onto the wound in the operating room (A). The dressing was removed 1 week postoperatively. The wound appears to be epithelialized, dry, and with minimal swelling (B).

an optimal healing environment and thus may benefit from a muscle flap that improves local blood supply and optimizes wound healing.[54] Optimal soft-tissue coverage of the elbow is vital to the success of any surgical procedure. In the postoperative period, the surgeon must be confident in the durability of the soft-tissue closure to allow early motion and thus the prevention of stiffness and contracture.

Prevention of wound dehiscence is ideal, as it prevents additional procedures and allows earlier return to function. Historically, soft-tissue defects of the elbow have been treated with a variety of local and distant flaps, such as a local fasciocutaneous flaps, radial forearm pedicle flap, latissimus dorsi muscle free flap, or free tissue rectus abdominis flap.[55–57] However, these flaps are performed once a soft-tissue defect already exists, rather than as a preemptive measure to prevent wound complications. In the setting of a posterior wound dehiscence or posterior wound infection, thorough wound debridement of necrotic skin edges is performed initially. If the wound is grossly contaminated, a flap procedure may be performed in a staged manner after the wound bed is clean.

Postoperatively, the elbow is placed in a well-padded splint with an anterior plaster slab to maintain the elbow in maximum extension. This position decreases the tension across the posterior skin incision. Active mobilization depends on the index procedure but usually is started on the second postoperative day. If there is a heightened concern for wound healing or in the setting of revision surgery, the elbow is splinted for 2 weeks, and motion is started after suture removal at the 2 week follow-up visit. Incisional wound vacuum-assisted devices have also been used in selected complex cases with posterior wound dissections in the authors' practice. These devices have diminished the amount of postoperative edema as well as the rate of wound complications (**Fig. 3**).

REFERENCES

1. Lindenhovius AL, Jupiter JB. The posttraumatic stiff elbow: a review of the literature. J Hand Surg 2007; 32:1605–23.

2. Doornberg JN, de Jong IM, Lindenhovius AL, et al. The anteromedial facet of the coronoid process of the ulna. J Shoulder Elbow Surg 2007;16:667–70.

3. Shukla DR, Pillai G, McAnany S, et al. Heterotopic ossification formation after fracture-dislocations of the elbow. J Shoulder Elbow Surg 2015;24:333–8.

4. O'Driscoll SW, Jupiter JB, Cohen MS, et al. Difficult elbow fractures: pearls and pitfalls. Instr Course Lect 2003;52:113–34.

5. Hastings H 2nd, Graham TJ. The classification and treatment of heterotopic ossification about the elbow and forearm. Hand Clin 1994;10:417–37.

6. Abrams GD, Bellino MJ, Cheung EV. Risk factors for development of heterotopic ossification of the elbow after fracture fixation. J Shoulder Elbow Surg 2012; 21:1550–4.

7. Garland DE. Surgical approaches for resection of heterotopic ossification in traumatic brain-injured adults. Clin Orthop Relat Res 1991;(263):59–70.

8. Thompson HC 3rd, Garcia A. Myositis ossificans: aftermath of elbow injuries. Clin Orthop Relat Res 1967;50:129–34.

9. Chen G, Liao Q, Luo W, et al. Triceps-sparing versus olecranon osteotomy for ORIF: analysis of 67 cases of intercondylar fractures of the distal humerus. Injury 2011;42:366–70.

10. Foruria AM, Augustin S, Morrey BF, et al. Heterotopic ossification after surgery for fractures and fracture-dislocations involving the proximal aspect of the radius or ulna. J Bone Joint Surg Am 2013;95:e66.

11. Foruria AM, Lawrence TM, Augustin S, et al. Heterotopic ossification after surgery for distal humeral fractures. Bone Joint J 2014;96-B:1681–7.

12. Ehsan A, Huang JI, Lyons M, et al. Surgical management of posttraumatic elbow arthrofibrosis. J Trauma Acute Care Surg 2012;72:1399–403.

13. Salazar D, Golz A, Israel H, et al. Heterotopic ossification of the elbow treated with surgical resection: risk factors, bony ankylosis, and complications. Clin Orthop Relat Res 2014;472:2269–75.

14. Brouwer KM, Lindenhovius AL, de Witte PB, et al. Resection of heterotopic ossification of the elbow: a comparison of ankylosis and partial restriction. J Hand Surg 2010;35:1115–9.

15. Everding NG, Maschke SD, Hoyen HA, et al. Prevention and treatment of elbow stiffness: a 5-year update. J Hand Surg 2013;38:2496–507 [quiz: 507].

16. O'Driscoll SW, Juipter J. Selected instructional course lectures: the unstable elbow. J Bone Joint Surg Am 2000;82-A:723–38.

17. Doornberg JN, Ring D. Coronoid fracture patterns. J Hand Surg 2006;31:45–52.

18. Hartzler RU, Llusa-Perez M, Steinmann SP, et al. Transverse coronoid fracture: when does it have to be fixed? Clin Orthop Relat Res 2014;472:2068–74.

19. Schneeberger AG, Sadowski MM, Jacob HA. Coronoid process and radial head as posterolateral rotatory stabilizers of the elbow. J Bone Joint Surg Am 2004;86-A:975–82.

20. Papatheodorou LK, Rubright JH, Heim KA, et al. Terrible triad injuries of the elbow: does the coronoid always need to be fixed? Clin Orthop Relat Res 2014;472:2084–91.

21. Park SM, Lee JS, Jung JY, et al. How should anteromedial coronoid facet fracture be managed? A surgical strategy based on O'Driscoll classification

and ligament injury. J Shoulder Elbow Surg 2015;24: 74–82.

22. Sanchez-Sotelo J, O'Driscoll SW, Morrey BF. Medial oblique compression fracture of the coronoid process of the ulna. J Shoulder Elbow Surg 2005;14: 60–4.

23. Lee SK, Ha K, Kim KJ, et al. Coronoid plate fixation of type II and III coronoid process fractures: outcome and prognostic factors. Eur J Orthop Surg Traumatol 2012;22:213–9.

24. Pollock JW, Brownhill J, Ferreira L, et al. The effect of anteromedial facet fractures of the coronoid and lateral collateral ligament injury on elbow stability and kinematics. J Bone Joint Surg Am 2009;91: 1448–58.

25. Chen HW, Liu GD, Wu LJ. Complications of treating terrible triad injury of the elbow: a systematic review. PLoS One 2014;9:e97476.

26. Fitzgibbons PG, Louie D, Dyer GS, et al. Functional outcomes after fixation of "terrible triad" elbow fracture dislocations. Orthopedics 2014;37: e373–6.

27. Ruch DS, Triepel CR. Hinged elbow fixation for recurrent instability following fracture dislocation. Injury 2001;32(Suppl 4):SD70–8.

28. Charalambous CP, Stanley JK. Posterolateral rotatory instability of the elbow. J Bone Joint Surg Br 2008;90:272–9.

29. Cheung EV. Chronic lateral elbow instability. Orthop Clin North Am 2008;39:221–8. vi, vii.

30. Charalambous CP, Stanley JK, Siddique I, et al. Posterolateral rotatory laxity following surgery to the head of the radius: biomechanical comparison of two surgical approaches. J Bone Joint Surg Br 2009;91:82–7.

31. O'Driscoll SW. Classification and evaluation of recurrent instability of the elbow. Clin Orthop Relat Res 2000;(370):34–43.

32. Schaeffeler C, Waldt S, Woertler K. Traumatic instability of the elbow - anatomy, pathomechanisms and presentation on imaging. Eur Radiol 2013;23: 2582–93.

33. Goodwin D, Dynin M, Macdonnell JR, et al. The role of arthroscopy in chronic elbow instability. Arthroscopy 2013;29:2029–36.

34. Ahmed I, Mistry J. The management of acute and chronic elbow instability. Orthop Clin North Am 2015;46:271–80.

35. Anakwenze OA, Kwon D, O'Donnell E, et al. Surgical treatment of posterolateral rotatory instability of the elbow. Arthroscopy 2014;30:866–71.

36. Lindenhovius AL, Brouwer KM, Doornberg JN, et al. Long-term outcome of operatively treated fracture-dislocations of the olecranon. J Orthop Trauma 2008;22:325–31.

37. Rasool MN. Dislocations of the elbow in children. J Bone Joint Surg Br 2004;86:1050–8.

38. Martin BD, Johansen JA, Edwards SG. Complications related to simple dislocations of the elbow. Hand Clin 2008;24:9–25.

39. Ristic S, Strauch RJ, Rosenwasser MP. The assessment and treatment of nerve dysfunction after trauma around the elbow. Clin Orthop Relat Res 2000;(370):138–53.

40. Endean ED, Veldenz HC, Schwarcz TH, et al. Recognition of arterial injury in elbow dislocation. J Vasc Surg 1992;16:402–6.

41. Marcheix B, Chaufour X, Ayel J, et al. Transection of the brachial artery after closed posterior elbow dislocation. J Vasc Surg 2005;42:1230–2.

42. Platz A, Heinzelmann M, Ertel W, et al. Posterior elbow dislocation with associated vascular injury after blunt trauma. J Trauma 1999;46:948–50.

43. Macko D, Szabo RM. Complications of tension-band wiring of olecranon fractures. J Bone Joint Surg Am 1985;67:1396–401.

44. Murphy DF, Greene WB, Dameron TB Jr. Displaced olecranon fractures in adults. Clinical evaluation. Clin Orthop Relat Res 1987;(224):215–23.

45. Athwal GS, Hoxie SC, Rispoli DM, et al. Precontoured parallel plate fixation of AO/OTA type C distal humerus fractures. J Orthop Trauma 2009;23:575–80.

46. Huang TL, Chiu FY, Chuang TY, et al. Surgical treatment of acute displaced fractures of adult distal humerus with reconstruction plate. Injury 2004;35: 1143–8.

47. Huang TL, Chiu FY, Chuang TY, et al. The results of open reduction and internal fixation in elderly patients with severe fractures of the distal humerus: a critical analysis of the results. J Trauma 2005;58: 62–9.

48. Korner J, Lill H, Muller LP, et al. Distal humerus fractures in elderly patients: results after open reduction and internal fixation. Osteoporos Int 2005;16(Suppl 2):S73–9.

49. Wildburger R, Mahring M, Hofer HP. Supraintercondylar fractures of the distal humerus: results of internal fixation. J Orthop Trauma 1991;5:301–7.

50. Throckmorton T, Zarkadas P, Sanchez-Sotelo J, et al. Failure patterns after linked semiconstrained total elbow arthroplasty for posttraumatic arthritis. J Bone Joint Surg Am 2010;92:1432–41.

51. Lawrence TM, Ahmadi S, Morrey BF, et al. Wound complications after distal humerus fracture fixation: incidence, risk factors, and outcome. J Shoulder Elbow Surg 2014;23:258–64.

52. Stadelmann WK, Digenis AG, Tobin GR. Physiology and healing dynamics of chronic cutaneous wounds. Am J Surg 1998;176:26s–38s.

53. Browne EZ Jr. Complications of skin grafts and pedicle flaps. Hand Clin 1986;2:353–9.

54. Calderon W, Chang N, Mathes SJ. Comparison of the effect of bacterial inoculation in

musculocutaneous and fasciocutaneous flaps. Plast Reconstr Surg 1986;77:785–94.

55. Choudry UH, Moran SL, Li S, et al. Soft-tissue coverage of the elbow: an outcome analysis and reconstructive algorithm. Plast Reconstr Surg 2007; 119:1852–7.

56. Jensen M, Moran SL. Soft tissue coverage of the elbow: a reconstructive algorithm. Orthop Clin North Am 2008;39:251–64, vii.

57. Stevanovic M, Sharpe F, Itamura JM. Treatment of soft tissue problems about the elbow. Clin Orthop Relat Res 2000;(370):127–37.

Soft-Tissue Coverage for Elbow Trauma

Brian P. Kelley, MD[a], Kevin C. Chung, MD, MS[b],*

KEYWORDS

- Elbow • Soft tissue • Reconstruction • Trauma • Wounds

KEY POINTS

- Durability, early motion, and ease of patient recovery are important considerations for elbow wound coverage.
- After debridement, small elbow wounds without exposure of vital structures may be closed primarily.
- Local or regional flap options are often available and may be adequate to accomplish wound closure. However, local flaps may be involved in the zone of injury.
- Fasciocutaneous flaps are preferable for coverage of tendons to provide a gliding surface. Muscle flaps are useful when filling empty space or if infection is a concern.
- When recipient vessels are intact, free tissue transfer may be an alternative if local or regional flaps are unavailable.

BACKGROUND

Elbow trauma may result in soft-tissue injury or loss. Reconstruction of subsequent defects can be complicated. Inadequate reconstruction of elbow soft-tissue defects can severely limit functional outcomes by restricting motion and impairing upper extremity function. Ideal tissues for reconstruction are soft, thin, pliable, and durable with repetitive motion. Appropriate debridement is critical, and the surgeon must balance removal of all nonviable tissue with preservation of critical structures. Timing of the reconstruction is important for preserving function and avoiding infection.

PRINCIPLES OF RECONSTRUCTION

Trauma is a common cause of soft-tissue defects of the elbow. Traumatic wounds are often complicated by exposure of or injury to bone, nerve, tendon, and vasculature. Reconstruction of each of these structures requires coverage that is supple and durable. Classically, the reconstructive ladder was used to suggest a course of action. However, a more complicated reconstruction may be a better option if it grants improved motion or a more durable construct. This escalation in complexity is known as the reconstructive elevator.

Patient health and the mechanism of injury change the surgical management of traumatic wounds. High-energy traumatic wounds are more complicated than those from low energy. High-energy wounds can have occult injuries that declare over time. These wounds need serial debridement and repeat examination before definitive coverage. Patient comorbidities or systemic injury may dramatically affect overall care. Smokers may have a predilection for peripheral

---

Research reported in this publication was supported by the National Institute of Arthritis and Musculoskeletal and Skin Diseases of the National Institutes of Health under Award Number 2 K24-AR053120-06. The content is solely the responsibility of the authors and does not necessarily represent the official views of the National Institutes of Health.

[a] Section of Plastic Surgery, The University of Michigan Health System, 1500 East Medical Center Drive, 2130 Taubman Center, SPC 5340, Ann Arbor, MI 48109-5340, USA; [b] Section of Plastic Surgery, The University of Michigan Medical School, The University of Michigan Health System, 1500 East Medical Center Drive, 2130 Taubman Center, SPC 5340, Ann Arbor, MI 48109-5340, USA
* Corresponding author.
E-mail address: kecchung@med.umich.edu

Hand Clin 31 (2015) 693–703
http://dx.doi.org/10.1016/j.hcl.2015.06.013

arterial disease and vasoconstriction. Other causes for healing impairment should be considered before reconstruction, including diabetes, irradiation, immunosuppression, or autoimmune disease. These conditions should be optimized at the earliest feasible point in care.

WOUND LOCATION

Reconstruction of the posterior elbow poses challenges different from that of anterior antecubital elbow. In general, the total area of the skin envelop on the posterior elbow is greater than that on the anterior elbow because the posterior elbow is tight when flexed. The elbow is capable of greater than 130° of motion, and coverage must be stable in both flexion and extension.[1] The skin overlying the olecranon and posterior elbow is thin and is at high risk for pressure injury. Therefore, protective sensation on the posterior elbow is useful to prevent further injury after reconstruction. The anterior and posterior antebrachial cutaneous nerves provide sensory innervation to the elbow. Primary closure, nerve repair, or innervated flap reconstruction may restore protective sensation to this area.

Reconstruction should not be delayed after the wound is clean and can tolerate coverage. A suggested reconstruction algorithm is provided (**Fig. 1**). Ideally, an isolated traumatic elbow wound should undergo immediate reconstruction. However, if the wound is grossly contaminated or tissue viability is questionable, serial debridement should be continued. For a complicated wound, the first priority is fracture fixation and vascular repair. In general, fracture fixation should precede other procedures to guard against injury to nerve or vessel repairs. In contaminated wounds, external fixation is preferred, as this preserves wound care options while not exposing the permanent fixation hardware to additional risk of infection. In cases of concomitant life-threatening injuries, amputation or delayed management should be considered. Early coverage of wounds, within the first 24 to 72 hours, decreases edema, lowers wound infection rates, improves scar healing, and improves limb function.[2,3]

PRIMARY, DELAYED PRIMARY, OR SECONDARY CLOSURE

Primary closure is the simplest option for clean, easily approximated, tension-free wounds. The presence of hardware or graft material should prompt the surgeon to consider other options. Nerve and vascular graft failure can result from erosion, infection, or pressure on the closure. Undermining skin edges is a common technique to aid in wound closure but should be done judiciously in early traumatic wounds. For contaminated wounds, primary closure may be an option if a delay is possible and local tissues are sufficient. Serial debridement and local wound care should be performed before definitive closure. If delayed primary closure is considered, there should be minimal tension on the repair and underlying vital anatomic structures should be well protected. Healing by secondary intention is reserved

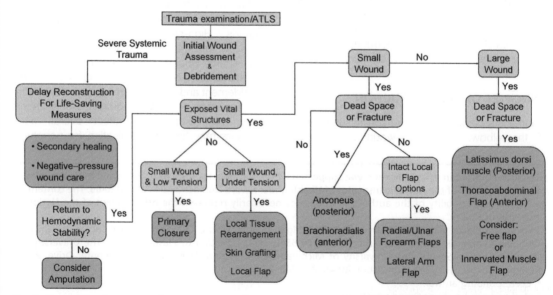

Fig. 1. Traumatic elbow wound reconstruction algorithm, suggested by the authors. ATLS, advanced trauma life support.

for small, structurally intact wounds. Secondary healing is also an option in patients whose wounds cannot be addressed because of other systemic issues. Tissue expanders have been used historically. Expanders require multiple procedures and are at risk for pressure injury, tissue thinning, infection, and extrusion.[4]

SKIN GRAFTING

Skin grafts are suitable reconstructive options in selective elbow injuries. Ideal wounds for skin grafting are those without exposed critical structures and an adequate vascular bed (**Fig. 2**). Grafts can be placed over intact fascia, paratenon, or periosteum with adequate revascularization but may result in unstable scarring. Over the olecranon, skin grafting may not be adequate to provide long-term durable coverage.

LOCAL RANDOM PATTERN FLAPS

Local flap reconstruction of the elbow provides more durable coverage than skin grafting and can be attempted in small wounds too large for primary repair. Use of local flaps at the elbow is limited because of a paucity of soft-tissue laxity. Local random flaps depend on dermal and subdermal blood supply, and healing is less consistent than in axial flaps. Examples of local tissue rearrangements include advancement flaps, Z-plasty, rhomboid flaps, or rotational flaps.[5–7] Secondary donor site defects may require skin

grafting. A 1:1 ratio of flap length to width is typically recommended. Narrow flaps are more prone to flap edge necrosis and delayed wound healing.[8]

AXIAL PATTERN FASCIOCUTANEOUS FLAPS

Axial pattern flaps are commonly used for upper extremity reconstruction. These flaps have well-defined blood supplies and can be designed as peninsular, island, or microvascular free flaps. The most common examples of axial pattern fasciocutaneous flaps in the upper extremity are the radial forearm, lateral arm, ulnar artery, antecubital fasciocutaneous, and posterior interosseous flaps.[9–19] Care must be taken to ensure patent vascular arcades at the wrist and palm to allow for retrograde flow to the flap or to ensure vessel patency to distal tissues. An Allen test should be documented preoperatively. If necessary, donor arteries can be repaired with vein grafting.

Radial forearm flap

Dominant arterial supply: Radial artery

Sensory innervation: Lateral antebrachial cutaneous nerve (volar radial forearm); Medial antebrachial cutaneous nerve (volar ulnar forearm)

Skin (length × width): Length 3 to 40 cm (up to 3 cm) × Width 2 to 15 cm (up to 2 cm)

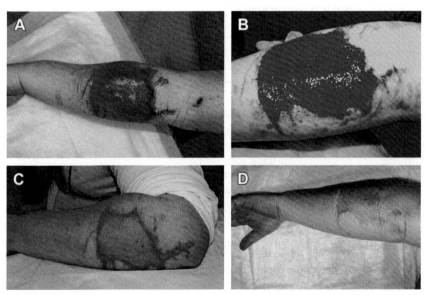

Fig. 2. Negative pressure wound care and skin grafting. (*A*) Ulnar-sided forearm/elbow wound without vital structure exposure. (*B*) Wound granulation after negative pressure therapy. (*C, D*) Early and long-term outcomes after skin grafting.

The radial forearm flap is a classic upper extremity workhorse flap.[20–23] The flap can be raised with sensory innervation and can be used as a composite flap with incorporation of distal radius bone. A patent palmar arch is mandatory to maintain hand perfusion, and this should be confirmed by Allen test.[24] If necessary, the radial artery can be reconstructed with saphenous vein graft. Thumb ischemia has been described in cases of an incomplete palmar arch after radial artery harvest.[25,26]

Donor site morbidity is high with the radial forearm flap, and the appearance of the donor forearm can be a major concern for patients. The forearm typically requires secondary reconstruction with skin grafting, as the skin laxity of the distal forearm is not amenable to primary repair. Furthermore, up to 13% of patients may develop exposed tendons, 19% have delayed donor site wound healing, and 32% have decreased sensation in the radial nerve distribution.[27] Bone harvest increases risk for radius fracture. Finally, cold intolerance, aching at the wrist, tendinous adhesions, and neuroma are also common donor site complications.[21] A suprafascial harvest has been described that may limit donor site morbidity.[22,28–30] However, subfascial dissection allows for ease of dissection, protection of subdermal vessels, and protection from shearing.

Lateral arm flap

Dominant arterial supply: posterior radial collateral artery

Sensory innervation: lateral brachial cutaneous nerve (distal: posterior antebrachial cutaneous nerve)

Skin (length × width): length 5 to 20 cm × width 3 to 12 cm (up to 6 cm)

The lateral arm flap is another common upper extremity workhorse flap (**Fig. 3**).[31] The lateral arm can be used as a free, pedicled, or contralateral cross-arm flap.[13,32–34] Composite flaps with sensation, muscle, or bone have been described.[35] The length can be extended up to 15 cm past the lateral epicondyle.[36]

PEDICLE MUSCLE OR MYOCUTANEOUS FLAPS

Muscle flaps are preferred over fasciocutaneous flaps in the setting of significant empty space or infection.[37,38] Neurotized muscle flaps can be used for restoration of motion. Local muscle flaps include the anconeus, brachioradialis, extensor carpi radialis longus, and flexor carpi ulnaris.[39–48] The most common distant pedicled muscle flap is the latissimus dorsi muscle. Local flaps may be limited by involvement in the zone of injury, whereas latissimus dorsi is often spared from localized trauma. Other than the latissimus, distant muscle flaps are rarely used, as they require a secondary operation, have high donor site morbidity, and may induce joint stiffness and free tissue transfer alternatives exist.[49]

Anconeus muscle

Dominant arterial supply: recurrent posterior interosseous and medial collateral artery[24]

Motor innervation: radial nerve

Muscle length: 2.5 × 7 cm (up to 10.6 cm)[24,50]

Pedicle length: 3.1 cm (range, 2.4–3.8 cm)

Mathes and Nahai class: type I versus type III[24,51]

The anconeus muscle is useful for coverage of small posterior elbow defects, and loss of anconeus function results in minimal patient morbidity.[6] It is particularly useful for injuries overlying the radiocapitellar joint, distal triceps tendon, or olecranon.[47] However, the anconeus is not dependable to cover defects greater than 5 to 7 cm², and the short arc of rotation makes it a poor choice for anterior or medial defects.

Brachioradialis muscle

Dominant arterial supply: radial recurrent artery and/or radial artery[45,52]

Motor innervation: radial nerve

Muscle dimensions: range, 8 × 15 cm (tapers distally)

Pedicle length: 3 cm from radial artery; located 7 to 10 cm distal to muscle origin

Mathes and Nahai class: type II

The brachioradialis muscle is used to cover small defects on the distal one-third to half of the arm or proximal forearm (**Fig. 4**). For the upper arm, it is best suited for anterolateral or posterolateral defects. The only relative contraindication to harvest is the absence of dominant elbow flexors, because of its function as a weak elbow flexor.

Flexor carpi ulnaris muscle
Dominant arterial supply: ulnar or recurrent ulnar arteries
Motor innervation: ulnar nerve
Muscle dimensions: range, 5 × 20 cm (tapers distally)
Pedicle location: 5.7 cm from medial epicondyle (range, 3–10 cm)[53]
Mathes and Nahai class: type II

The flexor carpi ulnaris muscle flap is useful for defects on the anterior, posterior, or medial elbow. Relative contraindications include a lack of other wrist flexors or lower morbidity alternatives for reconstruction.[54] Ulnar artery absence or ulnar hand dominance may also limit use of the flap. Loss of flexor carpi ulnaris results in weakened wrist flexion and ulnar deviation.

Latissimus dorsi muscle
Dominant arterial supply: thoracodorsal artery
Motor innervation: thoracodorsal nerve
Muscle (length × width): length 35 cm (range, 21–42 cm) × width 20 cm (range, 14–26 cm)
Skin (length × width): length 18 cm (up to 35 cm) × width 7 cm (up to 8–9 cm primarily)
Pedicle length: 8.5 cm (range, 6.5–12 cm)
Mathes and Nahai class: type V

The latissimus dorsi muscle is a robust flap used in both pedicle-based and free flap reconstruction. The flap can be designed to include a skin paddle or scapula. Furthermore, the muscle can remain innervated for functional innervated transfer to restore biceps or triceps function.[55–59] For elbow reconstruction, the pedicle flap can reach up to 6 to 8 cm distal to the olecranon.[60,61] The flap is particularly useful for large defects over the posterior upper arm or with a large zone of injury precluding local flap use.

Sacrifice of latissimus dorsi may result in shoulder weakness. Use may be contraindicated in patients with paraplegia or those requiring a life-long wheelchair or crutch use. Likewise, the latissimus dorsi should be used judiciously in patients at increased risk for breast cancer, as it is a common option for breast reconstruction. Preoperative vascular imaging should be considered if the patient has a history of axillary surgery. The most common complication is donor site seroma, but partial flap necrosis can occur at a high rate (>35%) when insetting beyond the olecranon.[62]

TWO-STAGE AXIAL FASCIOCUTANEOUS FLAPS

Distant axial fasciocutaneous flaps are a reliable option in hand and upper extremity reconstruction.[63–65] Thoracoabdominal flaps were first described in the 1940s, and options have expanded with the advent of perforator free tissue transfer.[66–68] Similar to distant muscle flaps, distant axial flaps often require a secondary procedure for flap inset and pedicle division. These flaps have been described for defects up to 22 cm in length.[63] The ideal use for these flaps is in the setting of a large defect, with the zone of injury eliminating local and regional reconstructive options. Two-stage flaps are a useful alternative when microsurgical techniques are unavailable. The main limitation for use is the need for prolonged immobilization and donor site morbidity. Perforator-based thoracoabdominal flaps include branches of the superior epigastric, inferior epigastric, deep circumflex iliac, intercostal (**Fig. 5**), and subcostal arteries.[68] However, thoracoabdominal angiosomes can be variable and large perforator-based fasciocutaneous flaps rely on a random pattern of perfusion near the flap edges.[69]

FREE TISSUE TRANSFER

Microsurgical free tissue transfer is the most robust reconstructive option for customized soft-tissue coverage at the elbow. Options for elbow coverage include muscle-only, myocutaneous, fasciocutaneous, omentum, vascularized bone, or composite flaps. The first indication for free tissue transfer is a large defect that exceeds the capability for local or regional flap coverage. Other indications include the need for multiple tissue types, specific flap orientation, and injury to local flap options. Free tissue transfer is also an alternative to multistage procedures. The only absolute contraindication to free tissue transfer is a vascular injury involving potential recipient vessels. Common free flaps used for elbow reconstruction include the anterolateral thigh (ALT), groin, scapular, parascapular, gracilis muscle, latissimus dorsi muscle, or fibular osteocutaneous flaps.[70–77] Free fasciocutaneous flaps can be harvested from the contralateral upper extremity, including the lateral arm and radial forearm flaps.

Donor site selection is a key benefit of free tissue transfer. Flaps that have minimal donor site morbidity can be chosen. For example, the ALT

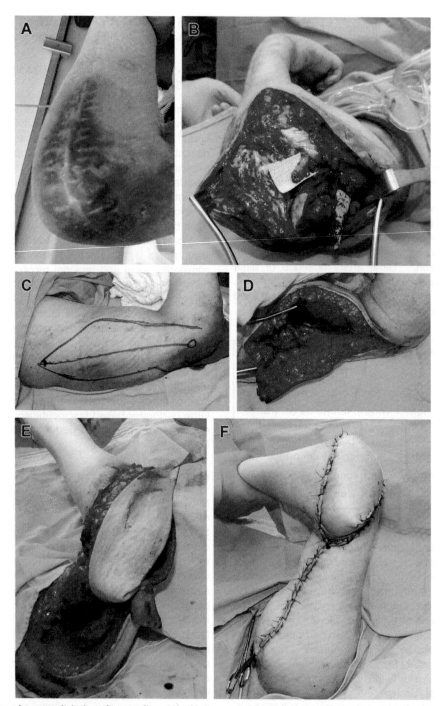

Fig. 3. Lateral arm pedicled perforator flap. (*A*) Chronic posttraumatic contracture and unstable elbow scarring. (*B*) Wound size after scar release; ulnar neuroma resection. (*C*) Preoperative marking for extended lateral arm flap. (*D*, *E*) Flap elevation with identification of the vascular pedicle; demonstration of flap mobility. (*F*) Flap inset.

and the gracilis muscle are both common flaps used from the lower extremity that can be closed primarily and result in minimal functional deficit. These tissues can also be neurotized for sensory or motor function. Reported risk of total flap loss in an experienced microsurgical center is less than 3%.[78] Risks for flap loss include elevated body mass index, technical difficulty, smoking, tamoxifen use, or anastomosis in the zone of injury.[79,80]

Anterolateral Thigh Flap

Dominant arterial supply: descending branch of the lateral circumflex femoral artery

Skin sensory innervation: lateral femoral cutaneous nerve

Motor innervation: branch to vastus lateralis from femoral nerve

Skin (length × width): length 16 cm (range, 4–35 cm) × width 8 cm (up to 8 cm primarily)

Pedicle length/diameter: 12 cm (range, 8–16 cm); 2.1 mm diameter

Muscle component: range, 2 to 20 cm of vastus lateralis muscle

The ALT flap is a fasciocutaneous flap that can include muscle and results in minimal donor site morbidity.[81] Typically, the donor site can be closed primarily. The perforator is found either septocutaneous or musculocutaneous, but the flap is noted to be highly reliable despite this variability.[77]

Gracilis muscle

Dominant arterial supply: medial femoral circumflex or branch of the profunda femoral artery

Motor innervation: anterior branch of the obturator nerve

Muscle (length × width): length two-thirds length of medial thigh × width 5 to 8 cm

Skin sensory innervation: medial cutaneous nerve of the thigh

Skin (length × width): length two-thirds of muscle length × width up to 4 to 6 cm primarily

Pedicle length/diameter: 7 cm (range, 6–8 cm); 1.5 mm (range, 0.5–2.0 mm)

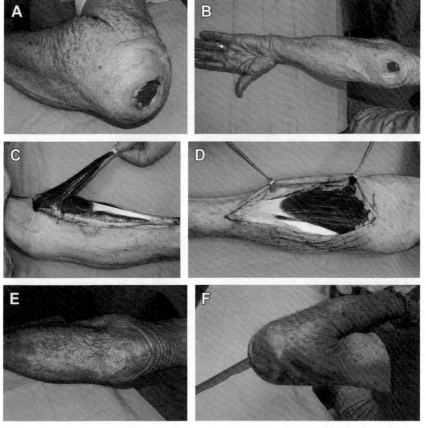

Fig. 4. Pedicled brachioradialis muscle flap. (*A, B*) Chronic traumatic wound overlying olecranon process, flexion and extension. (*C, D*) Brachioradialis harvest with demonstration of dissected vascular pedicle. (*E, F*) Long-term reconstructive result.

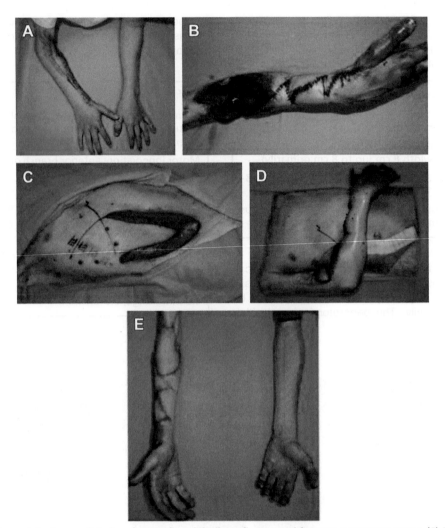

Fig. 5. Intercostal artery pedicled perforator flap. (*A*) Elbow flexion and forearm scar contractures. (*B*) Elbow and forearm wound after debridement and Z-plasty. (*C*) Flap design and elevation. (*D*) Flap inset. (*E*) Long-term result. (*From* Adkinson JM, Chung KC. Flap reconstruction of the elbow and forearm: a case-based approach. Hand Clin 2014;30(2):161; with permission.)

SUMMARY

Wounds of the elbow present unique anatomic and functional challenges for the reconstructive surgeon. The ultimate success of reconstruction relies on durable wound coverage and early motion of adjacent joints, muscles, and tendons. Therefore, management requires a thorough understanding of the advantages and limitations of coverage options. The choice of technique may change greatly with variation in patient comorbidities, wound size, or wound quality. Using the techniques discussed, reconstruction of the elbow can be accomplished in a directed, patient-specific manner.

REFERENCES

1. Patel KM, Higgins JP. Posterior elbow wounds: soft tissue coverage options and techniques. Orthop Clin North Am 2013;44(3):409–17, x.
2. Breidenbach WC 3rd. Emergency free tissue transfer for reconstruction of acute upper extremity wounds. Clin Plast Surg 1989;16(3):505–14.
3. Sherman R. Soft-tissue coverage for the elbow. Hand Clin 1997;13(2):291–302.
4. Meland NB, Smith AA, Johnson CH. Tissue expansion in the upper extremities. Hand Clin 1997; 13(2):303–14.
5. Hudson DA. Some thoughts on choosing a Z-plasty: the Z made simple. Plast Reconstr Surg 2000; 106(3):665–71.

6. Jensen M, Moran SL. Soft tissue coverage of the elbow: a reconstructive algorithm. Orthop Clin North Am 2008;39(2):251–64, vii.

7. Lister GD, Gibson T. Closure of rhomboid skin defects: the flaps of Limberg and Dufourmentel. Br J Plast Surg 1972;25(3):300–14.

8. Stevanovic M, Sharpe F, Itamura JM. Treatment of soft tissue problems about the elbow. Clin Orthop Relat Res 2000;(370):127–37.

9. Song R, Gao Y, Song Y, et al. The forearm flap. Clin Plast Surg 1982;9(1):21–6.

10. Muhlbauer W, Herndl E, Stock W. The forearm flap. Plast Reconstr Surg 1982;70(3):336–44.

11. Song R, Song Y, Yu Y, et al. The upper arm free flap. Clin Plast Surg 1982;9(1):27–35.

12. Cormack GC, Lamberty BG. Fasciocutaneous vessels in the upper arm: application to the design of new fasciocutaneous flaps. Plast Reconstr Surg 1984;74(2):244–50.

13. Katsaros J, Tan E, Zoltie N. The use of the lateral arm flap in upper limb surgery. J Hand Surg 1991;16(4):598–604.

14. Mathy JA, Moaveni Z, Tan ST. Perforator anatomy of the ulnar forearm fasciocutaneous flap. J Plast Reconstr Aesthet Surg 2012;65(8):1076–82.

15. Tao KZ, Chen EY, Ji RM, et al. Anatomical study on arteries of fasciae in the forearm fasciocutaneous flap. Clin Anat 2000;13(1):1–5.

16. Masquelet AC, Penteado CV. The posterior interosseous flap. Ann Chir Main 1987;6(2):131–9.

17. Orgill DP, Pribaz JJ, Morris DJ. Local fasciocutaneous flaps for olecranon coverage. Ann Plast Surg 1994;32(1):27–31.

18. Park JJ, Kim JS, Chung JI. Posterior interosseous free flap: various types. Plast Reconstr Surg 1997;100(5):1186–97 [discussion: 1198–9].

19. Blondeel N, Boeckx WD, Vanderstraeten GG, et al. The fate of the oblique abdominal muscles after free TRAM flap surgery. Br J Plast Surg 1997;50(5):315–21.

20. Bishop AT. Soft tissue loss about the elbow. Selecting optimal coverage. Hand Clin 1994;10(3):531–42.

21. Swanson E, Boyd JB, Manktelow RT. The radial forearm flap: reconstructive applications and donor-site defects in 35 consecutive patients. Plast Reconstr Surg 1990;85(2):258–66.

22. Timmons MJ. The vascular basis of the radial forearm flap. Plast Reconstr Surg 1986;77(1):80–92.

23. Tizian C, Sanner F, Berger A. The proximally pedicled arteria radialis forearm flap in the treatment of soft tissue defects of the dorsal elbow. Ann Plast Surg 1991;26(1):40–4.

24. Stevanovic M, Sharpe F. Soft-tissue coverage of the elbow. Plast Reconstr Surg 2013;132(3):387e–402e.

25. Heller F, Wei W, Wei FC. Chronic arterial insufficiency of the hand with fingertip necrosis 1 year after harvesting a radial forearm free flap. Plast Reconstr Surg 2004;114(3):728–31.

26. Jones BM, O'Brien CJ. Acute ischaemia of the hand resulting from elevation of a radial forearm flap. Br J Plast Surg 1985;38(3):396–7.

27. Richardson D, Fisher SE, Vaughan ED, et al. Radial forearm flap donor-site complications and morbidity: a prospective study. Plast Reconstr Surg 1997;99(1):109–15.

28. Webster HR, Robinson DW. The radial forearm flap without fascia and other refinements. Eur J Plast Surg 1995;18(1):11–3.

29. Chang SC, Miller G, Halbert CF, et al. Limiting donor site morbidity by suprafascial dissection of the radial forearm flap. Microsurgery 1996;17(3):136–40.

30. Wong CH, Lin JY, Wei FC. The bottom-up approach to the suprafascial harvest of the radial forearm flap. Am J Surg 2008;196(5):e60–4.

31. Culbertson JH, Mutimer K. The reverse lateral upper arm flap for elbow coverage. Ann Plast Surg 1987;18(1):62–8.

32. Ng SW, Teoh LC, Lee YL, et al. Contralateral pedicled lateral arm flap for hand reconstruction. Ann Plast Surg 2010;64(2):159–63.

33. Scheker LR, Kleinert HE, Hanel DP. Lateral arm composite tissue transfer to ipsilateral hand defects. J Hand Surg 1987;12(5 Pt 1):665–72.

34. Akinci M, Ay S, Kamiloglu S, et al. Lateral arm free flaps in the defects of the upper extremity–a review of 72 cases. Hand Surg 2005;10(2–3):177–85.

35. Shenaq SM. Pretransfer expansion of a sensate lateral arm free flap. Ann Plast Surg 1987;19(6):558–62.

36. Kuek LB, Chuan TL. The extended lateral arm flap: a new modification. J Reconstr Microsurg 1991;7(3):167–73.

37. Calderon W, Chang N, Mathes SJ. Comparison of the effect of bacterial inoculation in musculocutaneous and fasciocutaneous flaps. Plast Reconstr Surg 1986;77(5):785–94.

38. Chang N, Mathes SJ. Comparison of the effect of bacterial inoculation in musculocutaneous and random-pattern flaps. Plast Reconstr Surg 1982;70(1):1–10.

39. Fleager KE, Cheung EV. The "anconeus slide": rotation flap for management of posterior wound complications about the elbow. J Shoulder Elbow Surg 2011;20(8):1310–6.

40. Janevicius RV, Greager JA. The extensor carpi radialis longus muscle flap for anterior elbow coverage. J Hand Surg 1992;17(1):102–6.

41. Lalikos JF, Fudem GM. Brachioradialis musculocutaneous flap closure of the elbow utilizing a distal skin island: a case report. Ann Plast Surg 1997;39(2):201–4.

42. Lingaraj K, Lim AY, Puhaindran ME, et al. Case report: the split flexor carpi ulnaris as a local muscle flap. Clin Orthop Relat Res 2007;455:262–6.

43. Meals RA. The use of a flexor carpi ulnaris muscle flap in the treatment of an infected nonunion of the proximal ulna. A case report. Clin Orthop Relat Res 1989;(240):168–72.

44. Ohtsuka H, Imagawa S. Reconstruction of a posterior defect of the elbow joint using an extensor carpi radialis longus myocutaneous flap: case report. Br J Plast Surg 1985;38(2):238–40.

45. Rohrich RJ, Ingram AE Jr. Brachioradialis muscle flap: clinical anatomy and use in soft-tissue reconstruction of the elbow. Ann Plast Surg 1995;35(1):70–6.

46. Sanger JR, Ye Z, Yousif NJ, et al. The brachioradialis forearm flap: anatomy and clinical application. Plast Reconstr Surg 1994;94(5):667–74.

47. Schmidt CC, Kohut GN, Greenberg JA, et al. The anconeus muscle flap: its anatomy and clinical application. J Hand Surg 1999;24(2):359–69.

48. Wysocki RW, Gray RL, Fernandez JJ, et al. Posterior elbow coverage using whole and split flexor carpi ulnaris flaps: a cadaveric study. J Hand Surg 2008; 33(10):1807–12.

49. Sbitany U, Wray RC Jr. Use of the rectus abdominis muscle flap to reconstruct an elbow defect. Plast Reconstr Surg 1986;77(6):988–9.

50. Ng ZY, Lee SW, Mitchell JH, et al. Functional anconeus free flap for thenar reconstruction: a cadaveric study. Hand 2012;7(3):286–92.

51. Mathes SJ, Levine J. Chapter 5: Muscle flaps and their blood supply. In: Thorne CH, Beasley RW, Aston SJ, et al, editors. Grabb & Smith's Plastic Surgery. 6th edition. Philadelphia: Lippincott Williams & Wilkins; 2007. p. 42.

52. Leversedge FJ, Casey PJ, Payne SH, et al. Vascular anatomy of the brachioradialis rotational musculocutaneous flap. J Hand Surg 2001;26(4):711–21.

53. Sharpe F, Barry P, Lin SD, et al. Anatomic study of the flexor carpi ulnaris muscle and its application to soft tissue coverage of the elbow with clinical correlation. J Shoulder Elbow Surg 2014;23(1): 82–90.

54. Raskin KB, Wilgis EF. Flexor carpi ulnaris transfer for radial nerve palsy: functional testing of long-term results. J Hand Surg 1995;20(5):737–42.

55. Mordick TG 2nd, Britton EN, Brantigan C. Pedicled latissimus dorsi transfer for immediate soft-tissue coverage and elbow flexion. Plast Reconstr Surg 1997;99(6):1742–4.

56. Park C, Shin KS. Functioning free latissimus dorsi muscle transplantation: anterogradely positioned usage in reconstruction of extensive forearm defect. Ann Plast Surg 1991;27(1):87–91 [discussion: 92].

57. Pruzansky M, Kelly M, Weinberg H. Latissimus dorsi musculocutaneous flap for elbow extension. J Surg Oncol 1991;47(1):62–6.

58. Russell RC, Pribaz J, Zook EG, et al. Functional evaluation of latissimus dorsi donor site. Plast Reconstr Surg 1986;78(3):336–44.

59. Zancolli E, Mitre H. Latissimus dorsi transfer to restore elbow flexion. An appraisal of eight cases. J Bone Joint Surg Am 1973;55(6):1265–75.

60. Jutte DL, Rees R, Nanney L, et al. Latissimus dorsi flap: a valuable resource in lower arm reconstruction. South Med J 1987;80(1):37–40.

61. Stevanovic M, Sharpe F, Thommen VD, et al. Latissimus dorsi pedicle flap for coverage of soft tissue defects about the elbow. J Shoulder Elbow Surg 1999; 8(6):634–43.

62. Choudry UH, Moran SL, Li S, et al. Soft-tissue coverage of the elbow: an outcome analysis and reconstructive algorithm. Plast Reconstr Surg 2007; 119(6):1852–7.

63. Burstein FD, Salomon JC, Stahl RS. Elbow joint salvage with the transverse rectus island flap: a new application. Plast Reconstr Surg 1989;84(3): 492–7 [discussion: 498].

64. Fisher J. External oblique fasciocutaneous flap for elbow coverage. Plast Reconstr Surg 1985;75(1): 51–61.

65. Davis WM, McCraw JB, Carraway JH. Use of a direct, transverse, thoracoabdominal flap to close difficult wounds of the thorax and upper extremity. Plast Reconstr Surg 1977;60(4):526–33.

66. Brown JB, Cannon B, Graham WC, et al. Direct flap repair of defects of the arm and hand : preparation of gunshot wounds for repair of nerves, bones and tendons. Ann Surg 1945;122(4):706–15.

67. Cannon B, Trott AW. Expeditious use of direct flaps in extremity repairs. Plast Reconstr Surg (1946) 1949;4(5):415–9.

68. Adkinson JM, Chung KC. Flap reconstruction of the elbow and forearm: a case-based approach. Hand Clin 2014;30(2):153–63, v.

69. Farber GL, Taylor KF, Smith AC. Pedicled thoracoabdominal flap coverage about the elbow in traumatic war injuries. Hand 2010;5(1):43–8.

70. Chen HC, Tang YB, Mardini S, et al. Reconstruction of the hand and upper limb with free flaps based on musculocutaneous perforators. Microsurgery 2004; 24(4):270–80.

71. Kremer T, Bickert B, Germann G, et al. Outcome assessment after reconstruction of complex defects of the forearm and hand with osteocutaneous free flaps. Plast Reconstr Surg 2006;118(2):443–54 [discussion: 455–6].

72. Yildirim S, Taylan G, Eker G, et al. Free flap choice for soft tissue reconstruction of the severely damaged upper extremity. J Reconstr Microsurg 2006;22(8):599–609.

73. Manktelow RT, Zuker RM, McKee NH. Functioning free muscle transplantation. J Hand Surg 1984; 9A(1):32–9.

74. Manktelow RT, McKee NH. Free muscle transplantation to provide active finger flexion. J Hand Surg 1978;3(5):416–26.

75. Hamilton SG, Morrison WA. The scapular free flap. Br J Plast Surg 1982;35(1):2–7.

76. Urbaniak JR, Koman LA, Goldner RD, et al. The vascularized cutaneous scapular flap. Plast Reconstr Surg 1982;69(5):772–8.

77. Zhou G, Qiao Q, Chen GY, et al. Clinical experience and surgical anatomy of 32 free anterolateral thigh flap transplantations. Br J Plast Surg 1991;44(2):91–6.

78. Godina M. Early microsurgical reconstruction of complex trauma of the extremities. Plast Reconstr Surg 1986;78(3):285–92.

79. Kelley BP, Valero V, Yi M, et al. Tamoxifen increases the risk of microvascular flap complications in patients undergoing microvascular breast reconstruction. Plast Reconstr Surg 2012;129(2): 305–14.

80. Daniel RK, Weiland AJ. Free tissue transfers for upper extremity reconstruction. J Hand Surg 1982;7(1): 66–76.

81. Song YG, Chen GZ, Song YL. The free thigh flap: a new free flap concept based on the septocutaneous artery. Br J Plast Surg 1984;37(2):149–59.

Index

Note: Page numbers of article titles are in **boldface** type.

Hand Clin 31 (2015) 705–708
http://dx.doi.org/10.1016/S0749-0712(15)00116-X
0749-0712/15/$ – see front matter © 2015 Elsevier Inc. All rights reserved.

Printed and bound by CPI Group (UK) Ltd, Croydon, CR0 4YY

03/10/2024

01040377-0001